Respiratory Disease Series: Diagnostic Tools and Disease Managements

Series Editors

Hiroyuki Nakamura
Ibaraki Medical Center
Tokyo Medical University
Ibaraki, Japan

Kazutetsu Aoshiba
Ibaraki Medical Center
Tokyo Medical University
Ibaraki, Japan

This book series cover a variety of topics in respiratory diseases, with each volume providing an overview of the current state of knowledge, recent discoveries and future prospects for each disease. In each chapter the editors pose critical questions, which are often unresolved clinical issues. These are then discussed by the authors, providing insights and suggestions as to which developments need to be addressed. The series offers new information, which will inspire innovative ideas to further develop respiratory medicine.This collection of monographs is aimed at benefiting patients across the globe suffering from respiratory disease.

Edited by established authorities in the field and written by pioneering experts, this book series will be valuable to those researchers and physicians working in respiratory medicine. The series is aimed at a broad readership, and the books will also be a valuable resource for radiologists, emergency medicine physicians, pathologists, pharmacologists and basic research scientists.

More information about this series at http://www.springer.com/series/15152

Jiro Fujita
Editor

Influenza

Advances in Diagnosis and Management

Springer

Editor
Jiro Fujita
Department of Infectious, Respiratory, and Digestive Medicine
Graduate School of Medicine, University of the Ryukyus
Okinawa
Japan

ISSN 2509-5552 ISSN 2509-5560 (electronic)
Respiratory Disease Series: Diagnostic Tools and Disease Managements
ISBN 978-981-15-9108-2 ISBN 978-981-15-9109-9 (eBook)
https://doi.org/10.1007/978-981-15-9109-9

This Springer imprint is published by the registered company Springer Nature Singapore Pte Ltd.
The registered company address is: 152 Beach Road, #21-01/04 Gateway East, Singapore 189721, Singapore

Preface

We are going to publish a new textbook about influenza virus infection.

Influenza can be easily transmitted and is associated with increased morbidity and mortality, especially in immunocompromised inpatients. Therefore, it is important to take prompt measures to prevent droplet transmission of influenza virus. It is recommended that people receive vaccination for influenza. In addition, if the number of patients with influenza increases, it is recommended to wear surgical masks. Furthermore, understanding the pathogenesis, as well as complications, early diagnosis, and treatment, is essential to reduce the number of deaths caused by influenza virus infection.

In hospital settings, even when the staff are vaccinated against influenza virus, it is impossible to prevent all nosocomial influenza virus infections. Therefore, chemoprophylaxis for those who have had close contact with the index case can supplement the prerequisite vaccination to control influenza virus infection.

Although Japan is the largest consumer of neuraminidase inhibitors, the emergent oseltamivir-resistant influenza A(H1/N1) virus during the 2008–2009 season in Japan has not spread since the 2009–2010 season, and the frequency of neuraminidase inhibitor-resistant viruses has been quite low to date.

In March 2018, oral baloxavir marboxil, the first polymerase inhibitor licensed for the treatment of uncomplicated influenza, was introduced in Japan. Baloxavir marboxil is a prodrug that is metabolized into baloxavir acid that directly inhibits cap-dependent endonuclease activity of the polymerase acidic protein of influenza A and B viruses and suppresses the intracellular growth of influenza virus. In phase II and III trials on outpatients with uncomplicated influenza-like illness, baloxavir has been well tolerated in adults, adolescents, and high-risk patients with comorbidities such as asthma and chronic lung disease. With the widespread use of baloxavir, emergence of reduced baloxavir susceptibility has become a significant challenge. However, since the frequency of reduced baloxavir susceptibility before the treatment remains unclear, the clinical impact of this drug should be closely monitored.

This book consists of six parts. In Part I, the World Health Organization Global Strategy to control influenza viral infection is described. In Part II, there are five themes as follows: epidemiology in Japan, transmission at home, cellular and biochemical pathogenic processes, pathology of severe influenza virus pneumonia, and diagnosis and treatment. In Part III, there are four themes: rapid diagnosis, differential diagnosis, radiologic findings of influenza pneumonia, and oral findings. In Part IV, there are two themes as follows: classification of pneumonia complicated with influenza and influenza encephalopathy. Part V consists of seven themes: treatment guidelines, treatment strategy in adolescents, how to use zanamivir and oseltamivir, how to use laninamivir octanoate, how to use baloxavir marboxil, how to use peramivir, and prophylaxis for influenza.

The final topic covers three aspects, as follows: influenza vaccine efficacy/effectiveness, the new anti-influenza drug baloxavir marboxil, and viruses resistant to oseltamivir or baloxavir marboxil.

I sincerely hope that this book would be useful for every medical staff who take care of patients with influenza virus infection.

Okinawa, Japan Jiro Fujita

Contents

Part I Introduction

1 Global Strategy for Influenza Viral Infection: What Is the Latest Information from WHO? 3
Takeaki Imamura and Hitoshi Oshitani

Part II Definition, Epidemiology, and Pathogenesis

2 Epidemiology of Influenza with a Description of Recent Trends in Japan: What Are the Key Epidemiologic Features of Seasonal Influenza? 15
Yuzo Arima, Takuri Takahashi, Tomimasa Sunagawa, and Motoi Suzuki

3 Transmission of Influenza Virus in the Home: How Are They Transmitted in the Home? 27
Nobuo Hirotsu

4 Cellular and Biochemical Pathogenic Processes in Severe Influenza Virus Infection: How Does Cytokine Storm Play a Role? 37
Hiroshi Kido, Takashi Kimoto, and Etsuhisa Takahashi

5 Pathology of Severe Influenza Virus Pneumonia: What Is the Importance of Alveolar Mouths? 47
Yuji Ohtsuki and Jiro Fujita

6 Pathology, Diagnosis, and Treatment of Influenza Infections/Pneumonia: What Are the Mechanisms of Secondary Bacterial Pneumonia? 57
Masafumi Seki

Part III Diagnosis

7 **Rapid Diagnosis of Influenza Viral Infection: What Are the Rapid Diagnostic Tests and Molecular Diagnosis?** ... 69
Naoki Uno and Katsunori Yanagihara

8 **Differential Diagnosis Between Influenza and Other Respiratory Viral Infections: What Are the Differential Diagnoses?** ... 79
Takeshi Kinjo and Jiro Fujita

9 **Radiologic Findings of Influenza Pneumonia: What Are the Recent Radiological Findings?** ... 91
Takeshi Johkoh

10 **Oral Findings of Influenza Viral Infection: What Are the Characteristic Pharyngeal Findings of Influenza?** ... 101
Yuichiro Tamaki

Part IV Complication

11 **Classification of Pneumonia Complicated with Influenza Viral Infection: What Are the Patterns of Pneumonia?** ... 107
Yuji Fujikura

12 **Influenza Encephalopathy: What Is Encephalopathy?** ... 115
Mitsuru Tsuge, Masato Yashiro, Naoki Ohno, and Hirokazu Tsukahara

Part V Management

13 **Treatment Guidelines for Influenza Virus Infection: What Does the Recent Guideline State?** ... 129
Tadashi Ishida

14 **Treatment Strategy for Influenza Viral Infection in Adolescent: What Is the Current Adolescent Treatment?** ... 137
Yosuke Aoki

15 **How to Use Anti-influenza Drugs: Zanamivir and Oseltamivir** ... 149
Naoki Kawai

16 **How to Use Anti-influenza Drugs: Laninamivir Octanoate** ... 161
Hideyuki Ikematsu

17 **How to Use Anti-influenza Drugs: Baloxavir Marboxil** ... 171
Takeki Uehara

18 **How to Use Anti-influenza Drugs: Peramivir** ... 181
Yutaka Saisho

19 **Prophylaxis of Influenza Viral Transmission: What Is the Current Prophylaxis?** ... 191
Nobuhiro Asai and Hiroshige Mikamo

Part VI Topics

20 Influenza Vaccine Efficacy/Effectiveness: With Special Reference to Current Epidemiological Methodology 201
Wakaba Fukushima

21 The New Anti-influenza Drug Baloxavir Marboxil: Can Influenza Viruses with Reduced Susceptibility to Baloxavir Maintain Viral Fitness? 211
Masaki Imai and Yoshihiro Kawaoka

22 Viruses Resistant to Oseltamivir or Baloxavir: What Do the Data Reveal About Resistance? 221
Emi Takashita

Correction to: Influenza C1

Part I
Introduction

Chapter 1
Global Strategy for Influenza Viral Infection: What Is the Latest Information from WHO?

Takeaki Imamura and Hitoshi Oshitani

Abstract Influenza is a viral respiratory disease of great importance. Both seasonal and pandemic influenza pose serious burdens and threats to global public health. The current WHO strategy for influenza is based on the International Health Regulations revised in 2005 (IHR 2005), ensuring a core national public health capacity building alongside a systemic international response mechanism. Lessons and challenges from past threats such as highly pathogenic avian influenza outbreaks led to strengthening and reforms of the WHO strategy, including the expansion of the Global Influenza Surveillance and Response System, multi-sectoral collaboration with the One Health approach, adoption of the Pandemic Influenza Preparedness Framework, and the introduction of Emergency Risk Management for Health. In 2019, the WHO issued the Global Influenza Strategy to provide a framework aimed at strengthening the prevention and control of seasonal influenza and preparedness for future pandemics. Humankind managed to cope with the past global public health threats with WHO as the leader. However, the WHO faces mounting obstacles to fulfilling its purpose.

Keywords WHO · IHR · GISRS · PIP framework · ERMH

1 Introduction

More than 100 years have passed since the Spanish influenza H1N1pandemic from 1918 to 1919, which resulted in up to 50 million deaths [1, 2]. In the past 100 years, there have been three additional influenza pandemics: Asian influenza H2N2 in 1957–1958, resulting in 1–4 million deaths; Hong Kong influenza H3N2 in 1968–1969, resulting in 1–4 million deaths; and swine-origin H1N1 pandemic influenza in 2009–2010, resulting in 100,000–400,000 deaths [3, 4]. Annual

T. Imamura · H. Oshitani (✉)
Department of Virology, Tohoku University Graduate School of Medicine, Sendai, Japan
e-mail: oshitanih@med.tohoku.ac.jp

J. Fujita (ed.), *Influenza*, Respiratory Disease Series: Diagnostic Tools and Disease Managements, https://doi.org/10.1007/978-981-15-9109-9_1

economic losses from a global influenza pandemic are estimated to be about 500 billion US dollars per year [5]. The avian influenza virus and influenza viruses from other animal species are known to have sporadically caused spill-over transmissions to humans; furthermore, some highly pathogenic avian influenza (HPAI) virus strains may require only a few amino acid mutations to acquire efficient transmission capability among humans [6–9]. The next influenza pandemic is considered a matter of "when," not "if" [10].

Seasonal influenza, although often underestimated compared to pandemic influenza, also poses a serious burden on global health and the global economy. The estimation is that there are 1 billion influenza cases each year, among which are 3–5 million severe cases and 290,000–650,000 influenza-related respiratory deaths [11]. The highest mortality rates are estimated in sub-Saharan Africa, Southeast Asia, and among people aged 75 years or older [11–13]. Seasonal epidemics are also associated with economic burden resulting from direct medical costs and indirect costs of lost productivity [14, 15].

Nonpharmaceutical interventions, vaccines, antiviral drugs, and other treatments comprise measures against both seasonal and pandemic influenza. Nonpharmaceutical interventions range from hand washing on the personal level to social distancing policy at the community level, and they are the first line of defense against influenza [10]. The Global Influenza Surveillance and Response System (GISRS) comprises 147 WHO National Influenza Centers (NIC) and six WHO Collaborating Centers, as of July 2020 (Fig. 1.1) [16]. It is a global mechanism of surveillance,

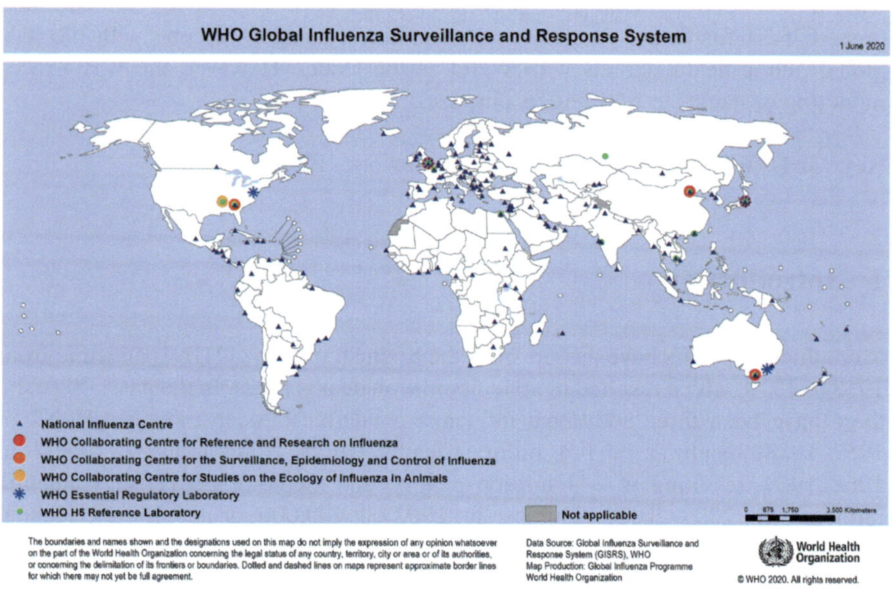

Fig. 1.1 WHO Global Influenza Surveillance and Response System (as of 1 June 2020). (Cited from https://www.who.int/influenza/gisrs_laboratory/GISRS_map.jpg?ua=1. Accessed 5 August 2020)

preparedness, and response to seasonal, pandemic, and zoonotic influenza. Annual WHO recommendations on the composition of the influenza vaccine for the following season are based on the analysis of surveillance data generated by GISRS. Based on the WHO's recommendations, each country produces seasonal influenza vaccines mainly using embryonated eggs. Research and development of more effective next-generation vaccines is being conducted worldwide, including studies of cell-based vaccine production, broadly protective influenza vaccines, and improved methods for predicting future epidemic strains [17, 18]. The WHO also issued guidelines for clinical and pharmaceutical management of influenza [19].

Influenza poses a threat to global public health, which requires preparedness and response at the international level. According to the International Health Regulations (IHR), as revised in 2005, the WHO has been strengthening the preparedness and response for global public health threats, including seasonal and pandemic influenza. The WHO has expanded the GISRS, engaged in multi-sectoral collaboration with the One Health approach, adopted the Pandemic Influenza Preparedness (PIP) Framework, and introduced Emergency Risk Management for Health (ERMH) [20–22]. Despite these achievements, the world is still "ill-prepared" against influenza and other global health emergencies. In 2019, the WHO issued the strategic plan for 2019–2030, aiming "to enhance global and national pandemic preparedness, to combat the ongoing threat of zoonotic influenza, and to improve prevention and control of seasonal influenza in all countries" (p. 4) [10].

2 International Health Regulations (IHR), 2005

Severe acute respiratory syndrome (SARS) was the first global public health emergency of the twenty-first century. SARS and sporadic human cases of HPAI H5N1 prompted the revision of the IHR adopted in 1969. The IHR (1969) covered six quarantinable diseases, including cholera, plague, yellow fever, smallpox, relapsing fever, and typhus. It was later amended, in 1973 and 1981, reducing the number of covered diseases to three: yellow fever, plague, and cholera [23]. As the frequency of the emergence or reemergence of international infectious disease threats and other public health risks increased due to the rising density of the human population, the expansion of agriculture and livestock production, greater human–wildlife interaction, and the growth of international travel and trade [24], the IHR (2005) was adopted in 2005 and entered into force in 2007.

The purpose of the IHR (2005) is "to prevent, protect against, control and provide a public health response to the international spread of disease in ways that are commensurate with and restricted to public health risks, and which avoid unnecessary interference with international traffic and trade" (p. 1) [25]. The IHR (2005) was characterized by not limiting its scope to specific diseases. Strengthening core public health capacities is deemed obligatory for countries. Countries are also required to notify the WHO of events that may constitute a public health emergency of international concern (PHEIC), and to establish national IHR focal points. The

IHR (2005) also describes the algorithm to determine a potential PHEIC. The Director-General of the WHO may declare PHEIC based on the recommendations of the emergency committee. When a PHEIC is declared, the WHO provides corresponding temporary recommendations.

3 Swine-Origin H1N1 Pandemic Influenza in 2009

The swine-origin H1N1 influenza pandemic in 2009 was the first declaration of a PHEIC [26]. The GISRS detected and characterized the virus in a timely fashion, and the first candidate reassortant vaccine virus was developed within a month after the declaration of the PHEIC. The WHO assisted affected countries and distributed more than three million courses of antiviral drugs. Despite these accomplishments, the 2009 pandemic exposed the WHO's defects in many areas. The most serious problem was the delayed distribution of influenza vaccine in low- and middle-income countries [26, 27]. Some middle-income countries had some vaccine production capacities and produced vaccines using virus samples shared with the WHO through GISRS. However, these capacities were not enough to cover their populations, and many middle-income countries and most low-income countries did not have any vaccine production capacities. The WHO and most low- and middle-income countries had to rely on "donations" of vaccines and financial support from manufacturers and high-income countries. Furthermore, the pledged donations were fulfilled only after the major wave of the pandemic had passed [28–30].

4 Pandemic Influenza Preparedness (PIP) Framework

The PIP Framework was developed in 2011, aiming for the strengthened sharing of influenza viruses with human pandemic potential and equitable access to vaccines and other benefits [21]. The establishment of the Framework reflected the negotiation of equitable access in influenza vaccines against HPAI H5N1, which led to the establishment of the Global Initiative for Sharing All Influenza Data (GISAID), and pandemic H1N1 in 2009 [27]. The PIP Framework was unique in imposing contractual obligations on participating governments, private partners, and other stakeholders, enforcing them to provide, with tiered pricing, a certain proportion of manufactured vaccines and antivirals to WHO [31]. However, the Framework harbors many deficiencies and challenges. One of the limitations of the PIP Framework is that it covers only influenza viruses with human pandemic potential; the Framework is not applied to seasonal influenza or non-influenza pathogens, including Ebola virus, Zika virus, Middle East respiratory syndrome coronavirus (MERS-CoV), SARS coronavirus 1 (SARS-CoV-1), or SARS coronavirus 2 (SARS-CoV-2) [32]. The pragmatic efficacy of the PIP Framework remains unclear, and equitable access to vaccines and other drugs is currently sought through activities of intergovernmental organizations and nongovernmental mechanisms [27]. The PIP

Framework's application to genetic sequencing data is not established despite the Framework's multiple revisions [33]. The relationship with competing international establishments needs to be clarified: the GISAID, and the Nagoya Protocol on Access to Genetic Resources and the Fair and Equitable Sharing [34, 35].

5 Emergency Risk Management for Health Approach

The swine-origin influenza pandemic in 2009 also exposed the need for a flexible, risk-based approach in the global response to rapidly changing pandemics, as decisions must be made with scientific evidence. WHO and member states had originally prepared for a pandemic of high severity and mortality, resulting in public confusion during the pandemic 2009, which, luckily, turned out to be a milder event [36]. The Pandemic Influenza Risk Management WHO Interim Guidance in 2013 proposed a risk-based approach to pandemic influenza risk management, the ERMH approach [22]. It utilizes three indices for assessing public health risk: transmissibility, seriousness of disease, and impact. Unlike the previous categorization of six pandemic phases, the 2013 guidance introduced the continuum of pandemic phases, interpandemic, alert, pandemic, and transition (Fig. 1.2). The guidance indicates WHO actions according to the continuum of pandemic phases but instructs that emergency risk management at the country level must be flexible in accommodating different consequences within individual countries [22].

6 Core Public Health Capacity Strengthening

The 2009 pandemic also revealed the lack of minimum core public health capacities in many countries, which is required by the IHR (2005) [4]. The WHO review committee concluded that "The world is ill-prepared to respond to a severe influenza pandemic or to any similarly global, sustained and threatening public health

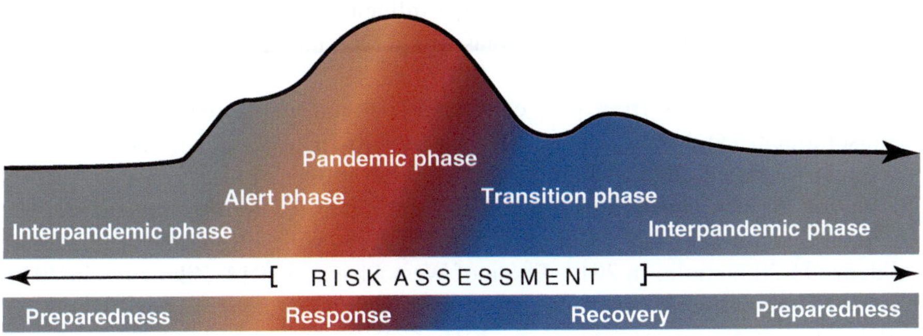

Fig. 1.2 The continuum of pandemic phases. (Cited from Pandemic Influenza Risk Management WHO Interim Guidance, 2013, World Health Organization)

emergency," and it recommended the accelerated implementation of core capacities required by the IHR (2005) [4]. The Joint External Evaluation (JEE) tool was developed in 2016 to assess member states' core public health capacities and to assist them in identifying the most urgent needs within their health systems [10, 37].

7 The Global Influenza Strategy for 2019–2030

In 2019, the WHO issued the Global Influenza Strategy for 2019–2030 to provide a framework for WHO countries and partners aiming for strengthening the prevention and control of seasonal influenza and their preparedness for future global pandemics [10]. The strategy focuses on the development of better global tools, such as vaccines, antivirals, and treatments. Another focus of the strategy is to establish stronger country capacities that are integrated within national health security planning and universal health coverage. The strategy identifies the following as ongoing challenges: improvement of epidemiological and virological surveillance systems; better understanding of influenza morbidity, mortality, and economic burden; development of pandemic preparedness on a national level; better education of nonpharmaceutical interventions against influenza; vaccines' improvement and the development of new vaccines; reinforcement of seasonal vaccination programs; proper stockpiling of antiviral drugs; further research on alternative treatments, therapies, and strategies; and development of consolidated guidelines for the clinical management of influenza-related illness.

8 Conclusion

The WHO has contributed to the prevention, detection, control, and treatment of influenza and other public health threats. As humankind make provision for future epidemics and pandemics, core public health capacity strengthening at the national level and international collaboration are both essential components of the world's preparedness against influenza. The Global Influenza Strategy for 2019–2030 provides a framework for strengthening seasonal prevention and control and preparedness for future global pandemics.

Despite the lessons from past experiences, the world remains "ill-prepared" against influenza and other public health threats [10]. The world is constantly under the threat to global public health [24, 38]. Avian influenza viruses are constantly circulating in wild birds and poultry, causing sporadic human infections. The Director-General previously declared six PHEICs: swine-origin H1N1 pandemic influenza in 2009, polio in 2014, Ebola of West Africa in 2014, Zika virus in 2016, Ebola of Democratic Republic of Congo and surrounding countries in 2018–2020, and the current coronavirus disease of 2019 (COVID-19) since 2019. Each of these events has provided various lessons and challenges, some of which are new, but most were indicated in past events. The necessity of core national capacity strengthening has been addressed since the adoption of the IHR (2005). Inequity in pathogen sharing and vaccine distribution remains a major issue, and the WHO lacks stable, sustainable funding. Furthermore, communication failures and mutual distrust among WHO members hinder global public health response capabilities.

The WHO is still the leader in addressing and managing issues of global health, but it is also evident that mounting obstacles exist that prevent the WHO from fully serving its purpose.

References

1. Johnson NP, Mueller J. Updating the accounts: global mortality of the 1918-1920 "Spanish" influenza pandemic. Bull Hist Med. 2002;76(1):105–15. https://doi.org/10.1353/bhm.2002.0022.
2. Spreeuwenberg P, Kroneman M, Paget J. Reassessing the global mortality burden of the 1918 influenza pandemic. Am J Epidemiol. 2018;187(12):2561–7. https://doi.org/10.1093/aje/kwy191.
3. Krammer F, Smith GJD, Fouchier RAM, Peiris M, Kedzierska K, Doherty PC, et al. Influenza. Nat Rev Dis Primers. 2018;4(1):3. https://doi.org/10.1038/s41572-018-0002-y.
4. World Health Organization. Implementation of the International Health Regulations (2005); 2011.
5. Fan VY, Jamison DT, Summers LH. Pandemic risk: how large are the expected losses? Bull World Health Organ. 2018;96(2):129–34. https://doi.org/10.2471/BLT.17.199588.
6. World Health Organization. Cumulative number of confirmed human cases of avian influenza A(H5N1) reported to WHO, 2003-2020. 10 July 2020. https://www.who.int/influenza/human_animal_interface/2020_10_07_tableH5N1.pdf?ua=1. Accessed 9 Aug 2020.
7. Widdowson MA, Bresee JS, Jernigan DB. The global threat of animal influenza viruses of zoonotic concern: then and now. J Infect Dis. 2017;216(Suppl. 4):S493–8. https://doi.org/10.1093/infdis/jix331.
8. Imai M, Watanabe T, Hatta M, Das SC, Ozawa M, Shinya K, et al. Experimental adaptation of an influenza H5 HA confers respiratory droplet transmission to a reassortant H5 HA/H1N1 virus in ferrets. Nature. 2012;486(7403):420–8. https://doi.org/10.1038/nature10831.
9. Herfst S, Schrauwen EJ, Linster M, Chutinimitkul S, de Wit E, Munster VJ, et al. Airborne transmission of influenza A/H5N1 virus between ferrets. Science. 2012;336(6088):1534–41. https://doi.org/10.1126/science.1213362.
10. World Health Organization. Global influenza strategy 2019–2030. Geneva: World Health Organization; 2019. https://apps.who.int/iris/bitstream/handle/10665/311184/9789241515320-eng.pdf?sequence=18&isAllowed=y. Accessed 9 Aug 2020.
11. Iuliano AD, Roguski KM, Chang HH, Muscatello DJ, Palekar R, Tempia S, et al. Estimates of global seasonal influenza-associated respiratory mortality: a modelling study. Lancet (London, England). 2018;391(10127):1285–300. https://doi.org/10.1016/S0140-6736(17)33293-2.
12. Troeger CE, Blacker BF, Khalil IA, Zimsen SRM, Albertson SB, Abate D, et al. Mortality, morbidity, and hospitalisations due to influenza lower respiratory tract infections, 2017: an analysis for the Global Burden of Disease Study 2017. Lancet Respir Med. 2019;7(1):69–89. https://doi.org/10.1016/S2213-2600(18)30496-X.
13. Wang X, Li Y, O'Brien KL, Madhi SA, Widdowson M-A, Byass P, et al. Global burden of respiratory infections associated with seasonal influenza in children under 5 years in 2018: a systematic review and modelling study. Lancet Glob Health. 2020;8(4):e497–510. https://doi.org/10.1016/s2214-109x(19)30545-5.

14. Peasah SK, Azziz-Baumgartner E, Breese J, Meltzer MI, Widdowson MA. Influenza cost and cost-effectiveness studies globally--a review. Vaccine. 2013;31(46):5339–48. https://doi.org/10.1016/j.vaccine.2013.09.013.
15. de Francisco Shapovalova N, Donadel M, Jit M, Hutubessy R. A systematic review of the social and economic burden of influenza in low- and middle-income countries. Vaccine. 2015;33(48):6537–44. https://doi.org/10.1016/j.vaccine.2015.10.066.
16. World Health Organization. National Influenza Centres. 28 July 2020. https://www.who.int/influenza/gisrs_laboratory/national_influenza_centres/National_Influenza_Centres_20200728_web.pdf?ua=1. Accessed 9 Aug 2020.
17. World Health Organization. WHO preferred product characteristics for next-generation influenza vaccines; 2017.
18. Yamayoshi S, Kawaoka Y. Current and future influenza vaccines. Nat Med. 2019;25(2):212–20. https://doi.org/10.1038/s41591-018-0340-z.
19. World Health Organization. WHO guidelines for pharmacological management of pandemic influenza A(H1N1) 2009 and other Influenza Viruses Part1. 2010. https://www.who.int/csr/resources/publications/swineflu/h1n1_guidelines_pharmaceutical_mngt.pdf?ua=1. Accessed 9 Aug 2020.
20. FAO-OIE-WHO. The FAO-OIE-WHO Collaboration: a Tripartite Concept Note Sharing responsibilities and coordinating global activities to address health risks at the animal-human-ecosystems interfaces. 2010. https://www.who.int/influenza/resources/documents/tripartite_concept_note_hanoi_042011_en.pdf?ua=1. Accessed 9 Aug 2020.
21. World Health Organization. Pandemic influenza preparedness framework for the sharing of influenza viruses and access to vaccines and other benefits. 2011. https://apps.who.int/iris/bitstream/handle/10665/44796/9789241503082_eng.pdf?sequence=1. Accessed 9 Aug 2020.
22. World Health Organization. Pandemic influenza risk management WHO Interim Guidance. 2013. https://www.who.int/influenza/preparedness/pandemic/GIP_PandemicInfluenzaRiskManagementInterimGuidance_Jun2013.pdf?ua=1. Accessed 9 Aug 2020.
23. World Health Organization. International Health Regulations (1969). 1983. https://apps.who.int/iris/bitstream/handle/10665/96616/9241580070.pdf?sequence=1. Accessed 9 Aug 2020.
24. Morse SS, Mazet JAK, Woolhouse M, Parrish CR, Carroll D, Karesh WB, et al. Prediction and prevention of the next pandemic zoonosis. Lancet. 2012;380(9857):1956–65. https://doi.org/10.1016/s0140-6736(12)61684-5.
25. World Health Organization. International Health Regulations 2005. 3rd ed; 2016.
26. Fineberg HV. Pandemic preparedness and response—lessons from the H1N1 influenza of 2009. N Engl J Med. 2014;370(14):1335–42. https://doi.org/10.1056/NEJMra1208802.
27. Fidler DP. Negotiating equitable access to influenza vaccines: global health diplomacy and the controversies surrounding avian influenza H5N1 and pandemic influenza H1N1. PLoS Med. 2010;7(5):e1000247. https://doi.org/10.1371/journal.pmed.1000247.
28. World Health Organization. Report of the WHO pandemic influenza A(H1N1) vaccine deployment initiative; 2012.
29. World Health Organization. Urgent support for developing countries' responses to the H1N1 influenza pandemic. 2009. https://reliefweb.int/sites/reliefweb.int/files/resources/47A26C749293325185257663005F6EE9-Full_Report.pdf. Accessed 9 Aug 2020.
30. World Health Organization. Main operational lessons learnt from the WHO Pandemic Influenza A(H1N1) Vaccine Deployment Initiative. 2011. https://apps.who.int/iris/bitstream/handle/10665/44711/9789241564342_eng.pdf?sequence=1&isAllowed=y. Accessed 9 Aug 2020.
31. Gostin LO, Phelan A, Stoto MA, Kraemer JD, Reddy KS. Virus sharing, genetic sequencing, and global health security. Science (New York, NY). 2014;345(6202):1295–6. https://doi.org/10.1126/science.1257622.
32. Gostin LO, DeBartolo MC, Katz R. The global health law trilogy: towards a safer, healthier, and fairer world. Lancet. 2017;390(10105):1918–26. https://doi.org/10.1016/s0140-6736(17)31261-8.

33. World Health Organization. Report of the 2016 PIP Framework Review Group. 2017. https://apps.who.int/gb/ebwha/pdf_files/WHA70/A70_17-en.pdf?ua=1. Accessed 13 Aug 2020.
34. Shu Y, McCauley J. GISAID: global initiative on sharing all influenza data - from vision to reality. Euro Surveill. 2017;22:13. https://doi.org/10.2807/1560-7917.ES.2017.22.13.30494.
35. World Health Organization. Implementation of the Nagoya protocol and pathogen sharing: public health implications. https://www.who.int/docs/default-source/documents/nagoya-protocol/nagoya-full-study-english.pdf?sfvrsn=ec2ab49d_12. Accessed 9 Aug 2020.
36. World Health Organization. Pandemic influenza risk management: a WHO guide to inform and harmonize national and international pandemic preparedness and response. 2017. https://apps.who.int/iris/bitstream/handle/10665/259893/WHO-WHE-IHM-GIP-2017.1-eng.pdf?sequence=1&isAllowed=y. Accessed 9 Aug 2020.
37. World Health Organization. Joint external evaluation tool second edition. 2018. https://extranet.who.int/sph/sites/default/files/document-library/document/9789241550222-eng.pdf. Accessed 9 Aug 2020.
38. Jones KE, Patel NG, Levy MA, Storeygard A, Balk D, Gittleman JL, et al. Global trends in emerging infectious diseases. Nature. 2008;451(7181):990–3. https://doi.org/10.1038/nature06536.

Part II
Definition, Epidemiology, and Pathogenesis

Chapter 2
Epidemiology of Influenza with a Description of Recent Trends in Japan: What Are the Key Epidemiologic Features of Seasonal Influenza?

Yuzo Arima, Takuri Takahashi, Tomimasa Sunagawa, and Motoi Suzuki

Abstract Influenza causes substantial morbidity and mortality each year globally, with periodic pandemics. For annually occurring seasonal influenza, influenza A and influenza B viruses are responsible for most of the burden. Both of these viruses are constantly evolving, and influenza A viruses have the ability to change dramatically, with pandemic potential. For seasonal influenza in Japan, usually a greater burden is due to influenza A, although influenza B detections increase later in the season and there have been some years where influenza B predominated with a large public health impact. Usually, seasonal influenza activity peaks in the winter and remains low during the summer; seasonality, however, varies by year and location (Okinawa shows less distinct seasonality), and pandemics have occurred outside the regular season. Compared to young adults, children and the elderly normally experience higher influenza morbidity. However, the relative burden for each age group may vary by season, and young adults may be considerably affected in a pandemic. These evolving and unpredictable epidemiologic features of influenza highlight the importance of continuous and timely surveillance, with careful assessments by time, place, person, and virus.

Keywords Respiratory · Seasonal · Pandemic · Surveillance · Zoonotic

Y. Arima (✉) · T. Takahashi · T. Sunagawa · M. Suzuki
Infectious Disease Surveillance Center, National Institute of Infectious Diseases, Tokyo, Japan
e-mail: arima@niid.go.jp

J. Fujita (ed.), *Influenza*, Respiratory Disease Series: Diagnostic Tools and Disease Managements, https://doi.org/10.1007/978-981-15-9109-9_2

1 Introduction

Humans have had a long history with influenza. Epidemiologic characteristics suggestive of influenza have been recorded for centuries, and a major influenza pandemic left its mark a century ago, with substantial mortality [1, 2]. Mass human movement during World War I was thought to have facilitated the 1918–1919 pandemic [1, 2], and in today's globalized society, the potential reach and impact of influenza is high. Moreover, as a zoonotic disease with avian reservoirs, influenza virus is constantly evolving and not eradicable [2–5]. These realities necessitate continuous monitoring of influenza. With its respiratory burden every winter, and with an increasingly aging Japanese population, influenza poses particular concerns for Japan. Within this context, we discuss the basic epidemiologic features of influenza, presenting an overview with reference to past pandemics, followed by a description of recent influenza trends in Japan based on national surveillance data.

2 Overview of Influenza

Influenza is an RNA virus containing envelope glycoproteins hemagglutinin (HA) and neuraminidase (NA). Among the three types of influenza viruses known to cause human disease (A, B, C), A and B are responsible for the majority of influenza morbidity [5]. Antigenic changes in HA and NA occur through "antigenic drift" (minor change) and "antigenic shift" (major change) [1, 5]. Among influenza A viruses, three subtypes of HA (H1, H2, and H3) and two subtypes of NA (N1 and N2) have circulated widely in humans; only influenza A viruses have caused pandemics [1, 5]. In contrast, influenza B viruses are described as two distinct lineages, B/Yamagata and B/Victoria, and influenza B viruses show less antigenic changes [1, 5].

Among influenza A viruses, antibody against one type/subtype confers limited or no protection against another type/subtype. Frequent emergence of antigenic variants through antigenic drift leads to seasonal epidemics, while antigenic shift has been associated with pandemics [1, 2, 5]. Each successive antigenic variant has replaced its predecessor—for instance, since the emergence of the pandemic A/H1N1 variant in 2009, the previously circulating A/H1N1 variant has not been detected [1, 2, 5, 6].

With regard to transmission, influenza virus spreads primarily via aerosols of respiratory secretions expelled by infected persons (e.g., during coughing or sneezing); exposure occurs via breathing in droplets that contain the virus (or contact, such as with contaminated hands). Once infected, the time to disease onset is usually a few days [2]. Given this human-to-human transmission mode—combined with influenza's short incubation period—influenza can be acutely outbreak-prone.

The majority of influenza infections result in mild syndromes (e.g., fever, cough/sore throat, muscle/joint pain, malaise); while treatment is often supportive, the use of the antiviral drug oseltamivir is prevalent in Japan. However, influenza can lead to severe respiratory illness and cardiopulmonary/circulatory complications with fatal consequences, especially among the vulnerable such as the elderly [1, 7]. Secondary bacterial pneumonia can contribute to poor outcomes, and this was believed to have contributed to the high mortality during the 1918–1919 pandemic [1]. During this pandemic, many young healthy adults also died, and pathologic findings indicated particularly severe pneumonia [1, 2].

3 Influenza Pandemics and the Zoonotic Link

In effect, a unique concern with influenza is its ability to cause pandemics, often resulting in substantial morbidity and mortality, societal disruption, and economic loss. Pandemics occur when a new or substantially different influenza A subtype is transmitted efficiently between individuals in a sustained manner on a global scale [1, 2, 5].

The 1918–1919 pandemic (A/H1N1) was very severe with high morbidity and mortality, particularly in young adults. There were some uniquely severe clinical features, and it is considered to be the influenza pandemic with greatest mortality in recent history. While often called the "Spanish Flu," the geographic origin of the pandemic is still debated [1, 2].

Believed to have started in southern China, an A/H2N2 virus with different HA and NA antigens from the formerly circulating A/H1N1 viruses was detected in 1957 (first isolated in Japan). The "Asian" A/H2N2 virus quickly spread worldwide, characterized by two waves (October 1957 and January 1958) resulting in excess mortality, with the highest attack rates in children [1, 2].

In 1968, "Hong Kong" influenza A/H3N2 emerged, with a different HA (H3) but sharing the same NA (N2) with previously circulating H2N2 viruses. It is believed to be a reassortant that derived HA and polymerase genes from an avian influenza virus and the remaining gene segments from the circulating human H2N2 virus. Attack rates were again highest in children. Notably, the pandemic's impact was likely reduced because much of the population had some pre-existing immunity to the N2 protein [1, 2].

As of this writing, the most recent influenza pandemic was first described in spring 2009 in Mexico and the southwestern United States. While H1N1 viruses have been circulating since 1977 (which were themselves similar to H1N1 viruses that had circulated during the early 1950s), the emergent "swine" influenza virus (A(H1N1)pdm09) was different—it was closely related to influenza A viruses that had been circulating in North American and Eurasian pigs [8, 9]. Relative to seasonal influenza, children and nonelderly adults suffered more serious outcomes, and pregnancy and obesity also appeared to be risk factors for severe outcomes [9].

These periodic pandemics have taught us important lessons. A recurrent theme with influenza virus is its ability to reassort genes from both human and animal viruses—such mixing can lead to novel viruses with pandemic potential. Notably, waterfowl are the natural reservoir of influenza A viruses [1, 8] and serve as an essentially uneradicable source. While the species barrier for human infection is believed to be large for avian influenza viruses, pigs are hypothesized to serve as an intermediate "mixing vessel" [1, 2].

A seminal event, however, occurred in Hong Kong in 1997 with influenza A/H5N1, resulting in 18 human cases (including 6 deaths). All gene segments were avian in origin and reassortment with human influenza A viruses had not occurred. Notably, there was a concurrent influenza outbreak in chickens in local live bird markets, and viruses isolated from the markets were identical to those isolated from human cases. While transmission appeared to be poultry-to-human with inefficient human-to-human spread, this event demonstrated that avian influenza A viruses could infect humans without passing through an intermediate host [1, 2].

Since then, while rare, multiple avian influenza virus infections in humans have been detected globally, particularly in Asia [10]. Swine influenza viruses circulating in North America have also sporadically infected humans [8, 11]. These realities have motivated global efforts to enhance coordination with the animal sector ("One Health" approach) [3–5]. While only H1, H2, and H3 are known to have caused human epidemics and pandemics to date, risk assessments for the other HA and NA subtypes circulating in animals are thus deemed critical [3, 4].

4 Epidemiology: Time, Place, Person, and Virus

4.1 Seasonal Influenza: Global Burden and Surveillance

While zoonotic influenza poses unpredictable threats and pandemics can result in substantial public health impact, the greatest cumulative global burden of influenza comes from its seasonal form. Importantly, with a large number of infections occurring yearly, even a relatively low case-fatality rate translates to large absolute number of deaths, and modelling studies have indicated the high population-level impact [7]. A hallmark of influenza has in fact been excess mortality. Moreover, mild respiratory illness can still pose a medical and societal concern, with health facilities becoming overwhelmed, worker/school absenteeism, and productivity loss.

Much of the understanding on the descriptive epidemiology of seasonal influenza comes from routine surveillance data (special studies, such as influenza vaccine effectiveness studies [11], can be used to answer questions not possible from routine surveillance) [12]. Routine surveillance systems allow for ongoing descriptive assessments, timely situational awareness, and informed response, including risk communication to clinicians and the public. Globally, the World Health Organization's Global Influenza Surveillance and Response System performs year-round influenza surveillance, based on syndrome-based (aggregate influenza-like illness (ILI) case) and virologic (circulating virus subtypes and lineages, proportion of ILI specimens tested that are influenza-positive, and antiviral resistance) data by week, region/country, and where possible by age group [13, 14].

4.2 Seasonal Influenza Surveillance in Japan

In Japan, influenza is monitored similarly, based on "time," "place," and "person" data, along with virologic details. A nationwide network of sentinel sites provides sustained, timely influenza data—under the National Epidemiological Surveillance of Infectious Diseases (NESID) system, ~5000 sentinel sites (~3000 pediatric and ~ 2000 internal medicine health facilities) report patients diagnosed with influenza on a weekly basis [6, 11]. Additionally, since 2011, the number of hospitalized influenza patients (i.e., severe outcomes) are monitored via ~500 sentinel hospitals nationwide [6, 11]. Monitoring these sentinel data on medically attended influenza patients provides useful indicators of the spread, tempo, and magnitude of transmission, and demonstrates the substantial morbidity attributable to seasonal influenza in Japan.

Virologically, laboratory-based surveillance allows for genetic and antigenic description of circulating strains. Importantly, these data are used to select virus strains for inclusion in the annual vaccine, and enable detection of unusual strains or changes in the distribution of circulating viruses [6, 11]. In addition, antiviral resistance monitoring for key antiviral drugs (e.g., oseltamivir, peramivir, and most recently baloxavir) facilitates timely communication and guidance regarding their use [5, 6, 15, 16].

Lastly, it is well acknowledged that understanding influenza epidemiology and activity level require multiple data sources [5, 12], and other surveillance/information systems are also monitored [6]. The following are routinely or periodically performed in Japan: daily event-based surveillance (e.g., monitoring various information sources for facility outbreaks); weekly ILI school absenteeism surveillance; weekly acute encephalitis surveillance; weekly excess mortality surveillance; and annual seroprevalence surveys [6, 11].

4.3 Recent Epidemiologic Features of Seasonal Influenza in Japan

Nationally, influenza activity usually starts to increase in September or October, surpassing the seasonal threshold that indicates the start of the influenza season (average of >1 influenza case per sentinel site per week, based on the ~5000 sentinel facilities) in November or December (range: week 46 to week 1 during 2010–2018) [6, 11]. The peak is usually in late January or early February, and activity returns to baseline levels in the spring (Fig. 2.1); similar temporal trends are observed in the

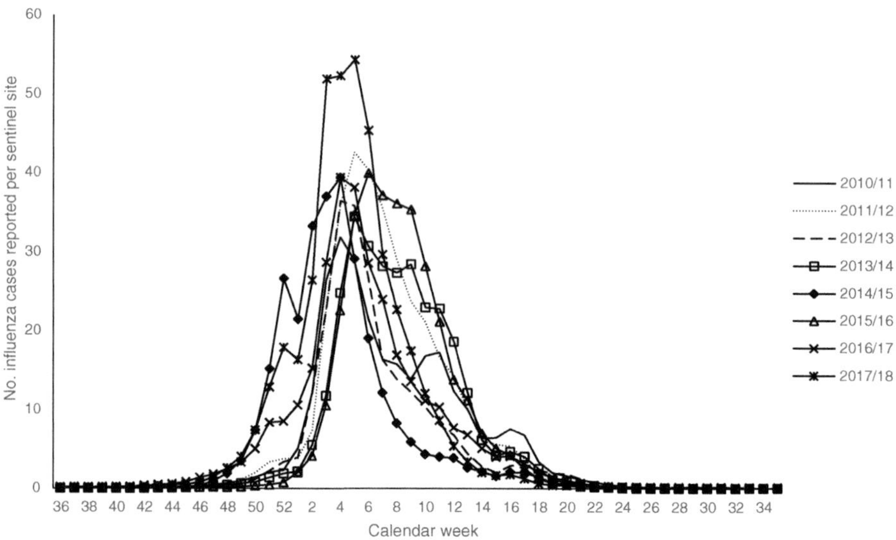

Fig. 2.1 Number of reported influenza cases per sentinel site, 2010/2011 to 2017/2018 seasons. (Source: National Institute of Infectious Diseases, https://www.niid.go.jp/niid/ja/idwr.html)

frequencies of hospitalized influenza and ILI school absenteeism. While this seasonality is predictable, there is heterogeneity in the timing of season start and peak week, with varying levels in magnitude (Fig. 2.1). For instance, while the season started early (week 46) and peaked early (week 4) in the 2016–2017 season, 2015–2016 season saw a later start (week 1) and peak (week 6). In terms of magnitude, the 2017–2018 season saw very high peak levels while low peaks were experienced in 2010–2011 and 2013–2014 seasons.

Seasonality of influenza also depends on "place." Relative to the rest of Japan, Okinawa, the southernmost prefecture in Japan, has a higher baseline level of influenza activity, with less pronounced seasonality [6, 11, 17]. This trend is consistent with that in other tropical/subtropical areas, where influenza seasonality is less well-defined, with more year-round circulation of influenza virus [18]. In addition, depending on the year, where influenza activity starts to increase can differ; some years see increase in activity start in the north, while other years see it begin in the south (or other areas) [6]. It is thus important to monitor influenza spatiotemporally.

Perhaps the most important variability for seasonal influenza is observed demographically. Attack rates for ILI are usually highest in children, who serve as vehicles of transmission in the community and the household—children are often the first group to be affected in the season, with increased school absenteeism serving as an indicator of increased influenza activity [5, 6]. In terms of severe outcomes, a U-shaped age distribution is often observed (Fig. 2.2), with influenza-associated hospitalizations greatest among young children and the elderly; for instance, in the 2017/18 season, while those aged <10 and >69 years respectively made up 23% and

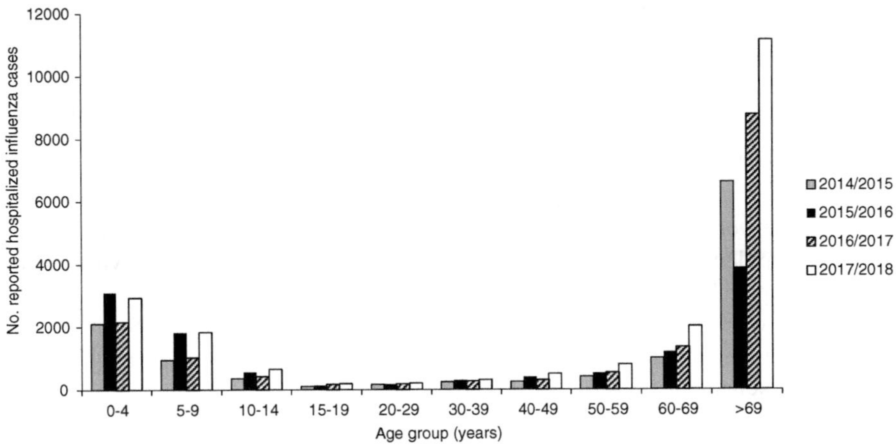

Fig. 2.2 Number of hospitalized influenza cases reported by sentinel hospitals, by age group, 2014/2015 to 2017/2018 seasons. (Source: National Institute of Infectious Diseases, https://www.niid.go.jp/niid/ja/flu-m/590-idsc/8107-fludoko-2017.html and https://www.niid.go.jp/niid/ja/flu-m/590-idsc/7323-fludoko-2016.html)

54% of the hospitalized influenza cases reported from sentinel hospitals, they accounted for 8% and 20% of the population, respectively [19].

Notably, some years are more severe for children, while others are more severe for the elderly. Depending on the year, influenza's age-specific impacts can differ—in recent years, this has been correlated with circulating influenza A subtypes, where H3N2-dominant years (e.g., 2016/2017) have been associated with greater burden in the elderly, while years with H1N1 predominance (e.g., 2015/2016) have been linked to increased burden in the young [6, 17, 20] (Figs. 2.2 and 2.3). Acute encephalitis surveillance also indicates relatively higher influenza encephalitis/encephalopathy attack rates in children when H1N1 predominates [20, 21]. Given such age-dependence and variation by year, assessment by age group is essential, and virological monitoring can offer insights regarding risk groups.

Indeed, extensive virological surveillance in Japan has shown that influenza is a moving target, with circulating subtypes, lineages, and strains changing during and across seasons. While influenza A tends to contribute much of the influenza burden each year, influenza B detections increase absolutely and in relative proportion later in the season [6, 17, 20, 22] (Fig. 2.3). Across seasons, for influenza A, H1 predominated in the 2013/2014 and 2015/2016 seasons, while H3 was predominant in the 2014/2015 and 2016/2017 seasons [6, 17, 20] (Fig. 2.3). For influenza B, while both lineages co-circulated during the 2016/2017 season, the vast majority were B/Yamagata in the 2017/2018 season [6, 17, 22]. Influenza B, in fact, has occasionally shown its ability to cause great burden [23], and B/Yamagata was responsible for an early and large impact in the 2017/2018 season [6, 22] (Fig. 2.3). In retrospect, updating the vaccine from a trivalent to a quadrivalent vaccine that includes both type B lineages beginning in the 2015/2016 season was prudent.

Fig. 2.3 Number of influenza viruses detected by subtype (influenza A) and lineage (influenza B), by week, 2014/2015 to 2017/2018 seasons: (a) 2014/2015 season; (**b**) 2015/2016 season; (**c**) 2016/2017 season; (**d**) 2017/2018 season. As NA typing has not always been performed, influenza A viruses are listed as A/H1pdm09 and A/H3. (Source: National Institute of Infectious Diseases, https://www.niid.go.jp/niid/ja/flu-m/590-idsc/8107-fludoko-2017.html)

Over the years, surveillance has taught us that a defining feature of seasonal influenza epidemiology is its variability over time, place, person, and virus. Even within "person," the association between influenza and gender is often age-dependent, with a higher male proportion among young children [24]. Such features preclude broad generalizations, and necessitate continuous surveillance, with stratified assessments and careful interpretations.

5 Conclusion

Influenza A and B viruses are responsible for much of the seasonal influenza burden, and influenza A viruses can undergo substantial antigenic changes to cause pandemics. For seasonal influenza in Japan, usually a greater burden is due to influenza A, although influenza B detections increase in the spring and some seasons have seen considerable burden from influenza B. Seasonal influenza activity increases in the fall, peaks in the winter, declines in the spring, and remains low during the summer; however, seasonality may vary by year and location, and pandemics can occur at any time. Children and the elderly usually experience disproportionate morbidity, but the relative burden for each age group varies by season, and young adults may be considerably affected in a pandemic. The evolving and varied epidemiologic features of influenza make ongoing and timely surveillance imperative, warranting careful assessments by person, place, time, and virus. For public health practitioners and clinicians, staying informed of influenza epidemiology can facilitate appropriate prevention and mitigation measures. To this end, epidemiologic monitoring will continue to serve as an important defense against this unpredictable virus.

What are the key epidemiologic features of seasonal influenza in terms of time, place, person, and virus (overall and in Japan)?

- Influenza A and influenza B viruses are responsible for the majority of the influenza burden in humans, and both are associated with seasonal influenza. Influenza A viruses have been associated with avian influenza infections in humans, are able to undergo large antigenic changes and capable of causing pandemics.

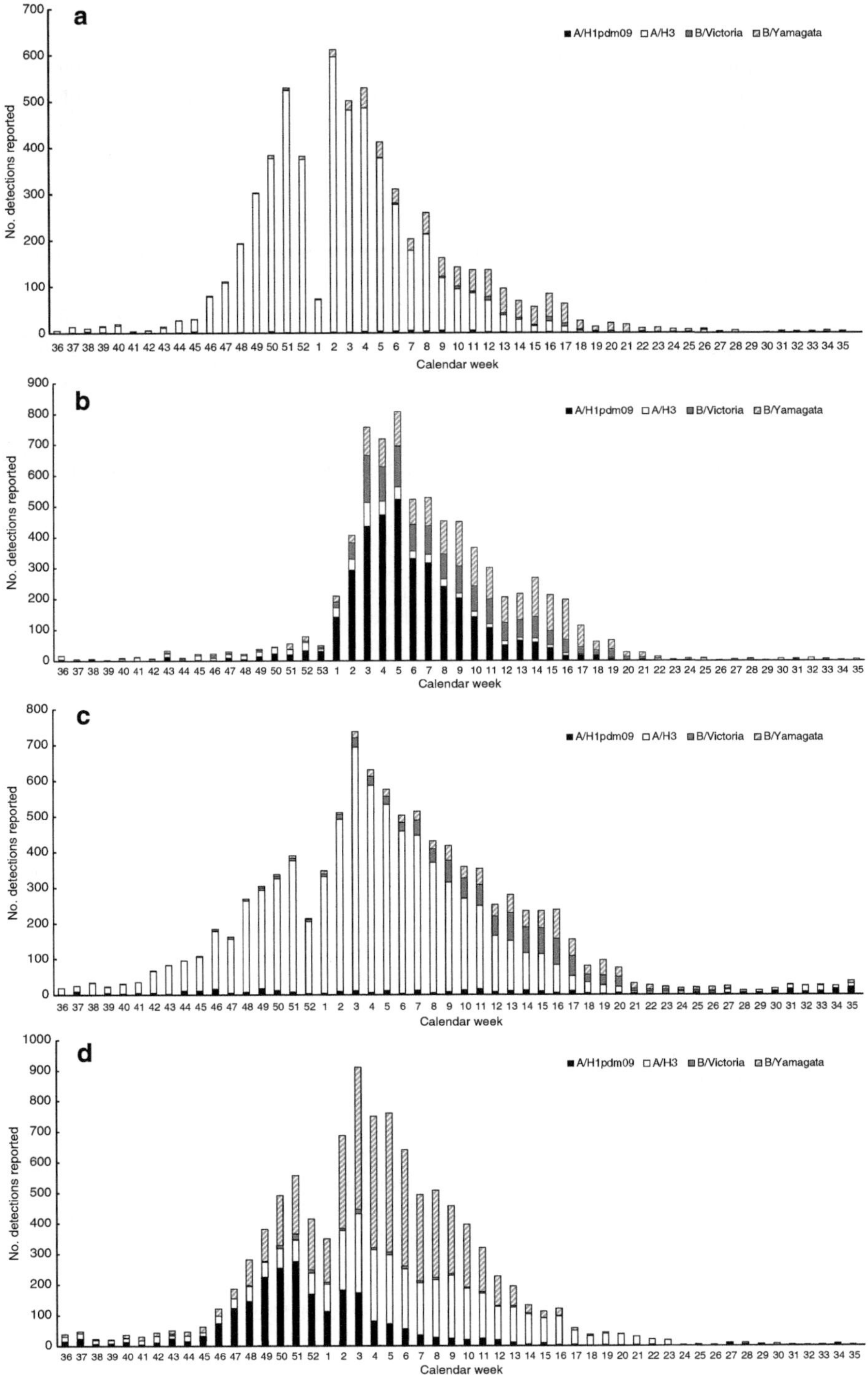
a
■ A/H1pdm09 □ A/H3 ■ B/Victoria ▨ B/Yamagata
No. detections reported
Calendar week
b
■ A/H1pdm09 □ A/H3 ■ B/Victoria ▨ B/Yamagata
No. detections reported
Calendar week
c
■ A/H1pdm09 □ A/H3 ■ B/Victoria ▨ B/Yamagata
No. detections reported
Calendar week
d
■ A/H1pdm09 □ A/H3 ■ B/Victoria ▨ B/Yamagata
No. detections reported
Calendar week

- For seasonal influenza in Japan, usually a greater burden is due to influenza A, although influenza B detections increase later in the season. There have also been some seasons where influenza B was predominant with considerable public health impact.
- Usually, seasonal influenza activity increases in the fall, peaks in the winter, declines in the spring, and remains low during the summer; however, seasonality may vary by year, and pandemics have occurred outside the regular season. Subtropical Okinawa shows less distinct seasonality, with more year-round circulation of influenza virus.
- Compared to young adults, children and the elderly usually experience higher morbidity for seasonal influenza. However, the relative burden for each age group may vary by season, and young adults may be considerably affected in a pandemic.
- The evolving features of influenza A and B viruses indicate the importance of continuous surveillance, with careful assessments by time, place, person, and virus.

Acknowledgements The authors are grateful to all the staff at local public health centers and prefectural and municipal public health institutes who contribute to influenza surveillance activities. They also greatly appreciate Hitomi Kinoshita, Mariko Tokunaga, Masae Yoshikawa, Osamu Takahara, and other members of the National Institute of Infectious Diseases involved in routine influenza surveillance.

References

1. Cox NJ, Subbarao K. Global epidemiology of influenza: past and present. Annu Rev Med. 2000;51:407–21. https://doi.org/10.1146/annurev.med.51.1.407.
2. Kimball AM. Risky trade : infectious disease in the era of global trade. Aldershot: Ashgate; 2006.
3. World Health Organization Global Influenza Programme. Tool for influenza pandemic risk assessment (TIPRA). Geneva: World Health Organization; 2016.
4. Burke SA, Trock SC. Use of influenza risk assessment tool for prepandemic preparedness. Emerg Infect Dis. 2018;24(3):471–7. https://doi.org/10.3201/eid2403.171852.
5. M'Ikanatha NM. Infectious disease surveillance. 2nd ed. Wiley-Blackwell: Chichester; 2013.
6. National Institute of Infectious Diseases. Influenza level map (comprehensive influenza surveillance information in Japanese). https://www.niid.go.jp/niid/ja/flu-map.html. Accessed 30 May 2020.
7. Iuliano AD, Roguski KM, Chang HH, Muscatello DJ, Palekar R, Tempia S, et al. Estimates of global seasonal influenza-associated respiratory mortality: a modelling study. Lancet. 2018;391(10127):1285–300. https://doi.org/10.1016/S0140-6736(17)33293-2.
8. Garten RJ, Davis CT, Russell CA, Shu B, Lindstrom S, Balish A, et al. Antigenic and genetic characteristics of swine-origin 2009 A(H1N1) influenza viruses circulating in humans. Science. 2009;325(5937):197–201. https://doi.org/10.1126/science.1176225.
9. Bautista E, Chotpitayasunondh T, Gao Z, Harper SA, Shaw M, Uyeki TM, et al. Clinical aspects of pandemic 2009 influenza A(H1N1) virus infection. N Engl J Med. 2010;362(18):1708–19. https://doi.org/10.1056/NEJMra1000449.

10. Hamid S, Arima Y, Dueger E, Konings F, Bell L, Lee CK, et al. From H5N1 to HxNy: an epidemiologic overview of human infections with avian influenza in the Western Pacific Region, 2003-2017. Western Pac Surveill Response J. 2018;9(5 Suppl 1):53–67. https://doi.org/10.3565/wpsar.2018.9.2.001.
11. National Institute of Infectious Diseases. Influenza 2018/19 season, Japan. Infect Agents Surveill Rep. 2019;40:177–9.
12. World Health Organization. WHO global epidemiological surveillance standards for influenza. Geneva: World Health Organization; 2014.
13. World Health Organization: FluID. https://www.who.int/influenza/surveillance_monitoring/fluid/en/. Accessed 30 May 2020.
14. World Health Organization: FluNet. https://www.who.int/influenza/gisrs_laboratory/flunet/en/. Accessed 30 May 2020.
15. Takashita E, Fujisaki S, Shirakura M, Nakamura K, Kishida N, Kuwahara T, et al. Influenza A(H1N1)pdm09 virus exhibiting enhanced cross-resistance to oseltamivir and peramivir due to a dual H275Y/G147R substitution, Japan, March 2016. Euro Surveill. 2016;21(24) https://doi.org/10.2807/1560-7917.ES.2016.21.24.30258.
16. Takashita E, Kawakami C, Ogawa R, Morita H, Fujisaki S, Shirakura M, et al. Influenza A(H3N2) virus exhibiting reduced susceptibility to baloxavir due to a polymerase acidic subunit I38T substitution detected from a hospitalised child without prior baloxavir treatment, Japan, January 2019. Euro Surveill. 2019;24(12) https://doi.org/10.2807/1560-7917.ES.2019.24.12.1900170.
17. National Institute of Infectious Diseases. Influenza 2016/17 season, Japan. Infect Agents Surveill Rep. 2017;38:209–11.
18. Ly S, Arashiro T, Ieng V, Tsuyuoka R, Parry A, Horwood P, et al. Establishing seasonal and alert influenza thresholds in Cambodia using the WHO method: implications for effective utilization of influenza surveillance in the tropics and subtropics. Western Pac Surveill Response J. 2017;8(1):22–32. https://doi.org/10.5365/WPSAR.2017.8.1.002.
19. Ministry of Health. Labour and welfare: vital statistics in Japan. 2018. https://www.mhlw.go.jp/toukei/saikin/hw/jinkou/kakutei17/index.html. Accessed 30 May 2020.
20. National Institute of Infectious Diseases. Influenza 2015/16 season, Japan. Infect Agents Surveill Rep. 2016;37:211–2.
21. Okuno H, Yahata Y, Tanaka-Taya K, Arai S, Satoh H, Morino S, et al. Characteristics and outcomes of influenza-associated encephalopathy cases among children and adults in Japan, 2010-2015. Clin Infect Dis. 2018;66(12):1831–7. https://doi.org/10.1093/cid/cix1126.
22. National Institute of Infectious Diseases. Influenza 2017/18 season, Japan. Infect Agents Surveill Rep. 2018;39:181–3.
23. Murakami Y, Hashimoto S, Kawado M, Ohta A, Taniguchi K, Sunagawa T, et al. Estimated number of patients with influenza A(H1)pdm09, or other viral types, from 2010 to 2014 in Japan. PLoS One. 2016;11(1):e0146520. https://doi.org/10.1371/journal.pone.0146520.
24. Peretz J, Hall OJ, Klein SL. Sex differences in influenza virus infection, vaccination, and therapies. In: Klein SRC, editor. Sex and gender differences in infection and treatments for infectious diseases. Cham: Springer; 2015. p. 183–90.

Chapter 3
Transmission of Influenza Virus in the Home: How Are They Transmitted in the Home?

Nobuo Hirotsu

Abstract Household transmission plays a significant role in the spread of influenza epidemics. Understanding of the viral transmission patterns in households is important for effective infection prevention measures. An investigation in the 2010/2011–2015/2016 seasons showed that household transmission of influenza A occurred in 18.5% of households, with a secondary infection rate of 8.0%. The present investigation assessed secondary infection rates by generation/age of household members (i.e., fathers, mothers, and offspring aged 0–6, 7–12, 13–18, and 19+ years). When the index case was an infant, the secondary infection rates were as high as 15.1% among infants and 18.2% among mothers, and infants were more infectious to overall household contacts (secondary infection rate, 12.4%) than were any other generations. For influenza B, the household secondary infection rate was lower than that for influenza A, and the number of secondary cases peaked 2 days later than that for influenza A.

Household transmission was also influenced by viral load kinetics following treatment. Initiation of treatment beyond 48 h after symptomatic onset increased the secondary infection rate to 16.6%. According to a prospective, observational study, effectiveness (antiviral potency) of anti-influenza drugs also affected the secondary infection rate. These results suggest that the difference in the secondary infection rates among different antivirals can be an index for selecting medications.

Keywords Influenza · Household transmission · Anti-influenza drugs

N. Hirotsu (✉)
Hirotsu Medical Clinic, Hisamoto, Takatsu-Ku, Kawasaki, Japan
e-mail: non-hirotsu@umin.ac.jp

J. Fujita (ed.), *Influenza*, Respiratory Disease Series: Diagnostic Tools and Disease Managements, https://doi.org/10.1007/978-981-15-9109-9_3

1 Introduction

Influenza viruses have some distinct characteristics compared with other viruses. Epidemics of influenza occur every year, though in varying epidemic scales. In addition, household transmission is common in any age groups. This is primarily because influenza virus strains change every year through antigenic drift (or occasionally shift), allowing repeated infections in the same person in different years. Once a household member is infected with influenza virus, the infection can spread among household members of any age, owing to the highly infectious nature of the virus, and this largely contributes to the spread of the epidemic in the society.

Understanding of the transmission patterns of influenza virus in households is important to allow for effective infection prevention measures. More specifically, it is important to investigate the transmission routes, the secondary infection rates by transmission route, and the directions of transmission (to know who are more infectious to whom) and the serial interval (to know the infectious duration).

Unfortunately, however, household transmission can occur even if all possible anti-infection measures are taken. Previously we reported a delay in initiation of treatment as a risk factor for increase of household transmission [1]. In addition, the effectiveness (antiviral potency) of anti-influenza drugs also affects household transmission rate. Currently in Japan, four neuraminidase inhibitors (NAIs) and a cap-dependent endonuclease inhibitor are used in clinical practice. Understanding of the effects of medications on household transmission provides important information for selecting medications.

2 Subjects and Methods

These epidemiological investigations to determine transmission routes among families and infection intervals, and the prospective, observational study to compare the household transmission rate between NA inhibitors [2] were conducted at Hirotsu Medical Clinic (Kanagawa, Japan) from the 2010/2011 season to the 2015/2016 season. The latter was joint research with Shionogi & Co., Ltd. based on a protocol approved by ethics committee of Shionogi & Co., Ltd. Household transmission of influenza was investigated among 1482 patients who had flu-like symptoms and a body temperature of 37.5 °C or higher with a diagnosis of influenza A documented by a rapid diagnostic test, as well as their 4631 household members in 1209 households where two or more persons including the patient resided together. The influenza A virus subtype was H3N2 in 1061 patients (in 872 households with 3332 household members) and H1N1pdm in 421 patients (in 337 households with 1299 household members). For the latter study, patients infected influenza A or B who meet the protocol's criterion were analyzed. As the latter was an observational study, patients were treated with an NAI (oseltamivir, zanamivir, laninamivir, or peramivir), or remained untreated (e.g., if patient visited clinic >48 h after onset of illness), at the discretion of the physician.

Influenza A and B were determined using ImmunoAce® Flu (Tauns Laboratories, Inc., Shizuoka, Japan), and influenza A/H1pdm and A/H3 subtypes were determined using LineJudge® (Tauns Laboratories, Inc.).

Written informed consent to accept data epidemiological analysis thereafter publication was obtained from the patients or their guardians. Informed consent to conduct the joint study to compare transmission rate among drugs was obtained using opt-out procedure.

2.1 *Data Collection*

Regarding the participants (i.e., index patients or secondary contacts) who provided consent to be in this study at Hirotsu Medical Clinic, demographic and baseline data were collected in terms of sex, age, number of people in the household, household composition, presence or absence of influenza vaccination, and a history of past infections. Clinical data were collected from medical records in terms of the clinical course from symptomatic onset to the diagnosis, and to drug administration. A questionnaire form, the diary was also used to capture data on the patient's medication adherence at home and changes in clinical symptoms up to resolution of fever and other symptoms. The questionnaire form data were retrieved at the patient's re-visit or by mail or fax, or checked by follow-up phone call.

If the same person repeatedly had influenza infections in different flu seasons during the study period, different occurrences were handled as different cases. Even if the patient (i.e., index patient or secondary contact) had visited another hospital, the patient could be included in this study as long as the required information for this study (e.g., re-testing data, medical interview at our medical clinic, additional information from other hospitals and household members) was obtained at the patient's visit to our clinic. Among the participants (i.e., index patients or secondary contacts), the initial consultation for the disease was made at this clinic in 92.2% and other hospitals in 7.8% (Fig. 3.1).

2.2 *Definition of Household Transmission*

Based on the collected data as stated above, a graph was prepared to depict the frequency of intervals of symptomatic onset in multiple patients in the same households (Fig. 3.2).

According to an analysis of the symptomatic onset over 1 month in index patients, the secondary transmissions in the same households are typically distributed during the first 8 days and then the incident decreased, irrespective of the influenza virus

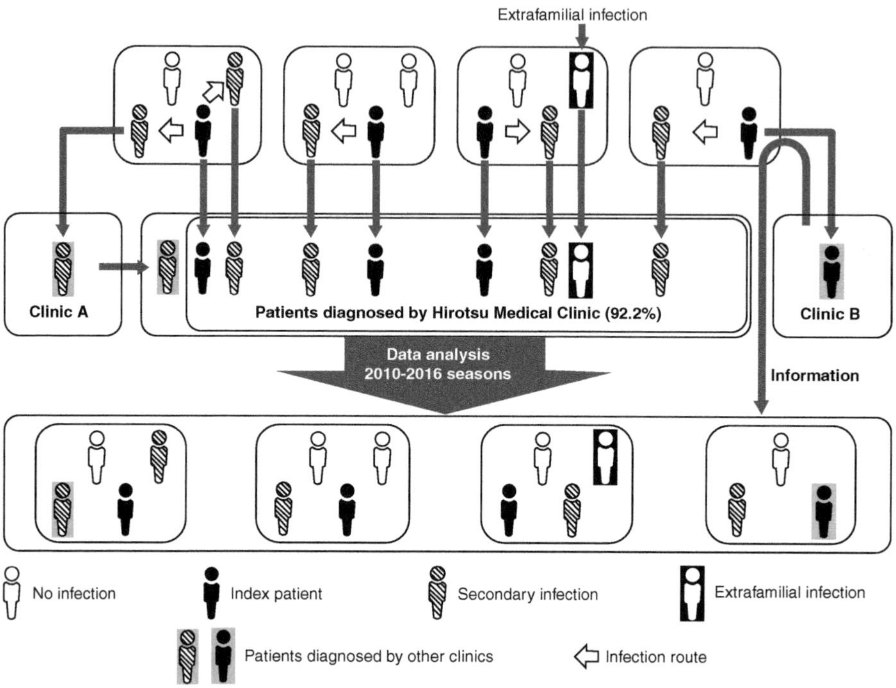

Fig. 3.1 Schematic depicting the source of index and secondary infection patients included in this analysis. Approximately 8% of data was obtained from their family and other medical clinics. Transmission rates were calculated using data of primary and secondary infections. Almost all patient's viral types and subtypes were checked and their consistency was confirmed among patients. Extrafamilial infections can be incorporated into analysis population to some extent but are considered the minority

type/subtype. Thus, household transmission could be regarded as symptomatic onset in a household contact within 8 days of symptomatic onset in the index patient. However, in light of the known influenza incubation period of approximately 24 h, symptomatic onset in a household contact within 24 h of symptomatic onset in the index patient implies another source of infection (which could be responsible for the infection in the index patient as well). Thus, household transmission was defined as symptomatic onset within 7 days after the day following the symptomatic onset in the index patient. Of note, influenza infection occurring in the last 3 weeks of follow-up indicated transmission from outside of the household (extra-familial transmission), which accounted for 15% of those regarded as secondary cases. Thus, even during the first week, although household transmission was likely, a possibility of extra-familial transmission could be considered in 5% (per 1 week) of those regarded as secondary cases (Fig. 3.2).

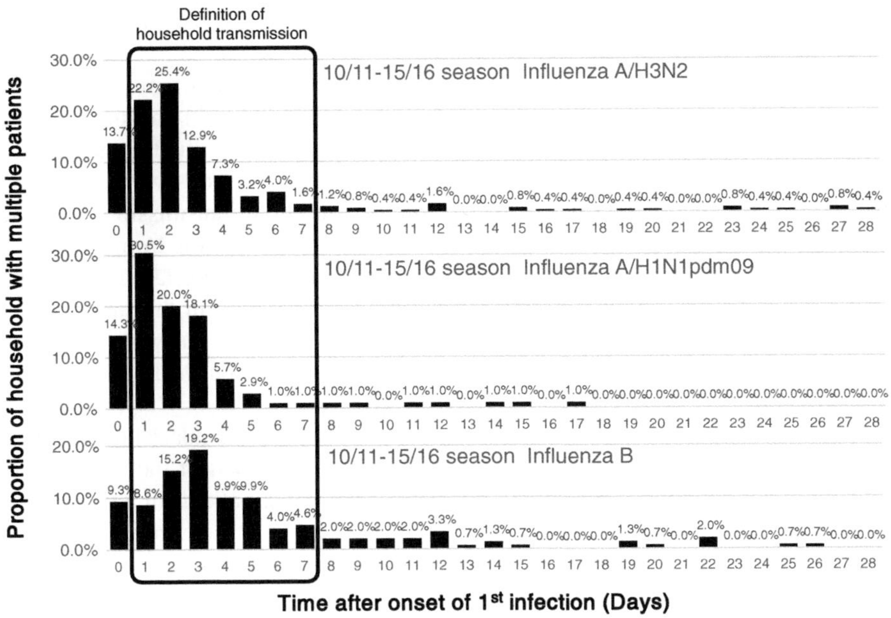

Fig. 3.2 Household secondary infection intervals(Definition of household transmission). Secondary infection patients were household members who were diagnosed with the same influenza type/subtype as the index patient between 24 h and 7 days after the onset of symptoms in the index patient

2.3 *Data Analysis*

The data were analyzed for the following three purposes: (1) to estimate the secondary infection rates with stratification of household members according to generation/age; (2) to evaluate any difference in household transmission in association with the time from symptomatic onset of influenza to the start of treatment; and (3) to compare the household secondary infection rates among different anti-influenza drugs.

2.3.1 Secondary Infection Rates with Stratification of Household Members According to Generation/Age

All persons with influenza infection were classified according to generation/age into grandfathers/grandmothers, fathers, mothers, and offspring, with the offspring further classified into the age groups of 0–6, 7–12, 13–18, and 19+ years, totaling eight strata of generation/age. In fact, however, in the grandfathers/grandmothers generation, there were no index cases and as few as two secondary cases. Thus, the analyses excluded the grandfathers/grandmothers stratum and used the remaining seven strata.

Then, for each influenza virus type/subtype in each season, among multiple patients in the same households who met the criteria for household transmission, the index patient and the person with secondary infection were identified as the persons with household transmission. If there were two or more persons with secondary infection, if the serial interval met the criteria for household transmission, all those with secondary infection were regarded as having the infection from the index patient. On the other hand, any persons who did not meet the criteria for household transmission among multiple persons with influenza infection in the same household were regarded as patients with extra-familial infection, as with the index patients who resided with one or more household members but had no household transmission.

Finally, for each of the seven strata of index patients, the secondary infection rate was determined, using the number of secondary cases in each of the seven strata divided by the number of household contacts of the index patient. In addition, the household transmission rate was determined, by calculating the number of households with household transmission divided by the total number of the households in the study.

2.3.2 Influence of Viral Load Kinetics on Household Transmission

As for the clinical practice regarding influenza in Japan, almost all patients with a confirmed diagnosis of influenza based on a rapid diagnostic test kit are treated with anti-influenza virus medication. As for influenza viral load kinetics during this period, the virus enters the cell and replicates and causes symptoms after the incubation period. As medication is administered, the viral replication is inhibited, and the virus is eliminated by the patient's immune system. Virus transmission is influenced by the viral load, which is influenced by the time to the start of medication and the antiviral potency of the drug. For this reason, influence of the time from symptomatic onset to the start of treatment on the household secondary infection rate was evaluated, with comparison of the antiviral potency between different drugs.

For the former, the time of symptomatic onset of influenza was defined as the time of onset of fever of 37.5 °C or higher, and the household secondary infection rate was calculated for each 24-h period between the fever onset and the start of treatment.

3 Analysis Results

The household secondary infection rate (it is expressed that rate of household members with secondary infection in previous report [3]) was calculated as the number of infected persons divided by the number of household contacts, based on the number of household members at the time of symptomatic onset in the index patient. The household transmission rate (it is expressed that proportion of households with secondary infection in previous report [3]) was calculated as the number of households with at least one case of household transmission divided by the total number of the households (with one index patient and one or more uninfected persons) in the study.

3.1 Household Transmission Rate

Of a total of 1209 households (involving 4631 household members) in this study, household transmission occurred in 224 households (household transmission rate, 18.5%).

By age/generation of index patients, household transmission occurred in 93 (28.2%) of 330 households of index patients aged 0–6 years, in 65 (18.5%) of 357 households of index patients aged 7–12 years, in 15 (15.0%) of 100 households of index patients aged 13–18 years, 6 (7.6%) of 79 households of index patients aged 19 years or older, 22 (10.5%) of 209 households of index patients as mothers, and 23 (17.2%) of 134 households of index patients as fathers (Fig. 3.3).

3.2 Household Secondary Infection Rate

Secondary transmission occurred in 273 of 3422 household contacts (secondary infection rate, 8.0%) of the 224 index patients (in 1209 households). The secondary infection rate by generation/age of index patients and secondary patients is shown in Fig. 3.3.

There were 330 index patients aged 0–6 years, which led to secondary transmission in 116 (12.4%) of 936 household contacts. Notably, by generation/age stratum, when the index patient was aged 0–6 years, household transmission was noted in 60 (18.2%) of 330 mothers and 20 (6.2%) of 324 fathers. When the index patient was a mother, household transmission was noted in 14 (11.1%) of 126 children aged 0–6 years and 4 (2.0%) of 204 fathers. When the index patient was a father, household transmission was noted in 14 (15.9%) of 88 children aged 0–6 years and 12 (9.0%) of 133 mothers.

3.3 Effect of NAIs on Daily Secondary Infection Rate

The daily secondary infection rate (SIR) differed according to the NAI used by index and secondary infection patients (Fig. 3.4). Daily SIRs for all influenza subtypes were highest for patients treated with oseltamivir compared with other NAIs

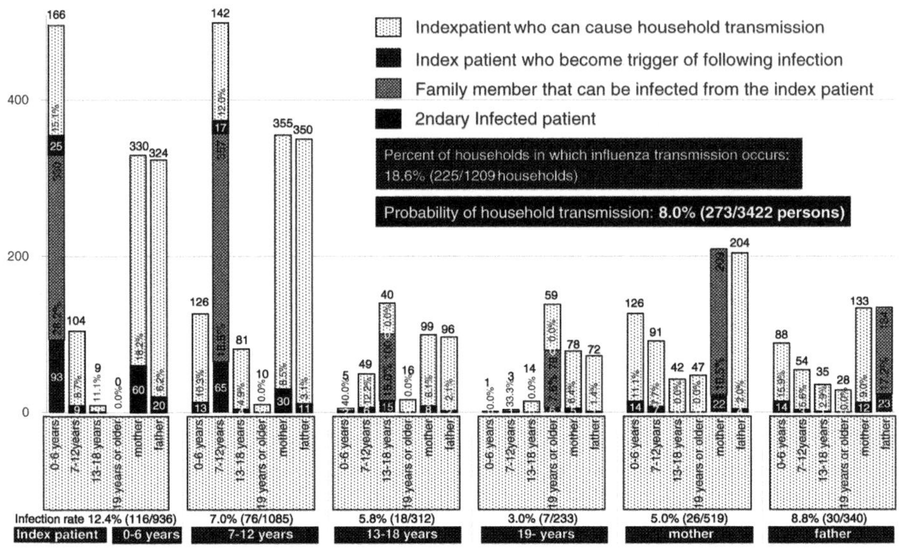

Fig. 3.3 Transmission routes and transmission rates among families. The bottom row shows the family composition of the primary patient in the family, and the transmission rate of each is shown above. And above the row, it shows the family member that can be affected, and the graph shows the number of primary patients, index patients and the number of their families, also the transmission rate per infection route

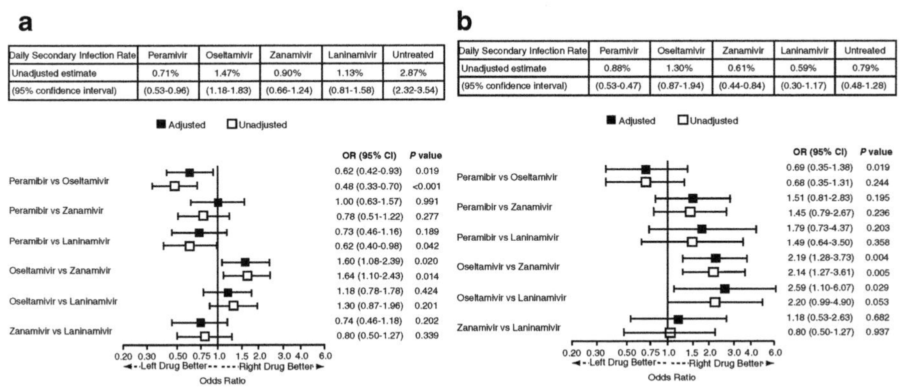

Fig. 3.4 Daily household secondary infection rates for influenza A (**a**), and B (**b**). Shown are unadjusted estimates and 95% confidence intervals (CI) when patients (index and secondary infection) were treated with peramivir, oseltamivir, zanamivir, or laninamivir, or when patients were untreated, and unadjusted and adjusted odds ratios (OR) of pairwise comparisons between neuraminidase inhibitors

[3]. Pairwise comparisons of the daily SIR indicated that household transmission of influenza A was lower with peramivir or zanamivir than with oseltamivir (Fig. 3.4a). Transmission of influenza B was also lower with zanamivir or laninamivir than with oseltamivir (Fig. 3.4b). Compared with no treatment, all NAIs reduced the daily SIR of influenza A, with the extent of daily SIR reduction ranging from 49% (reduced from 2.87 to 1.47%) with oseltamivir to 75% (reduced from 2.87 to 0.71%) with peramivir [3].

4 Discussion

Transmission in households and schools plays a significant role in the spread of influenza epidemics. In particular, a household represents a group of persons of different ages who live together and thus are inevitably in close contact with each other in time and space. In such a setting, droplet transmission of influenza virus is difficult to avoid, but it is important to prevent the spread of transmission. In Japan, almost all patients with influenza receive a definite diagnosis soon after symptomatic onset. This allows a chance for early isolation and early initiation of treatment, but infection control is not satisfactory. The study results indicated difficult isolation of index infants from their mothers, but also indicated very careful contact with infants by index mothers. As for fathers, infant-to-father transmission was uncommon but father-to-infant transmission was very common, and father-to-mother transmission was more common than mother-to-father transmission. The study found that not all household contacts were equally susceptible and persons in particular roles in the household were more infectious to all other contacts, suggesting the importance of aggressive control of the pathogen spread for infection prevention measures, rather than passive infection prevention.

The author previously reported that a delay in starting treatment promotes the spread of influenza transmission, and serves as a risk factor for household transmission [1]. Residual virus increases household transmission. In a randomized controlled study in pediatric patients aged 4–12 years who had influenza infection, four NAIs were compared, showing that the time to virus clearance was significantly shorter with peramivir than with oseltamivir (adjusted p-value = 0.035), thus documenting differences in the antiviral potency between different drugs [2]. In that article, the household transmission data were obtained from a prospective observational study (present study) conducted around the same time [3]. Based on the results of these two studies, the antiviral efficacy varied among different NAIs, suggesting the importance of selecting appropriate medication from the viewpoint of household transmission as well. A cap-dependent endonuclease inhibitor of baloxavir marboxil has been added to available drugs. Given that the median time to virus clearance was as short as 24 h with baloxavir, compared with 72 h with oseltamivir [4], baloxavir is also expected to reduce household transmission.

Regarding influenza B, the household secondary infection rate and the household transmission rate were lower than those for influenza A, and the number of secondary cases peaked 2 days later than that for influenza A (Fig. 3.2). For both influenza A and B, household transmission was most common with oseltamivir among the four NAIs.

5 Conclusions

The study results regarding household transmission indicate that mothers caring for infants with influenza can be inevitably at high risk, but the high infectiousness of fathers to infants and mothers suggests room for improvement through efforts to prevent the spread of infection. In addition, the use of drugs can reduce household transmission, thereby supplementing the efforts to prevent the spread of influenza epidemics.

To reduce household transmission, and in light of the effect of controlling the spread of influenza infection on public health, clinicians should consider starting treatment early with selection of most effective medication.

References

1. Hirotsu N, Wada K, Oshitani H. Risk factors of household transmission of pandemic (H1N1) 2009 among patients treated with antivirals: a prospective study at a primary clinic in Japan. PLoS One. 2012;7:e31519.
2. Hirotsu N, Saisho Y, Hasegawa T, et al. Clinical and virologic effects of four neuraminidase inhibitors in influenza A virus-infected children (aged 4–12 years): an open-label, randomized study in Japan. Expert Rev Anti-Infect Ther. 2018;16:173–82.
3. Hirotsu N, Saisho Y, Hasegawa T. The effect of neuraminidase inhibitors on household transmission in Japanese patients with influenza A and B infection: a prospective, observational study. Influenza Other Respir Viruses, 2019;13(2):123–132. https://doi.org/10.1111/irv.12590. Epub 2018 Dec 28.
4. Hayden F, Sugaya N, Hirotsu N, et al. Baloxavir Marboxil for uncomplicated influenza in adults and adolescents. N Engl J Med. 2018;376:913–2.

Chapter 4
Cellular and Biochemical Pathogenic Processes in Severe Influenza Virus Infection: How Does Cytokine Storm Play a Role?

Hiroshi Kido, Takashi Kimoto, and Etsuhisa Takahashi

Abstract Influenza A virus is one of the most common infectious pathogen and associated with significant morbidity and mortality. Infected patients with underlying diseases show rapid progression in disease severity. The initial pathogenic process of influenza virus infection is characterized by the induction of various proinflammatory cytokines as well as host cellular trypsin-type viral envelope-processing proteases in the airway, which enhance viral multiplication. This process has been termed the "influenza virus–cytokine–trypsin" cycle. In the advanced stage of infection, the cytokine storm induces disorders of glucose and lipid metabolism in the mitochondria, resulting in ATP crisis and various functional disorders particularly in organs and cells with high ATP consumption, such as vascular endothelial cells and cardiomyocytes. This process has been termed interconnection of the "metabolic disorders–cytokine" cycle with the "influenza virus–cytokine–trypsin" cycle. The interconnection exacerbates mitochondrial ATP crisis and could lead to multiple organ failure with severe edema. Breaking these cycles and interconnection is a promising therapeutic approach against severe influenza. In this review, we discuss the pathogenesis of severe influenza viral infection based on animal experiments and the potential therapeutic options.

Keywords Influenza A virus · Cytokine storm · Multiple organ failure · ATP crisis Pyruvate dehydrogenase kinase 4

H. Kido (✉) · T. Kimoto · E. Takahashi
Division of Enzyme Chemistry, Institute for Enzyme Research, Tokushima University, Tokushima, Japan
e-mail: kido@tokushima-u.ac.jp

J. Fujita (ed.), *Influenza*, Respiratory Disease Series: Diagnostic Tools and Disease Managements, https://doi.org/10.1007/978-981-15-9109-9_4

1 Introduction

Influenza A virus (IAV), a single-stranded negative-sense RNA virus, of the *Orthomyxoviridae* family, is the most common infective pathogen in human, causing significant morbidity and mortality in infants and elderly particularly those with underlying diseases, such as chronic lung disease, cardiac disease, renal disease, and diabetes mellitus [1–3]. In the advanced stage of IAV infection, multiple organ failure (MOF) with vascular hyperpermeability is usually associated with marked increases in the levels of proinflammatory cytokines, such as tumor necrosis factor (TNF)-α, interleukin (IL)-6, and IL-1β, coined the cytokine storm, and the most common cause of mortality. The hypercytokinemia alters the cellular redox state through different cytokine receptors and reduces the expression of four complex I subunits, oxygen consumption [4, 5], and ATP synthesis in the mitochondria. We have advanced previously the hypothesis of the "influenza virus–cytokine–trypsin" cycle interconnected with the "metabolic disorder–cytokine" cycle as one of the key mechanisms in the pathogenesis of severe IAV infection [6, 7].

All animal experiments described in this review were conducted according to the Guide for the Care and Use of Laboratory Animals (NIH Publication No. 85-23, 1996), and all the studies were approved by the Animals Care Committee of the University of Tokushima.

2 Cellular Trypsin-Type Viral Envelope-Processing Proteases, Essential Factors for Initial Viral Infection and Viral Multi-Replication Cycle

An important pre-requisite for IAV infection and multi-replication is the proteolytic breakdown of the viral envelope fusion glycoprotein hemagglutinin precursor (HA0) into HA1 and HA2 subunits [8]. However, IAV cannot process HA0 by itself as it lacks HA-processing protease(s) in its genome. Thus, the host cellular trypsin-type processing proteases, such as tryptase Clara, ectopic trypsin, TMPRSS2, and HAT [9], determine the IAV infectious tropism and its pathogenicity. In this regard, the initial IAV infection in the airway is followed by marked upregulation of ectopic trypsin in various organs and endothelial cells through the induction of proinflammatory cytokines [10, 11], particularly IL-1β [12], and the induced ectopic trypsin subsequently stimulates viral replication in various organs.

The mechanisms of vascular hyperpermeability and tissue destruction involved in the "influenza virus–cytokine–trypsin" cycle in IAV infection are illustrated in Fig. 4.1. The cytokine storm reduces ATP synthesis in the mitochondria through increased production of reactive oxygen species and intracellular calcium concentration $[Ca^{2+}]_i$ [13]. The resultant ATP depletion subsequently causes the dissociation of zonula occludens-1 (ZO-1), an intracellular tight junction component, from the actin cytoskeleton, thus increasing junctional permeability [14]. The cytokine

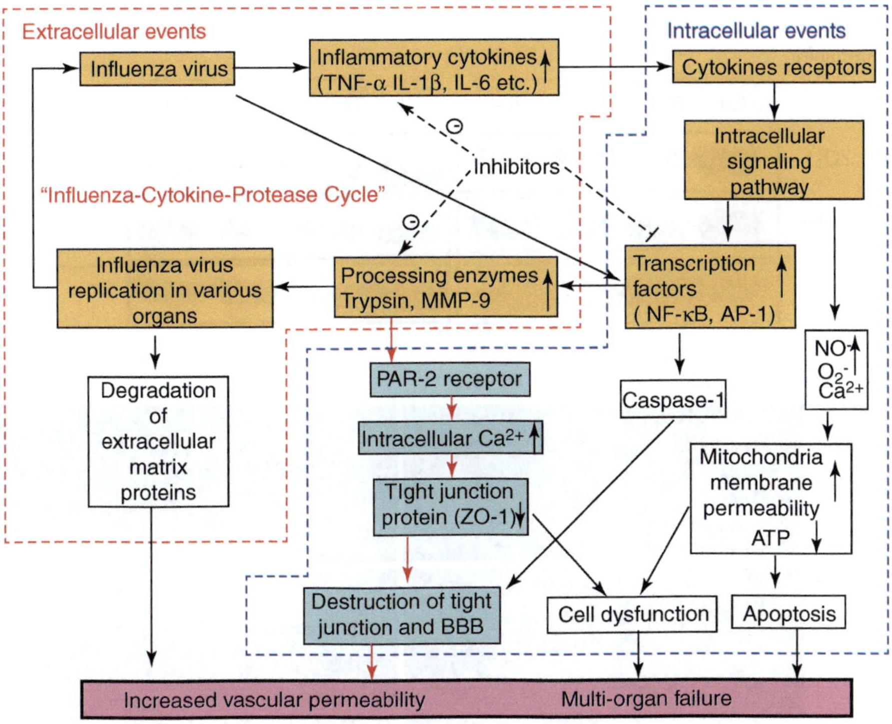

Fig. 4.1 The hypothesis of influenza virus–cytokine–trypsin cycle on the pathogenic processes of vascular hyperpermeability and tissue destruction in severe influenza. *AP-1* activator protein 1, *BBB* blood-brain barrier, *PAR-2* protease-activated receptor 2, *ZO-1* zonula occludens-1. (Reproduced with permission from Ref. [7]. Copyright 2016 The Japanese Respiratory Society)

storm also upregulates ectopic trypsin and matrix metalloproteinase-9 (MMP-9) in vascular endothelial cells and various organs through the activation of nuclear factor-kappa B (NF-κB) and activator protein 1 (AP-1) [10]. The upregulated trypsin also increases $[Ca^{2+}]_i$ and Cl^- and K^+ secretion via the protease-activated receptor (PAR)-2, resulting in loss of ZO-1 in endothelial cells and severe edema in the airways and colon [15].

Figure 4.2 shows tight-junction loss and hyperpermeability in vascular endothelial cells, which were both induced by proinflammatory cytokines, and the prevention of these two pathological processes by treatment with trypsin inhibitor aprotinin [10]. The addition of TNF-α, IL-6, and IL-1β to the cell culture for 12 h induced marked downregulation of ZO-1, and the loss was abrogated by aprotinin treatment (Fig. 4.2a). The cytokines also disrupted the continuous and linear arrangement of ZO-1, whereas aprotinin inhibited the disruption (Fig. 4.2b). Among these cytokines, IL-1β and TNF-α especially tended to increase endothelial cell monolayer permeability, and this effect was blocked by aprotinin ($P < 0.05$) (Fig. 4.2c). The loss of ZO-1 was also inhibited by PAR-2 antagonist [10].

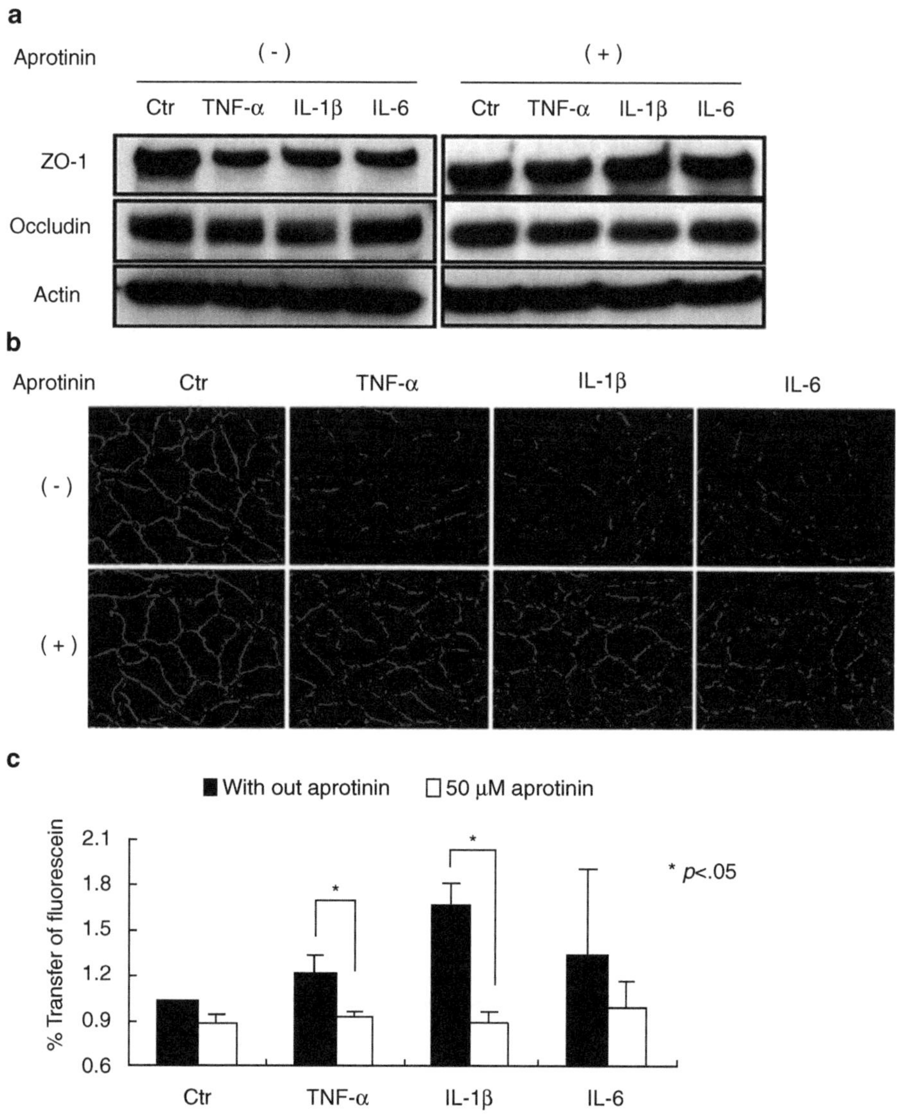

Fig. 4.2 Cytokines induce loss of tight junctions but this action can be abrogated by trypsin inhibitor. (**a**) Western blotting analysis of tight-junction proteins, zonula occludens (ZO)-1 and occludin, after treatment of the cells with cytokines for 12 h in the absence and presence of 50 μM aprotinin. Actin was used as an internal control (Ctr). (**b**) Representative example (from three separate experiments) of immunofluorescence showing decreased ZO-1 expression following cytokine treatment and its restoration by aprotinin. (**c**) Increased permeability of cells treated with cytokines and its rescue by aprotinin ($n = 3$). Data are mean ± SEM. *$P < 0.05$, with and without aprotinin. (Reproduced with permission from Ref. [6]. Copyright 2015 The Japan Academy)

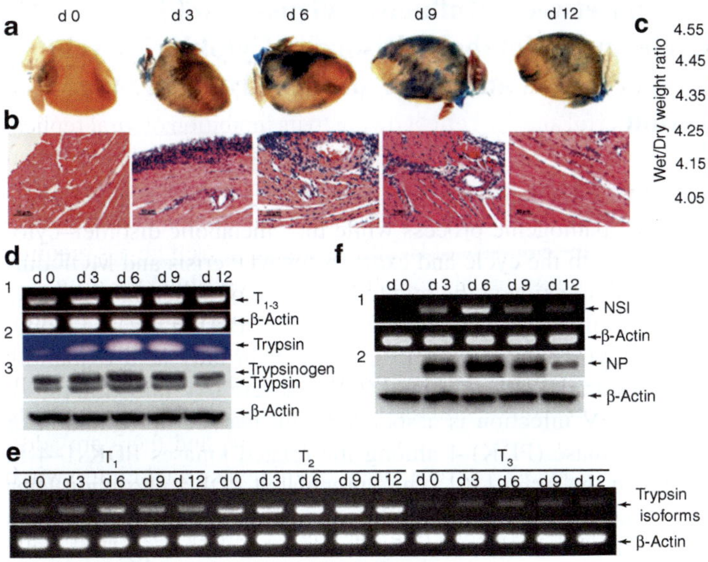

Fig. 4.3 IAV infection can progress to result in acute myocarditis, characterized by vascular hyperpermeability, tissue edema, inflammatory cell infiltration, based on upregulation of trypsin in the myocardium. (**a**) Vascular hyperpermeability monitored by Evans' blue extravasation during the course of infection from day 0 (d 0) to 12 (d 12). (**b**) Hematoxylin and eosin staining. Bar = 50 μm. (**c**) Cardiac edema determined by the wet/dry weight ratio. Data are mean ± SD of 10 mice in each group. $^{**}P < 0.01$ vs. d 0; $^{††}P < 0.01$ vs. d 9. (**d1**, **e**, and **f1**) RT-PCR-based detection of trypsin$_{1-3}$, trypsin isoforms T_1, T_2 and T_3 and IAV NS1 gene in the hearts from day 0 to 12 post-infection. (**d2**) Detection by zymography of trypsin activity, (**d3**) by western immunoblotting of trypsinogen and trypsin and (**f2**) viral nucleoprotein (NP). Each result is a representative of three experiments. (Reproduced with permission from Ref. [6]. Copyright 2015 The Japan Academy)

Figure 4.3 illustrates the pathological process of acute influenza myocarditis marked by increased vascular permeability and inflammatory cell infiltration [11]. In our experiments, inflammatory infiltrates started to appear in the subepicardium at day 3 post-infection, followed by extensive infiltration across the interstitium and perivascular areas deep into the myocardium, accompanied by extracellular matrix destruction at days 6 and 9, though resolution was evident at day 12 (Fig. 4.3a–c). Coronary vascular permeability (monitored by Evan's blue extravasation) and tissue edema (assessed by wet/dry weight ratio) increased at day 3, reaching peak values at days 6 and 9, and then decreased significantly at day 12. Notably, trypsinogen and its active form trypsin were upregulated, with peak levels noted at days 6 and 9 (Fig. 4.3d, e). IAV levels reached peak at day 6, as monitored by the NS1 gene and nucleoprotein (NP) (Fig. 4.3f).

3 Interconnection Between "Influenza Virus–Cytokine–Trypsin" Cycle and "Metabolic Disorder-Cytokine" Cycle Exacerbates ATP Crisis and MOF in the Advanced Stage of IAV Infection

At the early stages of IAV infection, the "influenza virus–cytokine–trypsin" cycle plays a central role in the pathogenic process while the "metabolic disorder–cytokine" cycle interconnects with the cycle and exacerbates ATP crisis and MOF during the progression of IAV infection at the mid to late phase of infection [6, 9, 16].

Two mitochondrial enzymes, pyruvate dehydrogenase (PDH) in glucose oxidation and carnitine palmitoyltransferase (CPT) in long-chain fatty acid oxidation, play key roles in mitochondrial ATP crisis and MOF in severe IAV infection [6, 9]. We reported that severe IAV infection is associated with marked upregulation of pyruvate dehydrogenase kinase (PDK) 4 among the related kinases PDKs1–4 in various organs, but not in the brain [16]. The upregulated PDK4 phosphorylates PDH, a mitochondrial gate keeper enzyme of glucose oxidation, and suppresses its activity, resulting in marked downregulation of glucose-mediated energy homeostasis, culminating in ATP crisis. Figure 4.4 shows that sublethal dose of IAV PR/8/34(H1N1) infection affects glucose oxidation and reduces energy metabolism in skeletal muscles, liver, lung, and heart, but not the brain, by reducing mitochondrial pyruvate dehydrogenase (PDH) activity [16]. In our animal models, the

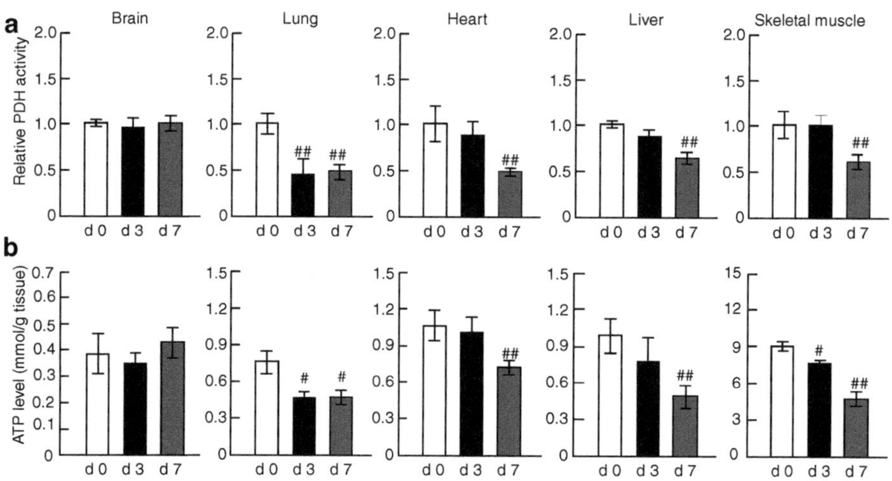

Fig. 4.4 Serial changes in PDH activity and ATP levels in skeletal muscles, heart, lung, liver, and brain of IAV-infected mice. Mice were infected with IAV/PR/8/34(H1N1) at 120 plaque-forming units (PFU) intranasally and the levels of PDH activity (**a**) and ATP (**b**) were analyzed at days 0 (d0), 3 (d3), and 7 (d7) post-infection. PDH activity levels after IAV infection relative to the values at day 0. Data are mean ± SD of 5 mice per group. $^{\#}P < 0.05$, $^{\#\#}P < 0.01$ vs. day 0, by one-way analysis of variance (ANOVA) with Tukey post-hoc test. (Reproduced with permission from Ref. [16]. Copyright 2014 Yamane et al.)

earliest reduction in PDH activity occurred at day 3 post-infection in the lungs, then spread at day 7 to the skeletal muscles, liver, and heart. Similar patterns of changes were noted in ATP levels in these organs. Changes in PDK4 protein expression levels in these organs clearly showed marked upregulation with peak values at day 3 in the lungs and at day 7 in skeletal muscles, heart, and liver. These results suggest that PDK4 is a suitable target molecule for the treatment of severe IAV infection. Among the known inhibitors of PDK, the pyruvate analog dichloroacetate (DCA) is the most common classic inhibitor [17], although it has clinically symptomatic side effects of peripheral neuropathy. In a recent publication, we reported that diisopropylamine dichloroacetate (DADA), which has been used for over 50 years for the treatment of chronic liver diseases without any adverse reaction, is a selective and safe inhibitor of PDK4 [16].

Figure 4.5 shows the effects of treatment with DADA on PDH activity and ATP levels in various organs in mice infected with sublethal dose of IAV [16]. The infection resulted in marked suppression of PDH activities and ATP levels at day 7 in the skeletal muscles, liver, lungs, and heart, compared with the non-infection control. DADA significantly prevented the suppression and restored PDH activities and ATP levels similar to those before infection. In addition, DADA also corrected the hypoglycemia, increased levels of blood lactate, free fatty acids, and β-hydroxybutyric acid [16].

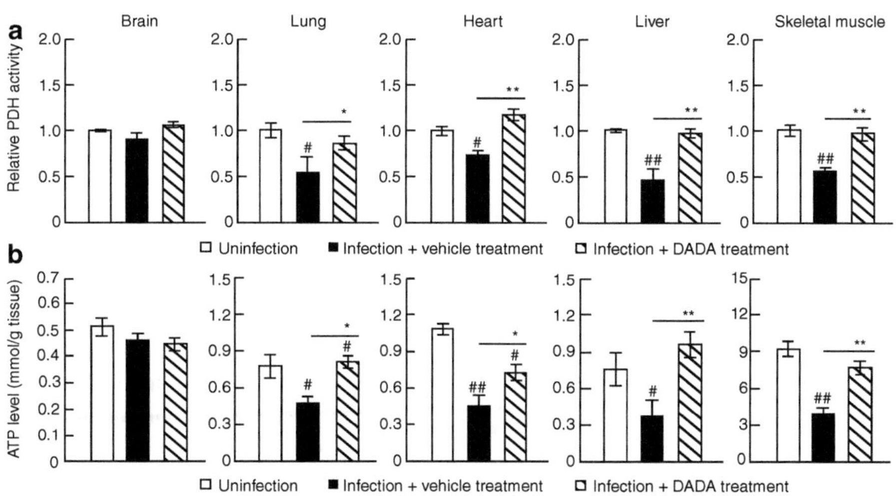

Fig. 4.5 Treatment with DADA restored suppressed PDH activity and ATP levels in skeletal muscle, heart, lung, and liver of IAV-infected mice. Mice infected with IAV at 120 PFU were treated orally with DADA at 50 mg/kg or vehicle at 12-h intervals for 14 days, and the levels of PDH activity (**a**) and ATP (**b**) were measured at day 7 post-infection. PDH activity levels are expressed relative to the values of the control (no-infection). Values are mean ± SD of 5 mice per group. $^{\#}P < 0.05$, $^{\#\#}P < 0.01$, vs. no-infection, $^{*}P < 0.05$, $^{**}P < 0.01$, vs. infected group treated with vehicle, by one-way analysis of variance (ANOVA) and Tukey post-hoc test. (Reproduced with permission from Ref. [16]. Copyright 2014 Yamane et al.)

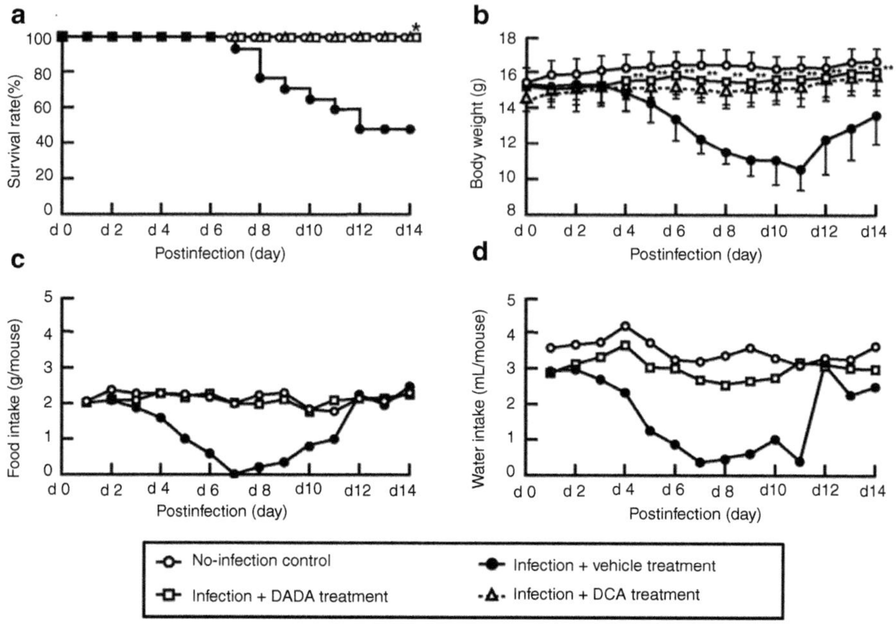

Fig. 4.6 Effects of DADA on survival rate, body weight, and food and water intake. Mice infected with 60 PFU IAV/PR/8/34(H1N1), representing 50% lethal dose, were treated with oral DADA at 50 mg/kg, vehicle, or administered DCA intraperitoneally at 28 mg/kg at 12-h intervals for 14 days. The survival rate, body weight, food intake, and water intake of infected mice were monitored. Survival rate (**a**) analyzed by Kaplan-Meier and log-rank tests. Changes in body weight (**b**), food intake (**c**), and water intake (**d**) for each group. Data are mean ± SD of 15 mice per group. $*P < 0.05$, $**P < 0$ 0.01, vs. infected group treated with vehicle, by two-way ANOVA. (Reproduced with permission from Ref. [16]. Copyright 2014 Yamane et al.)

Figure 4.6 shows a typical example of the effects of DADA on the survival rate, body weight, and food and water intake of mice infected with a semi-lethal dose of IAV up to post-infection day 14 [16]. The infected animals showed progressive avoidance of food and water during days 2–7 post-infection, and then started to die after day 7. However, the infected and DADA-treated mice showed no significant decrease in food and water intake as well as no significant reduction in body weight during the 14-day experimental period. While the survival rate of the infected untreated mice was 50%, it was 0% in the DADA-treated mice during the experimental period.

Another potentially effective therapeutic target is fatty acid oxidation in the mitochondria. Bezafibrate is another treatment option used to prevent fatty acid-mediated energy metabolic disorders induced by IAV infection. IAV-associated encephalopathy (IAE) is a pediatric complication of severe IAV infection, characterized by sudden onset of febrile convulsions and MOF during hyperpyrexia [18, 19]. We reported previously that a large proportion of patients with severe IAE exhibit a thermolabile phenotype of compound homo−/heterozygous variants for [1055 T > G/F352C] and [1102G > A/V368I] of CPT II and mitochondrial energy crisis during high fever [18, 19]. The thermolabile variants are inactivated during high fever, resulting in secondary CPT II deficiency, leading to an impaired mitochondrial fuel utilization state, and mitochondrial ATP crisis. Bezafibrate is a hypolipidemic pan-peroxisome proliferator-activated receptor (PPAR)-β/γ agonist known to stimulate carnitine palmitoyltransferase (CPT) II expression and promote mitochondrial energy crisis dissipation [20]. Treatment of fibroblasts of these IAE patients with bezafibrate and CPT II stabilizer L-carnitine, transcriptionally upregulated CPT II, filled up depleted enzyme activity and restored mitochondrial ATP levels even under hyperthermia at 41 °C [21].

4 Conclusion

The major pathogenic process of MOF in the advanced stage of IAV pneumonia and IAE, particularly in patients with underlying risk factors, is cell energy metabolic disorders associated with cellular dysfunction in various cells and tissues. The "influenza virus–cytokine–trypsin" cycle is involved in the initial stages of IAV infection, including viral multiplication, but the cycle can be inhibited by treatment with antiviral neuraminidase inhibitors. In the advanced stages of IAV infection, the "metabolic disorders–cytokine" cycle interconnects with the "influenza virus–cytokine–trypsin" cycle and worsens the severity of tissue damage and ATP crisis. In IAV-infected mice, treatment with DADA can normalize blood glucose levels and lipid metabolism through PDK4 inhibition observed during the "metabolic disorders–cytokine" cycle, as well as restore ATP levels in the mitochondria, and cytokine and trypsin levels in various organs, with resultant improvement in the clinical status and survival rate. Lipid metabolism-related energy disorders also induce mitochondrial ATP crisis, particularly in vascular endothelial cells of IAE patients with thermolabile CPT II variants. Treatment with the combination of bezafibrate, a PPAR-β/δ agonist, and L-carnitine significantly restores ATP levels in the fibroblasts of IAE children.

Acknowledgments Our studies were supported in part by Grants-in-Aid (24249059) from the Ministry of Education, Culture, Sports, Science and Technology of Japan; by Health and Labor Sciences Research Grants (Grant #12103307) from the Ministry of Health, Labor and Welfare of Japan.

References

1. Lipatov AS, Govorkova EA, Webby RJ, Ozaki H, Peiris M, Guan Y, et al. Influenza: emergence and control. J Virol. 2004;78:8951–9.
2. Kim HM, Brandt CD, Arrobio JO, Murphy B, Chanock RM, Parrott RH. Influenza A and B virus infection in infants and young children during the years 1957-1976. Am J Epidemiol. 1979;109:464–79.

3. Chowell G, Ayala A, Berisha V. Viboud C, Schumacher M. Risk factors for mortality among 2009 A/H1N1 influenza hospitalizations in Maricopa county, Arizona, April 2009 to March 2010. Comput Math Methods Med 2012;2012:914196.
4. Spraque AH, Khalil RA. Inflammatory cytokines in vascular dysfunction and vascular disease. Biochem Pharmacol. 2009;78:539–52.
5. Mariappan N, Elks CM, Fink B, Francis J. TNF-induced mitochondrial damage: a link between mitochondrial complex I activity and left ventricular dysfunction. Free Radic Biol Med. 2009;46:462–70.
6. Kido H. Influenza virus pathogenicity regulated by host cellular proteases, cytokines and metabolites, and its therapeutic options. Proc Jpn Acad Ser B Phys Biol Sci. 2015;91:351–68.
7. Kido H. Energy metabolic disorder is a major risk factor in severe influenza virus infection: proposals for new therapeutic options based on animal model experiments. Respir Investig. 2016;54:312–9.
8. Klenk H-D, Rott R, Orlich M, Blödom J. Activation of influenza A viruses by trypsin treatment. Virology. 1975;68:426–39.
9. Kido H, Takahashi E, Kimoto T. Role of host trypsin-type serine proteases and influenza virus–cytokine–trypsin cycle in influenza viral pathogenesis. Pathogenesis-based therapeutic options. Biochimie. 2019;166:203–13.
10. Wang S, Le TQ, Kurihara N, Chida J, Cisse Y, Yano M, et al. Influenza virus–cytokine–protease cycle in the pathogenesis of vascular hyperpermeability in severe influenza. J Infect Dis. 2010;202:991–1001.
11. Pan HY, Yamada H, Chida J, Wang S, Yano M, Yao M, et al. Up-regulation of ectopic trypsins in the myocardium by influenza A virus infection triggers acute myocarditis. Cardiovasc Res. 2011;89:595–603.
12. Indalao IL, Sawabuchi T, Takahashi E, Kido H. IL-1β is a key cytokine that induces trypsin upregulation in the influenza virus−cytokine−trypsin cycle. Arch Virol. 2017;162:201–11.
13. Mizuguchi M, Yamanouchi H, Ichiyama T, Shiomi M. Acute encephalopathy associated with influenza and other viral infection. Acta Neurol Scand Suppl. 2007;186:45–6.
14. Denker BM, Nigam SK. Molecular structure and assembly of the tight junction. Am J Phys. 1998;274:F1–9.
15. Palmer ML, Lee SY, Maniak PJ, Carlson D, Fahrenkrug SC, O'Grady SM. Protease-activated receptor regulation of Cl- secretion in Calu-3 cells requires prostaglandin release and CFTR activation. Am J Physiol Cell Physiol. 2006;290:C1189–98.
16. Yamane K, Indalao IL, Chida J, Yamamoto Y, Hanawa M, Kido H. Diisopropylamine dichloroacetate, a novel pyruvate dehydrogenase kinase 4 inhibitor, as a potential therapeutic agent for metabolic disorders and multiorgan failure in severe influenza. PLoS One. 2014;9:e98032.
17. Bersin RM, Stacpoole PW. Dichloroacetate as metabolic therapy for myocardial ischemia and failure. Am Heart J. 1997;134:841055.
18. Chen Y, Mizuguchi H, Yao D, Ide M, Kuroda Y, Shigematsu Y, et al. Thermolabile phenotype of carnitine palmitoyltransferase II variations as a predisposing factor for influenza-associated encephalopathy. FEBS Lett. 2005;579:2040–4.
19. Yao D, Mizuguchi H, Yamaguchi M, Yamada H, Chida J, Shikata K, et al. Thermal instability of compound variants of carnitine palmitoyltransferase II and impaired mitochondrial fuel utilization in influenza-associated encephalopathy. Hum Mutat. 2008;29:718–27.
20. Bonnefont JP, Bastin J, Laforêt P, Aubey F, Mogenet A, Romano S, et al. Long-term follow-up of bezafibrate treatment in patients with the myopathic form of carnitine palmitoyltransferase 2 deficiency. Clin Pharmacol Ther. 2010;88:101–8.
21. Yao M, Yao D, Yamaguchi M, Chida J, Yao D, Kido H. Bezafibrate upregulates carnitine palmitoyltransferase II expression and promotes mitochondrial energy crisis dissipation in fibroblasts of patients with influenza-associated encephalopathy. Mol Genet Metab. 2011;104:265–72.

Chapter 5
Pathology of Severe Influenza Virus Pneumonia: What Is the Importance of Alveolar Mouths?

Yuji Ohtsuki and Jiro Fujita

Abstract Alveolar mouths (AMs) are very important points for the formation of Masson bodies (MBs) and hyaline membranes (HMs), which are considered serious complications of influenza virus pneumonia. MBs arise by injury, caused by influenza virus infection of AMs, which cover the epithelial and endothelial cells of AMs. Resulting exudates of AMs, mesenchymal cells, fibroblasts, and myofibroblasts proliferate, forming polyp-like MBs which protrude into air spaces. These structures are very sensitive to steroid therapy and are absorbed rapidly after steroid administration. However, if the MBs contain fibrin, as seen in acute fibrinous organizing pneumonia (AFOP), and myofibroblast proliferation, absorbed MBs remain in the septal and luminal spaces as pulmonary fibrosis. Massive MBs cause serious disturbance to respiratory function in peripheral airways. In HM formation, following injury to the epithelial cells of AMs irregular shaped fluffy fragmented substances form at AMs, becoming larger and flat in shape and forming membranous HM structures that disturb peripheral gas exchange. These HMs are immunopositive for cytokeratins, epithelial membrane antigen, KL-6, surfactant protein A, and Factor VIII-related antigens, but never fibrin. Following HM and MB formation, peripheral airways including alveolar orifices, such as respiratory bronchioles, alveolar ducts, alveolar sacs, and alveoli lose their gas-exchange capacity. Moreover, HMs form rapidly at AMs in the structurally retained pulmonary parenchyma, leading to acute respiratory insufficiency and numerous associating MBs in the peripheral airways.

Keywords Alveolar mouth · Influenza viral pneumonia · Organizing pneumonia
Masson body · Hyaline membrane · Diffuse alveolar damage

Y. Ohtsuki (✉)
Department of Diagnostic Pathology, Tottori Prefectural Kousei Hospital, Kurayoshi, Tottori, Japan

Emeritus Professor, Kochi University, Kochi, Japan
e-mail: y-ohtsuki@hi3.enjoy.ne.jp

J. Fujita
Department of Infectious, Respiratory, and Digestive Medicine,
Graduate School of Medicine, University of the Ryukyus,
Okinawa, Japan

J. Fujita (ed.), *Influenza*, Respiratory Disease Series: Diagnostic Tools and Disease Managements, https://doi.org/10.1007/978-981-15-9109-9_5

1 Introduction

Alveolar mouths (AMs) in influenza virus pneumonia infections have not yet been emphasized [1–5], except in our previous report [6]. AMs are not only important in the initiation of HMs [7] but are also the essential points for MBs [6], some resulting in respiratory insufficiency, due to decreased respiratory capacity. AMs are located at alveolar orifices of peripheral airways, such as respiratory bronchioles (RB), alveolar ducts (AD), alveolar sacs (AS), and alveoli. Epithelial cells which cover AMs are easily injured during the early stage of influenza viral infection [6] and by many other kinds of stimuli [7]. AMs are therefore the *locus minoris resistentiae* of the lungs [7]. Both MB and HM arise from injured AMs, in which the epithelial and endothelial cells of capillaries are injured and destroyed by influenza virus [8–10]. The most serious complications for patients with influenza virus pneumonia are massive MB formation, diffuse alveolar damage (DAD), and most importantly hyaline membrane (HM) formation, which may cause death [2, 3]. Maintaining the initial structures of AMs is particularly important for the respiratory function of peripheral airways, including RB, AD, AS, and alveoli. Both influenza virus A and B cause viral pneumonia [11, 12]. In this column, the importance of AMs in retaining the respiratory function of peripheral airways in influenza virus pneumonia is addressed.

2 Location and Structure of Alveolar Mouths (AMs) (Fig. 5.1)

AMs are located at the orifices of alveoli in RB, AD, AS, and alveoli. AMs are composed of surface epithelial cells with thin cytoplasm, type II alveolar cells, and connective tissues consisting of elastic fibers, collagen fibers, smooth muscle cells, endothelial cells, and capillaries [7]. Due to the distance of surface epithelial cells from capillary lumina, thin cytoplasm of epithelial cells in AMs are susceptible to minor stimuli, and constitute a *locus minoris resistentiae*, resulting in the formation of MBs or fragmented/flat membranous HMs [7]. HM or MBs are formed where epithelial cells of AMs have been damaged. HMs are composed of destroyed epithelial cell debris, EMA, KL-6, SP-A, and factor VIII-related antigens [7, 13] which allow for minor stimuli to induce fibromuscular or muscular hyperplasia in AMs during long or chronic infections. This causes deformity and narrowing of peripheral airways, producing respiratory insufficiency [6, 7]. Influenza virus infects and destroys pulmonary type II epithelial cells while it increases permeability and/or hemorrhaging of endothelial cells [4, 5, 8–10, 14, 15]. Hemorrhages are also frequent complications of influenza virus pneumonia [3]. As mentioned, AMs are the

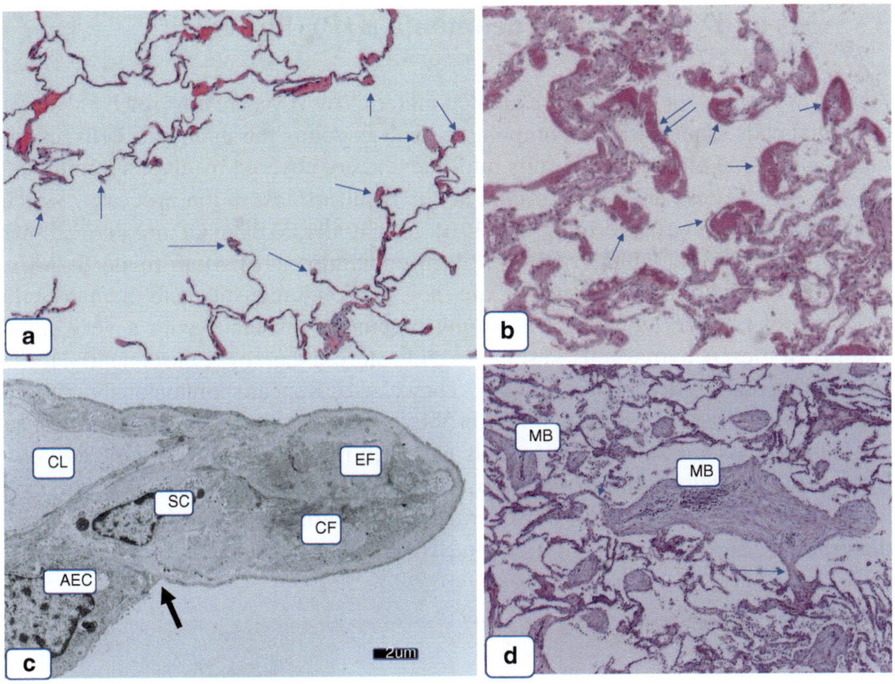

Fig. 5.1 Structure of alveolar mouths, hyaline membrane, and Masson body formation. (**a**) Longitudinal section of alveolar duct revealing many alveolar mouths (arrows) in free edges of alveoli. HE stain, ×100. (**b**) Fragmented irregular hyaline membrane (HM) formation at AMs of alveolar duct. Arrows indicate fragmented HMs at AMs. Double arrow indicates membranous HM in form. HE stain, ×200. (**c**) Ultrastructural findings of AMs, revealing capillary lumen, and elastic and collagen fibers. Arrow indicates the transitionl part from type II alveolar epithelial cells to covering epithelial cells of AMs. *CL* capillary lumina, *EF* elastic fibers, *CF* collagen fibers, *AEC* alveolar type II epithelial cells, *SC* stromal cell. Bar indicates 2 μm. (**d**) Masson bodies (MB) containing abundant myxoid substance are observed. Arrows indicate the connection between MBs and AMs. HE stain, ×100

key structures of the peripheral airway. AMs are covered by type II epithelial cells which have a very thin cytoplasm, like those of capillaries and are located separately from the capillary lumen. Structurally, they are similar to type I alveolar epithelial cells, but can extend to the surface of newly formed MBs and proliferate in MBs. In the stroma of AMs, elastic and collagenous fibers as well as capillaries have been detected. In summary, the initial targets of influenza virus during infection of peripheral airways are AMs, particularly their epithelial and endothelial cells, intervening macrophages, dendritic cells, and lymphocytes [16, 17]. Together with the structural weakness of AMs, this initiates ischemic changes in AMs, followed by MBs and/or HM formation.

3 AMs and Organizing Pneumonia (OP) (Fig. 5.2)

After AMs injury, the surface of exudated materials at AMs are covered by alveolar epithelial cells. Then, stromal components such as young mesenchymal cells, capillaries, and some inflammatory cells infiltrate and are covered by alveolar epithelial cells at AMs. These are MBs, formed as the result of absorption processes which occur in influenza virus, forming OP [1, 6]. Essentially, MBs in OP are divided into two types, fibrin containing and non-fibrin containing [18]. Both relate to AMs. Non-fibrin-containing MBs, which are not phosphotungustic acid hematoxylin (PTAH)-positive, are composed of young mucinous substance with a very small number of mesenchymal cells, respond well to steroid therapy. Consequently, these MBs disappear rapidly without fibrosis. They also disappear spontaneously without therapy with time. In contrast, myofibroblasts proliferate centrally inside fibrin-containing MBs and inflammatory cells gather in the center of MBs, covering distinct epithelial cells with thin cytoplasm. After inflammatory signs resolve, fibrosis and/or collagen bodies reveal peripheral airway deformities that lead to air flow disturbance [6]. In the case of AFOP, massive MBs are formed and organized [19,

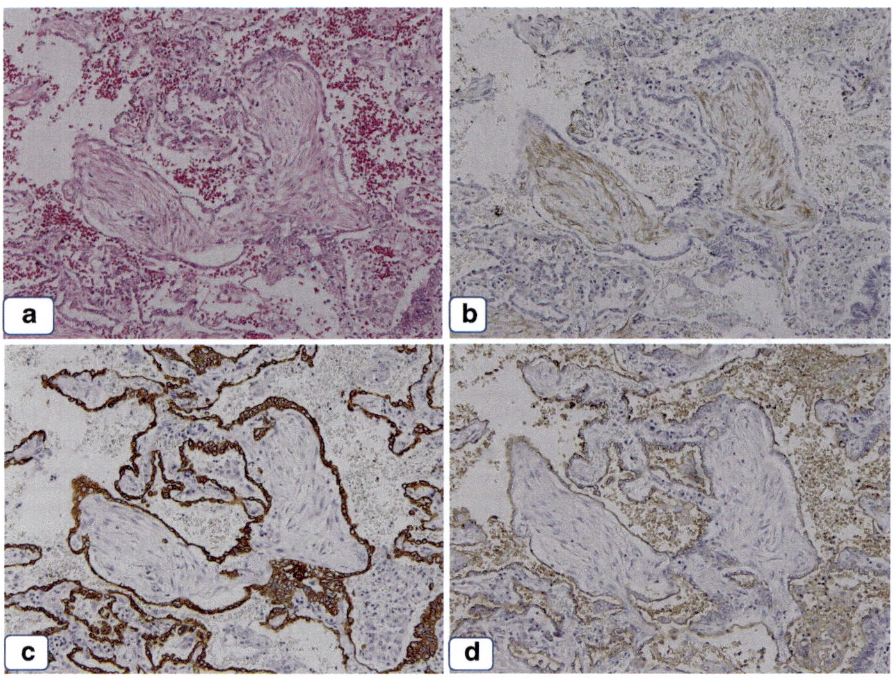

Fig. 5.2 Immune stains of MBs in influenza virus pneumonia. (**a**) MBs are completely epithelialized. HE stain, ×200. (**b**) Myofibroblastic cell proliferation is detected in MBs. Alpha-smooth muscle actin immune stain, ×200. (**c**) MBs are completely covered by epithelial cells. Pancytokeratin immune stain, ×200. (**d**) Linear expression of KL-6 positivity in MBs is detected. KL-6 immune stain, ×200 (cited from Ref. 6 with permission)

20]. Marked myofibroblast proliferation fills peripheral air spaces, especially RB, AD, AS, and acute respiratory insufficiency is rapidly induced.

MBs are connected with AMs, of which epithelium is considered the *locus minoris resistentiae* in peripheral airways, as shown in the early phase of HM formation [7]. Moreover, epithelial cells covering MBs are newly extended alveolar epithelial cells immunopositive for AE1/AE3 (pancytokeratins), but negative for SP-A and SP-D. These epithelial cells of MBs are derived from the divided alveolar type II epithelium of AMs. MBs fundamentally do not contain elastic fibers, but after absorbing fibrin-containing MBs, some deformities may remain due to interstitial myofibrosis or fibrosis [6]. KL-6 [21] is expressed very early in development in the premature lung [22] and on the surface of MBs. The blood supply of MBs is maintained through AMs by continuation of the septal blood vessels as revealed by immunopositive CD34, collagen Type IV, and Factor VIII-related antigen. The maturation of these newly formed epithelium covering MBs then occurs directly on MBs.

The pathological examination of AMs in the lung, especially RB, AD, AS, and alveoli, should be considered to be a very important morphological checkpoint for the assessment of pulmonary respiratory function in the peripheral airways.

4 AMs and Hyaline Membranes (HMs) (Fig. 5.3)

HMs at AMs are very important in the initial formation of fragmented HMs.

HMs are composed of both surface and deeper layers. The former is composed of SP-A, epithelial membrane antigen (EMA), and KL-6; the latter contains cell debris and fragmented cytokeratins as revealed by immunohistochemistry [6, 7] and ultrastructural findings (Ohtsuki et al., unpublished data). Ultrastructurally, HMs contain minute fragments of destroyed epithelial cells, including membranous, microtubular, granular, or fibrillar components (Ohtsuki et al., non-published data). During HM formation, basal laminae of alveoli are retained with no damage and are not positive for fibrin, but positive for SP-A, KL-6 and EMA, and cytokeratins (CK) [7] (Table 5.1). In particular, CK 19 is positive at the base of HM, revealing gradational positivity from the basal stromal side to the surface portion of HMs, consisting of fragmented cytokeratins derived from degraded alveolar epithelial cells. Influenza virus infections destroy alveolar epithelial cells. Fibrin exudation however is not absolutely involved. If fibrinous pneumonia occurs near HM formation, fibrin clots occurred secondary to HMs. The exudated fibrin however is not the fundamental component of HMs. Usually, HMs contain no fibrin at all, as shown by fibrin stains that were negative for HMs. If HMs are formed very rapidly, alveolar epithelial cells revealing p53 positive nuclei are detected beneath HMs. Its fundamental components are epithelial cell debris and intermingled Factor VIII antigen, associating surface components of alveoli, namely surfactant proteins, EMA, and KL-6, which are immunopositive for HMs. The immunopositivity varies depending on location. Even in the same lung section, positive and/or negative HMs are detected [23, 24]. The reasons for these varied immune reactions are unclear. HMs organize

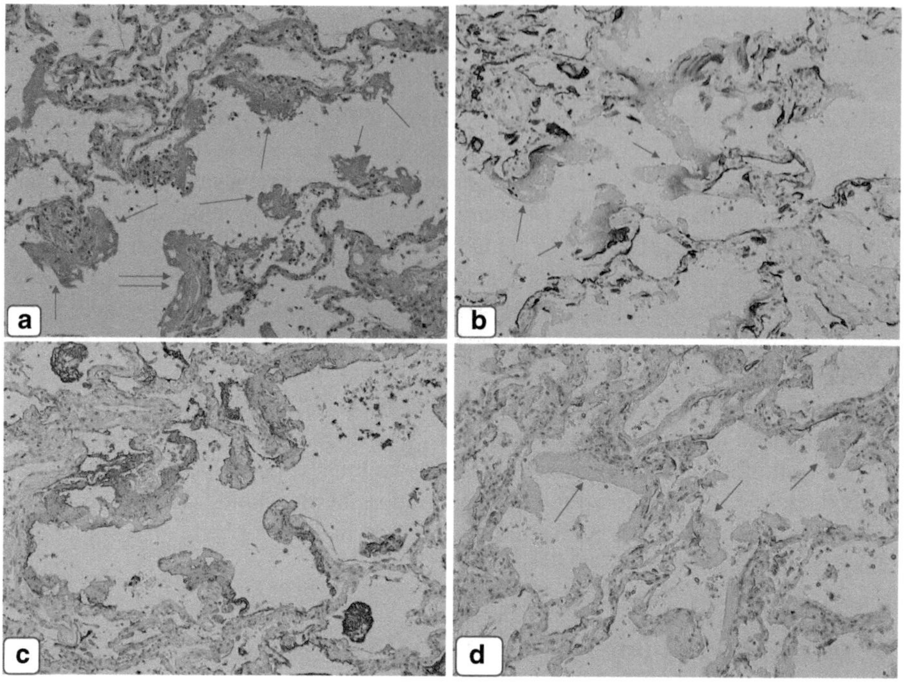

Fig. 5.3 Immune stain of hyaline membranes in influenza virus pneumonia. (**a**) Fragmented HMs are found at AMs (arrows). Double arrow indicate membranous form. HE stain, ×200. (**b**) Gradational positivity with pancytokeratin AE1/AE3 is detected (arrows). AE1/AE3 immune stain, ×200. (**c**) Surfactant protein A (SP-A) is positive with HMs. SP-A immune stain, ×200. (**d**) KL-6 is negative for HMs (arrows) in this influenza virus pneumonia. KL-6 immune stain, ×200 (cited from Ref. 6 with permission)

Table 5.1 Immunohistochemical stains of hyaline membrane

Antigens	General results
Pancytokeratins (AE1/AE3)	Diffusely positive with some negative cases
Cytokeratin 19 (CK19)	Diffusely positive featuring gradation from basal to surface area
Surfactant protein A (SP-A)	Diffusely positive
Epithelial membrane antigen (EMA)	Diffusely positive
[a]KL-6	Diffusely positive, but negative in influenza virus pneumonia in this report
Factor VIII related antigen	Diffusely positive
Fibrin stain ([b]PTAH)	Absolutely negative

These are the results of hyaline membrane immunostaining, including influenza virus pneumonia, and primary and secondary interstitial pneumonias. In influenza virus pneumonia, KL-6 is mostly negative. Whether this is the real characteristic finding of influenza virus pneumonia or not needs to be further investigated

[a]*KL-6* (Krebs von den Lungen 6) (provided by Eisai co., LTD, Tokyo, Japan)

[b]*PTAH* phosphotungustic acid hematoxylin stain for fibrin

by myofibroblasts which are derived from alveolar septa, then young granulation tissues replace HMs, and finally fibrous tissues are formed at alveolar septa appearing as deformities in the peripheral respiratory airflow. If these events occur rapidly, then respiratory failure is caused by HMs at diffuse alveolar damage (DAD). In direct viral infections of alveolar epithelial cells resulting in alveolar epithelial cell destruction, the cytoskeleton is destroyed by the virus infection, then the infected cells are broken into fragments. This debris is one of the important components of HMs as revealed by the positive immunoreactivity of HMs with cytokeratin antibodies, such as AE1/AE3, and CK 19 [6]. This immunoreactivity varies from the basal side to the apical side of HMs. This destruction occurs in various degrees in each part of the lungs. In fact, HMs stain both positive and negative for cytokeratins, often in the same location [23, 24].

With respect to cytokines during influenza virus infection, TNFalpha, IL-6, and IL-8 increase not only in the respiratory and central nervous systems, but also in extra-respiratory tissues including pancreas, liver, spleen, and jejunum, contributing to systemic cytokine responses [25]. Keratinocyte growth factor also accelerates the injury and death of alveolar type II cells after virus infection [26, 27].

5 Diffuse Alveolar Damage (DAD)

The initial target of influenza viruses is believed to be alveolar type II cells [8, 15]. In some reports, type I cells are also very important for virus infections in type II cells [17]. Alveolar macrophages and lymphocytes may assist with infection of epithelial cells [16]. Macrophages and lymphocytes are frequently implicated in the spread of virus infections. Lung dendritic cells also play a role as antigen presenting cells to alveolar epithelial cells [17]. Widespread virus infection in pulmonary epithelial cells induces DAD with HM formation. Bacterial coinfection is associated with a poor prognosis for influenza virus pneumonia, which targets endothelial cells and causes hemorrhaging in alveolar spaces. These bacterial infections and alveolar hemorrhage, as well as OP and HM-forming DAD, are serious complications in influenza-infected hosts throughout the course of disease [3, 6]. Among these complications, DAD is the most serious, given its association with acute respiratory distress syndrome (ARDS). In acute cases of exacerbation, DAD is detected in the parenchymal lung, presumably retaining effective respiratory function [28].

6 Conclusions

Both MBs and HMs formed at AMs are the main serious complications of influenza virus pneumonia. The epithelial cells of AMs are injured by virus infection, followed by exudation and destruction of epithelial cells. After influenza viral infection, exudates are the origin of MBs and destroyed epithelial cells is one of the key components of HMs. Both arising from AMs are the main serious causes of acute respiratory insufficiency in influenza virus pneumonia, causing disturbance of airflow and malfunction of peripheral airways at RB, AD, AS, and alveoli. Clinically, ARDS is a recognized result of these processes. AMs are therefore the key points of OP and DAD in pneumonia, caused by influenza virus infection.

Acknowledgement *We would like to thank Editage* (www.editage.com) *for English language editing.*

References

1. Torrego A, Pajares V, Mola A, Lerma E, Franquet T. Influenza A (H1N1) organizing pneumonia. BMC Case Rep. 2010. pil:bcr1220092531.
2. Sheng Z-M, Chertow DS, Ambroggio X, McCall S, McCall S, Pizygodzki RM, et al. Autopsy series of 68 cases of dying before and during the 1918 influenza pandemic peak. Proc Natl Acad Sci U S A. 2011;108(39):16416–21.
3. Nakajima N, Sato Y, Katano H, Hasegawa H, Kumasaka T, Hata S, et al. Histopathological and immunohistochemical findings of 20 autopsy cases with 2009 H1N1 virus infection. Mod Pathol. 2012;25(1):1–13.
4. Peteranderi C, Herold S, Schmoldt C. Human influenza virus infections. Semin Respir Care Med. 2016;37(4):487–500.
5. Miura TA. Respiratory epithelial cells as master communicators during viral infections. Curr Clin Microbiol Rep. 2019;6(1):10–7.
6. Fujita J, Ohtsuki Y, Higa H, Azuma M, Yoshinouchi T, Haranaga S, et al. Clinicopathological findings of four cases of pure influenza virus A pneumonia. Intern Med. 2014;53:1333–42.
7. Ohtsuki Y, Fujita J, Yoshinouchi T, Enzan H, Iguchi M, Lee GH, et al. Early stages of hyaline membrane formation detected in alveolar mouths in diffuse alveolar-damage-associated diseases: a detailed immunohistochemical study. Int J Surg Pathol. 2015;23:524–30.
8. Stegemann-Koniszewski S, Jeron A, Gereke M, Geffers R, Kroger A, Gunzer M, et al. Alveolar type II epithelial cells contribute to the anti-Influenza A virus response in the lung by integrating pathogen-and microenvironment-derived signals. MBio. 2016;7(3). pii:e00276-16.
9. Tundup S, Kandasamy M, Perez JT, Mena N, Steel J, Nagy T, et al. Endothelial cell tropism is a determinant of H5N1 pathogenesis in mammalian species. PLoS Pathog. 2017;13(3):e1006270.
10. Short KR, Kuiken T, van Riel D. Role of endothelial cells in the pathogenesis of influenza in humans. J Infect Dis. 2019;220(11):1859–60.
11. Kato S, Fujisawa T, Enomoto N, Inui N, Nakamura Y, Suda T. Severe respiratory failure associated with influenza B virus infection. Respirol Case Rep. 2015;3(2):61–3.
12. Asai N, Yokoi T, Nishiyama N, Koizumi Y, Sakanashi D, Kato H, et al. Secondary organizing pneumonia following viral pneumonia caused by severe influenza B: a case report and literature. BMC Infect Dis. 2017;17(1):572. https://doi.org/10.1186/s12879-017-2677-1.
13. Ohtsuki Y, Fujita J, Hachisuka Y, Uomoto M, Okada Y, Yoshinouchi T, et al. Immunohistochemical and immunoelectron microscopic studies of the localization of KL-6 and epithelial membrane antigen (EMA) in presumably normal pulmonary tissue and in interstitial pneumonia. Med Mol Morphol. 2007;40:198–02.
14. Short KR, Kasper J, van der Aa S, Andeweq AC, Zaaraoui-Boutahar F, Goeijienbier M, et al. Influenza virus damages the alveolar alveolar barrier by disrupting epithelial cell tight junctions. Eur Respir J. 2016;47:954–66.
15. Atkin-Smith GK, Duan M, Chen W, Poon IKH. The induction and consequences of influenza A virus-induced cell death. Cell Death Dis. 2018;9(10):1002. https://doi.org/10.1038/s41419-018-1035-6.

16. Londrigan SL, Tate MD, Brooks AG, Reading PC. Cell-surface receptors on macrophages and dendritic cells for attachement and entry of influenza virus. J Leukoc Biol. 2012;92(1):97–106.
17. Cardani A, Boulton A, Kim TS, Braciale TJ. Alveolar macrophages prevent lethal influenza pneumonia by inhibiting infection of type-l alveolar epithelial cells. PLoS Pathog. 2017;13(1):e1006140.
18. Yoshinouchi T, Ohtsuki Y, Kubo K, Shikata Y. Clinicopathological study on two types of cryptogenic organizing pneumonitis. Respir Med. 1995;89:271–8.
19. Beasley MB, Franks TJ, Galvin JR, Gochuico B, Travis WD. Acute fibrinous and organizing pneumonia: a histological pattern of lung injury and possible variant of diffuse alveolar damage. Arch Pathol Lab Med. 2002;126:1064–70.
20. Otto C, Huzly D, Kemna L, Huttel A, Benk C, Rieg S. Acute fibrinous and organizing pneumonia associated with influenza A/H1N1 pneumonia after lung transplantation. BMC Pulm Med. 2013;13:30. https://doi.org/10.1186/1471-2466-13-30.
21. Kohno N, Akiyama M, Kyoizumi S, Hakoda M, Kobuke K, Yamakido M. Detection of soluble tumor-associated antigens in sera and effusions using novel monoclonal antibodies, KL-3 and KL-6, against lung adenocarcinoma. Jpn J Clin Oncol. 1988;18:203–16.
22. Sun AP, Ohtsuki Y, Fujita J, Ishida T, Yoshinouchi T, Kohno N. KL-6, a human MUC1 mucin, is expressed early in premature lung. Respir Med. 2003;97:964–9.
23. Sun AP, Ohtsuki Y, Fujita J, Ishida T, Yoshinouchi T, Kohno N. Immunohistochemical characterisation of pulmonary hyaline membrane in various types of interstitial pneumonia. Pathology. 2003;35:120–4.
24. Peres e Serra A, Parra ER, Ehler E, Capellozzi VL. Nonhomogeneous immunostaining of hyaline membranes in different manifestations of diffuse alveolar damage. Clinics (Sao Paulo). 2006;61:497–02.
25. Short KR, Veeeris R, Leijten LM, van den Brand JM, Jong VL, Stittelaar K, et al. Proinflammatory cytokine responses in extra-respiratory tissue during severe influenza. J Infect Dis. 2017;216:829–33.
26. Camp JV, Jonsson CB. A role for neutrophils in viral respiratory disease. Front Immunol. 2017;8:550, eCollection 2017.
27. Nikolaidis NM, Noel JG, Pitstick LB, Gardner JC, Uehara Y, Wu H, et al. Mitogenic stimulation accelerates influenza-induced mortality by increasing susceptibility of alveolar type II cells to infection. Proc Natl Acad Sci U S A. 2017;114(32):E6613–22.
28. Ambrosini V, Cancellieri A, Chilosi M, Zompatori M, Trisolini R, Saragoni L, et al. Acute exacerbation of idiopathic pulmonary fibrosis: report of a series. Eur Respir J. 2003;22:821–6.

Chapter 6
Pathology, Diagnosis, and Treatment of Influenza Infections/Pneumonia: What Are the Mechanisms of Secondary Bacterial Pneumonia?

Masafumi Seki

Abstract Matrix with reports of aggravation of influenza mainly in elderly people in recent years, studies have focused particularly on the treatment of patients with pneumonia.

The guidelines established specifically emphasize the importance of accurate severity assessment, administration of anti-influenza/antibacterial agents, and preventive efforts centered on vaccinations in the world. Furthermore, Baloxavir/Marboxil (Xofluza), a novel anti-influenza agent, became commercially available in Japan from 2018. It is expected to be indicated also for the treatment of patients with severe influenza and those with associated pneumonia.

Keywords Anti-influenza agents · Antibiotics · Infection control · Antimicrobial stewardship · Vaccine

1 Introduction

Influenza is one of the most important respiratory infections because outbreaks occur each winter not only in Japan, but also all over the world, and the excess mortality rate increased greatly in the pandemic years [1–3].

In Japan, the "Nursing and Healthcare-Associated Pneumonia (NHCAP) Guideline" published by the Japanese Respiratory Society in 2011 also listed for the first time "secondary bacterial pneumonia associated with influenza," along with

M. Seki (✉)
Division of Infectious Diseases and Infection Control, Tohoku Medical and Pharmaceutical University Hospital, Sendai City, Miyagi, Japan
e-mail: m-seki@tohoku-mpu.ac.jp; seki@hosp.tohoku-mpu.ac.jp

J. Fujita (ed.), *Influenza*, Respiratory Disease Series: Diagnostic Tools and Disease Managements, https://doi.org/10.1007/978-981-15-9109-9_6

"aspiration pneumonia," as contributing factors and again confirmed that the elderly accounted for the majority of cases [2]. As such, there is a particular need for specific measures to treat adult patients with severe influenza and those with associated pneumonia, mainly among the elderly.

In addition, the neuraminidase inhibitors (NAI), oseltamivir, zanamivir, peramivir, and laninamivir are approved for therapeutic or prophylactic treatment of influenza virus infection, and favipiravir, a viral RNA-dependent RNA polymerase inhibitor, is approved and stockpiled for use against novel influenza virus infections in Japan should existing antivirals be ineffective [4, 5]. Furthermore, the novel cap-dependent endonuclease inhibitor (CEI) baloxavir marboxil (baloxavir; S-033188) was approved during 2018 to treat influenza A and B virus infections and has recently become available [6].

The present paper discusses the pathology and treatment of influenza pneumonia, as well as the trends of treatment, based on these guidelines also concerned with new anti-influenza agents.

2 Pathology and Classification of Influenza-Related Pneumonia

Influenza virus-associated pneumonia can be largely classified into:

1. Pneumonia caused by viral infections per se (primary influenza virus)
2. Pneumonia caused by the involvement of bacterial infections (influenza virus-associated bacterial pneumonia) [7–9].

Known risk factors for these forms of pneumonia or susceptibility to aggravation include aging, underlying pulmonary disease, diabetes, obesity, and pregnancy, which are also listed in the several guidelines (Table 6.1) [1–3].

Primary influenza viral pneumonia is usually caused by viruses alone and is commonly referred to as pure viral pneumonia. It manifests in the form of so-called severe interstitial pneumonia with alveolar flood and is very serious, since it can be further complicated by bacterial infections, leading to a high mortality rate [4, 10].

Influenza virus-associated bacterial pneumonia is caused by the involvement of bacterial infections and, importantly, is more prevalent than primary influenza viral pneumonia [7, 11, 12].

The most important causative bacteria for such pneumonias are the same as those that cause community-acquired pneumonia, namely pneumococci and *Haemophilus influenzae*. We have also confirmed the aggravation of such infections in an experiment conducted using a mouse model of coinfection by pneumococci and *Haemophilus influenzae* [8, 13–15].

Moreover, influenza virus-associated bacterial pneumonia is characterized by a high prevalence of coinfection by *Staphylococcus aureus* [2, 3]. This is thought to

Table 6.1 Risk factors for aggravation of influenza pneumonia [1]

• Age 65 years or older
• Chronic respiratory disease (asthma or COPD)
• Cardiovascular disease (excluding hypertension alone)
• Chronic renal, hepatic, hematologic, or metabolic (e.g., *diabetes*) disease
• Neuromuscular disease (motor paralysis, convulsion, dysphagia)
• Immunosuppressed condition (including HIV infection or drug-induced immunosuppression)
• Pregnancy
• Residency in a long-term care facility
• Marked obesity
• Long-term treatment with aspirin
• Tumor-bearing

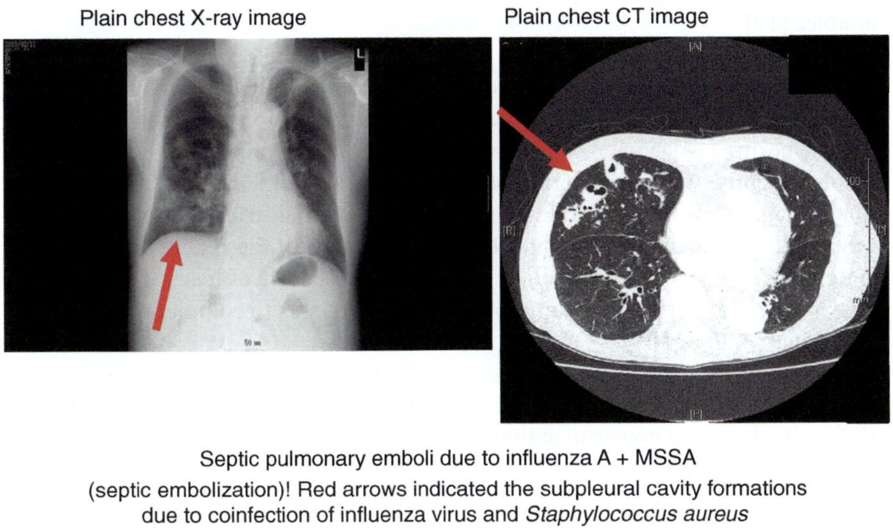

Fig. 6.1 A typical case of a pulmonary lesion associated with influenza (80 years old, male)

be attributable to the bacterial protease of *Staphylococcus aureus*, which promotes the cleavage of surface protein hemagglutinin (HA) on influenza virus, leading to viral activation [16].

However, clinically, pneumonia caused by *Staphylococcus aureus* involves primarily hematogenous infection rather than infection through the respiratory tract and is characterized by manifesting in the form of septic embolization more frequently than the common pneumonia (Fig. 6.1). In particular, aggravation and mortality are common, thus warranting more rigorous management and aggressive treatment.

3 Treatments: Anti-Influenza Agents and Antibiotics

First, it is important to assess the severity of the patient in order to decide the appropriate site to give treatment.

The Japanese Association for Infectious Diseases recommends that the age, dehydration, respiratory failure, orientation disturbance, pressure (A-DROP) scoring system used by the Japanese Respiratory Society be introduced in clinical practice for the management of influenza pneumonia [2, 17, 18].

The A-DROP scoring system is useful in that it allows accurate prognosis using only five variables, including age and main physical findings. The A-DROP scores are classified into categories ranging from mild to extremely severe, based on which a decision is made on whether to provide outpatient treatment with oral medication or inpatient treatment with primarily intravenous medication. Another tool used frequently in recent years and worthy of consideration is the quick Sequential Organ Failure Assessment (qSOFA), which classifies the severity of sepsis with only three variables [19].

The treatment of influenza per se has seen remarkable advances with the availability of oseltamivir (Tamiflu®), zanamivir (Relenza®), and other anti-influenza agents; it is far different from the past when conventional symptomatic treatments were the norm [1, 4].

Subsequently, with a pandemic of a new strain of influenza in 2009, new anti-influenza agents were approved for use one after another, ushering in a new phase in the field of influenza treatment. The biggest feature of these new drugs is that a single intravenous dose or inhalation is sufficient to achieve efficacy; thus, the challenge is how best to prescribe antibiotics and other agents to complement the use of these drugs [4, 20, 21].

In addition, recent recommendation for the management of influenza also provides the clinical indications for favipiravir (trade name: Avigan) [22]. Favipiravir exhibits an extremely powerful antiviral effect owing to its inhibition of viral replication. It has further attracted attention because of reports of its indication for the treatment of Ebola hemorrhagic fever and SARS-CoV-2 which is caused by an RNA virus as well. However, with some unresolved issues in terms of adverse drug reactions such as hyperuricemia, the Ministry of Health, Labour and Welfare has required particularly strict adherence to its clinical indication when prescribing the drug.

The availability in 2018 of baloxavir marboxil (trade name: Xofluza), an anti-influenza agent with a novel mechanism, is also an important topic (Table 6.2) [6]. While the emergence of low-sensitive viruses has been a concern, its overwhelming antiviral activity has been demonstrated. The key is how to use the drug in severe cases of influenza, particularly those with pneumonia, and there are additional challenges in the treatment of severe cases of influenza, including switch therapy [23].

Moreover, for the management of the common cold syndrome, a symptomatic treatment-based approach is recommended, with no antibiotics required [1, 3]. Influenza viral infection, nevertheless, is often complicated by bacterial

Table 6.2 Development and characteristics of recent anti-influenza agents

Genetic name	Laninamivir	Peramivir Hydrate	Favipiravir	Baloxavir Marboxil
Development code	CS-8958	S-021812	T-705	S-033188
Compound originator	Daiichi Sankyo	Bio Cryst	Toyama Chemical	Shionogi (Japan)
Development/ modeling	Daiichi Sankyo	Shionogi (Japan) Bio Cryst (U.S.)	Toyama Chemical	Shionogi (Japan)
Route of administration	Inhalation	Injection	Oral	Oral
Number of dose	1	1	Twice daily ×5 days	1
Mechanism of action	Neuraminidase inhibition (LANI)[a]	Neuraminidase inhibition (LANI)[a]	RNApolymerase inhibition	CAP-dependent endonuclease (CEN) inhibition
Marketing authorization (trade name)	Oct. 2010 (Inavir)	Jan. 2010 (Rapiacta)	Mar. 2014 conditional approval (Avigan)	Mar. 2018 (Xofluza)

[a]*LANI* long acting neuraminidase inhibitors

pneumonia; particularly in cases where the patient is elderly, aggressive concomitant use of antibiotics should be considered in addition to prescribing antiviral agents [11, 24]. However, rather than administering antibiotics aimlessly, selection of appropriate antibiotics that target potential causative bacteria that are detected at a high frequency is desirable. In such cases, despite some residual concerns about their antimicrobial activities against resistant *Streptococcus pneumoniae* and other bacteria, penicillins are the first-line agents, with the use of a relatively high dose recommended [2, 11].

In cases of the common cold and pneumonia, "judicious use of antibacterial drugs" was especially emphasized considering the risk of resistant bacteria. With regard to influenza treatment, while emphasizing the aggressive use of antiviral agents to prevent aggravation, there is no doubt that a cautious approach has been adopted with respect to the concomitant use of antibiotics. In these respects, to reiterate, the principles of and the actual actions taken with respect to Antimicrobial Stewardship (AS) or Antiviral Stewardship are extremely important [25].

4 Preventions: Vaccines and Infection Control

A pillar of prevention against influenza viral infections and associated pneumonia would be vaccination. Vaccination should be considered essential for high-risk patients, such as the elderly, especially those with a chronic lung disease, from the

Table 6.3 Comparison between a 13-valent conjugated vaccine (Prevnar) and a 23-valent capsular polysaccharide vaccine (Pneumovax)

	Prevnar	Pneumovax
Covered serotypes	Slightly narrow (13)	Broad (23)
Price	Slightly high (¥11,000)	Inexpensive (¥6000 → ¥3000\¥8000 → ¥4000)
Periodic vaccination	Not available	Available
Immunity induction	Strong (with conjugates)	Slightly weak (without conjugates)
Route of administration	Intramuscular injection (subcutaneous injection for pediatric population)	Intramuscular or subcutaneous injection

Generally, Pneumovax ⇔ in large hospitals (immunosuppression), Prevnar
However, initial vaccination with Prevnar → booster with Pneumovax is ideal

perspective of controlling aggravation and reducing mortality, rather than preventing onset [2, 3].

In recent years, the pneumococcal vaccine has become common in Japan as well, and revaccination for those aged 65 years or older has been approved. Reports indicating that there are synergistic effects with influenza vaccines have greatly increased the opportunities for their use.

In Japan, the 23-valent vaccine was first approved for periodic vaccination in 2014, and the 13-valent vaccine that has been used for the pediatric population has received approval for adult use as well (Table 6.3). Although the 13-valent vaccine covers a slightly narrower range of pneumococcal serotypes, the conjugates it contains make stronger immunostimulation possible [26–28].

Therefore, assessments are ongoing on a regimen consisting of an initial 13-valent vaccination followed by a booster 23-valent vaccination. Keeping in mind the proper use of the 23-valent vaccine for the general patient population and the 13-valent vaccine for transplant patients, particularly those in whom immunodeficiency is a concern, the 13-valent vaccine, as with the 23-valent vaccine, is also expected to receive approval for periodic vaccination.

5 Conclusions

The influenza epidemic each winter has resulted in a large number of victims, who are mostly elderly, and has become a major social problem. Countermeasures to control nosocomial and institutional infections are urgently needed. As mentioned in the guidelines, pneumonia is particularly important as a key complication. It is clear that coinfection by influenza virus and bacteria leads to a synergistic worsening, and measures to control both are urgently needed.

In the future, aggressive treatment of influenza (including not only H5N1 but also H7N9 avian influenza) and associated pneumonia, extracorporeal membrane oxygenation (ECMO) and other intensive care management strategies, and preventive measures will become more important.

Acknowledgements This work was supported by a Grant-in-Aid for Scientific Research (17K09623 to M.S.) from the Japanese Society for the Promotion of Science.

References

1. Uyeki TM, Bernstein HH, Bradley JS, Englund JA, File TM, Fry AM, Gravenstein S, Hayden FG, Harper SA, Hirshon JM, Ison MG, Johnston BL, Knight SL, McGeer A, Riley LE, Wolfe CR, Alexander PE, Pavia AT. Clinical practice guidelines by the Infectious Diseases Society of America: 2018 update on diagnosis, treatment, chemoprophylaxis, and institutional outbreak management of seasonal influenza. Clin Infect Dis. 2019;68:e1–e47.
2. Kohno S, Imamura Y, Shindo Y, Seki M, Ishida T, Teramoto S, Kadota J, Tomono K, Watanabe A. Clinical practice guidelines for nursing- and healthcare-associated pneumonia (NHCAP). Respir Investig. 2013;51:103–26.
3. Metlay JP, Waterer GW, Long AC, Anzueto A, Brozek J, Crothers K, Cooley LA, Dean NC, Fine MJ, Flanders SA, Griffin MR, Metersky ML, Musher DM, Restrepo MI, Whitney CG. Diagnosis and treatment of adults with community-acquired pneumonia. An official clinical practice guideline of the American Thoracic Society and Infectious Diseases Society of America. Am J Respir Crit Care Med. 2019;200:e45–67.
4. Oikawa N, Seki M. Clinical differences in hospitalized adult influenza patients between the A(H1N1) pdm09 and the A (H3N2) seasons in Japan. J Infect Dis Ther. 2018;6:1–6.
5. Takashita E, Ichikawa M, Morita H, Ogawa R, Fujisaki S, Shirakura M, Miura H, Nakamura K, Kishida N, Kuwahara T, Sugawara H, Sato A, Akimoto M, Mitamura K, Abe T, Yamazaki M, Watanabe S, Hasegawa H, Odagiri T. Human-to-human transmission of influenza A(H3N2) virus with reduced susceptibility to Baloxavir, Japan, February 2019. Emerg Infect Dis. 2019;17:25.
6. Hayden FG, Shindo N, Hirotsu N, Lee N, de Jong MD, Hurt AC, Ishida T, Sekino H, Yamada K, Portsmouth S, Kawaguchi K, Shishido T, Arai M, Tsuchiya K, Uehara T, Watanabe A, Baloxavir Marboxil Investigators Group. Baloxavir Marboxil for uncomplicated influenza in adults and adolescents. N Engl J Med. 2018;379:913–23.
7. Seki M, Yanagihara K, Higashiyama Y, Fukuda Y, Kaneko Y, Ohno H, Miyazaki Y, Hirakata Y, Tomono K, Kadota J, Tashiro T, Kohno S. Immunokinetics in severe pneumonia due to influenza virus and bacteria coinfection in mice. Eur Respir J. 2004;24:143–9.
8. Seki M, Fuke R, Oikawa N, Hariu M, Watanabe Y. Association of influenza with severe pneumonia/empyema in the community, hospital, and healthcare-associated setting. Respir Med Case Rep. 2016;19:1–4.
9. Seki M, Kohno S, Newstead MW, Zeng X, Bhan U, Lukacs NW, Kunkel SL, Standiford TJ. Critical role of IL-1 receptor-associated kinase-M in regulating chemokine-dependent deleterious inflammation in murine influenza pneumonia. J Immunol. 2010;184:1410–8.
10. Seki M, Suyama N, Hashiguchi K, Hara A, Kosai K, Kurihara S, Nakamura S, Yamamoto K, Imamura Y, Izumikawa K, Kakaya H, Yanagihara K, Yamamoto Y, Mukae H, Tashiro T, Kohno S. A patient with fulminant influenza-related bacterial pneumonia due to Streptococcus pneumoniae followed by Mycobacterium tuberculosis infection. Intern Med. 2008;47:2043–7.

11. Seki M, Kosai K, Yanagihara K, et al. Disease severity in patients with simultaneous influenza and bacterial pneumonia. Intern Med. 2007;46:953–8.
12. Seki M, Higashiyama Y, Tomono K, Yanagihara K, Ohno H, Kaneko Y, Izumikawa K, Miyazaki Y, Hirakata Y, Mizuta Y, Tashiro T, Kohno S. Acute infection with influenza virus enhances susceptibility to fatal pneumonia following Streptococcus pneumoniae infection in mice with chronic pulmonary colonization with Pseudomonas aeruginosa. Clin Exp Immunol. 2004;137:35–40.
13. Kosai K Seki M, Yanagihara K, Nakamura S, Kurihara S, Izumikawa K, Kakeya H, Yamamoto Y, Tashiro T, Kohno S. Elevated levels of high mobility group box chromosomal protein-1 (HMGB-1) in sera from patients with severe bacterial pneumonia coinfected with influenza virus. Scand J Infect Dis. 2007;40:338–42.
14. Seki M, Oikawa N, Hariu M, Watanabe Y. Methylprednisolone for antibiotic-refractory Haemophilus influenzae infection. J Infect Pulm Dis. 2017;3:1–3.
15. Seki M, Hashiguchi K, Kosai K, Higashiyama H, Yanagihara K, Kurihara S, Izumikawa K, Miyazaki M, Hirakata Y, Tashiro T, Kohno S. A patient with fulminant primary influenza pneumonia which developed into secondary bacterial pneumonia. Acta Med Nagasaki. 2006;51:121–4.
16. Tashiro M, Ciborowski P, Klenk HD, Pulverer G, Rott R. Role of Staphylococcus protease in the development of influenza pneumonia. Nature. 1987;325:536–7.
17. Seki M, Watanabe A, Mikasa K, Kadota J, Kohno S. Revision of the severity rating and classification of hospital-acquired pneumonia in the Japanese Respiratory Society guidelines. Respirology. 2008;13:880–5.
18. Seki M, Kosai K, Yanagihara K, Higashiyama Y, Kurihara S, Izumikawa K, Miyazaki Y, Hirakata Y, Tashiro T, Kohno S. Disease severity in patients with simultaneous influenza and bacterial pneumonia. Intern Med. 2007;46:953–8.
19. Singer M, Deutschman CS, Seymour CW, Shankar-Hari M, Annane D, Bauer M, Bellomo R, Bernard GR, Chiche JD, Coopersmith CM, Hotchkiss RS, Levy MM, Marshall JC, Martin GS, Opal SM, Rubenfeld GD, van der Poll T, Vincent JL, Angus DC. The third international consensus definitions for sepsis and septic shock (sepsis-3). JAMA. 2016;315:301–10.
20. Ison MG, Hui DS, Clezy K, O'Neil BJ, Flynt A, Collis PJ, Simon TJ, Alexander WJ. A clinical trial of intravenous peramivir compared with oral oseltamivir for the treatment of seasonal influenza in hospitalized adults. Antivir Ther. 2013;18:651–61.
21. Ison MG, Fraiz J, Heller B, Jauregui L, Mills G, O'Riordan W, O'Neil B, Playford EG, Rolf JD, Sada-Diaz E, Elder J, Collis P, Hernandez JE, Sheridan WP. Intravenous peramivir for treatment of influenza in hospitalized patients. Antivir Ther. 2014;19:349–61.
22. Kiso M, Lopes TJS, Yamayoshi S, Ito M, Yamashita M, Nakajima N, Hasegawa H, Neumann G, Kawaoka Y. Combination therapy with neuraminidase and polymerase inhibitors in nude mice infected with influenza virus. J Infect Dis. 2018;217:887–96.
23. Seki M, Sakai-Tagawa Y, Yasuhara A, Watanabe Y. Adult influenza A (H3N2) with reduced susceptibility to baloxavir or peramivir cured after switching anti-influenza agents. IDCases. 2019;18. eCollection 2019. https://doi.org/10.1016/j.idcr.2019.e00650.
24. Kakeya H, Seki M, Izumikawa K, Kosai K, Morinaga Y, Kurihara S, Nakamura S, Imamura Y, Miyazaki T, Tsukamoto M, Yanagihara K, Tashiro T, Kohno S. Efficacy of combination therapy with oseltamivir phosphate and azithromycin for influenza: a multicenter, open-label, randomized study. PLoS One. 2014;14:e91293.
25. Dellit TH, Sakai-Tagawa Y, McGowan JE Jr, Gerding DN, Weinstein RA, Burke JP, Huskins WC, Paterson DL, Fishman NO, Carpenter CF, Brennan PJ, Billeter M, Hooton TM. Infectious Diseases Society of America and the Society for Healthcare Epidemiology of America guidelines for developing an institutional program to enhance antimicrobial stewardship. Clin Infect Dis. 2007;44:159–77.

26. Maruyama T, Taguchi O, Niederman MS, Morser J, Kobayashi H, Kobayashi T, D'Alessandro-Gabazza C, Nakayama S, Nishikubo K, Noguchi T, Takei Y, Gabazza EC. Efficacy of 23-valent pneumococcal vaccine in preventing pneumonia and improving survival in nursing home residents: double blind, randomised and placebo controlled trial. BMJ. 2010;340:c004. https://doi.org/10.1136/bmj.c004.
27. van Deursen AMM, van Houten MA, Webber C, Patton M, Scott D, Patterson S, Jiang Q, Gruber WC, Schmoele-Thoma B, Grobbee DE, Bonten MJM, Sanders EAM. The impact of the 13-Valent pneumococcal conjugate vaccine on pneumococcal carriage in the Community Acquired Pneumonia Immunization Trial in Adults (CAPiTA) study. Clin Infect Dis. 2018;67:42–9.
28. Seki M, Chang B, Ohshima K, Watanabe Y. Two cases of acute pneumococcal purulent arthritis. IDCases. 2018;12:13–5.

Part III
Diagnosis

Chapter 7
Rapid Diagnosis of Influenza Viral Infection: What Are the Rapid Diagnostic Tests and Molecular Diagnosis?

Naoki Uno and Katsunori Yanagihara

Abstract Influenza is self-limited in otherwise healthy individuals but associated with increased morbidity and mortality in patients at high risk. Diagnosis of influenza infection can be made clinically without laboratory testing in patients who are not at risk and do not require hospital admission during an outbreak that has already been determined to be caused by influenza. However, influenza testing is indicated for patients at high risk for influenza complications, because test results are anticipated to influence clinical management. Influenza testing is also helpful in identifying the cause of outbreaks of respiratory illness. Rapid influenza diagnostic tests (RIDTs), which detect viral antigens in respiratory specimens, are commonly used in clinical practice but problematic because of their limited sensitivity. RIDTs will be replaced by molecular assays to minimize false-negative results.

Keywords Rapid influenza diagnostic tests · Molecular assays for diagnosis of influenza virus infection

1 Introduction

Rapid influenza diagnostic tests (RIDTs) have been traditionally used to make a diagnosis of influenza infection. RIDTs are point of care testing (POCT) performed by immunochromatography allowing to detect influenza viral proteins within approximately 15 min. RIDTs are actually fast and easy to perform. These advantages facilitated its general use. However, sensitivities of RIDTs are limited [1].

N. Uno (✉) · K. Yanagihara
Department of Laboratory Medicine, Graduate School of Biomedical Sciences, Nagasaki University, Nagasaki, Japan
e-mail: nuno@nagasaki-u.ac.jp

J. Fujita (ed.), *Influenza*, Respiratory Disease Series: Diagnostic Tools and Disease Managements, https://doi.org/10.1007/978-981-15-9109-9_7

False-negative RIDT results could result in improper clinical management such as withholding of necessary antiviral treatment, inappropriate use of antibiotics, unnecessary laboratory testing for other etiologies, and increase in influenza transmission. Food and Drug Administration (FDA) requires that all RIDTs achieve 80% or higher sensitivity compared with reverse transcription-polymerase chain reaction (RT-PCR). Infectious Diseases Society of America (IDSA) recommend use of molecular assays because of their high sensitivity [2].

2 Influenza Testing Methods

2.1 Rapid Influenza Diagnostic Tests (RIDTs)

RIDTs are commonly used for detection of influenza virus in clinical practice. Many tests are commercially available and used to assist in clinical decision making. RIDTs detect viral antigens in respiratory specimens collected generally by nasopharyngeal swab with 50–70% sensitivity and 90–95% specificity. The low sensitivity is always argued, because false-negative results are common especially when influenza is circulating in the population being tested. Positive RIDT results ensure appropriate use of antiviral medications, reduce unnecessary antibiotic use and laboratory testing for other etiologies, and implement infection prevention. However, negative RIDT results should be interpreted with caution because false-negative results are likely to occur during periods of high influenza activity (Fig. 7.1). IDSA no longer recommend RIDTs. Instead, they recommend molecular assays because of high sensitivity. Nevertheless, RIDTs are still used probably because they are actually simple and provide results quickly at the point of care, whereas molecular assays are not always available and not always as easy and fast as RIDTs. Some molecular platforms require special and often expensive instruments or devices. When rapid molecular assays are in widespread use, RIDTs will be replaced by them.

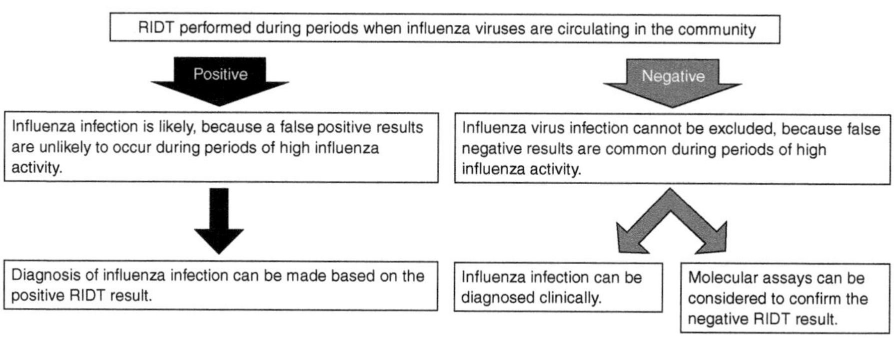

Fig. 7.1 Diagnostic procedure when RIDTs are used during periods of high influenza activity

We previously compared the results of a RIDT and RT-PCR using same clinical specimens when influenza viruses were circulating in the community [3]. The RIDT was based on immunochromatographic assay allowing detection of influenza viral antigens. A commercially available RIDT was used in routine clinical practice, whereas RT-PCR was developed in our clinical laboratory for research use. Clinical specimens were collected by a nasopharyngeal swab and resuspended in solution that was come with the RIDT product according to the manufacture's instruction. We extracted RNA from the suspension remaining after use of immunochromatographic strip and carried our quantitative RT-PCR. Twenty-six samples out of 77 RIDT negative samples tested positive by RT-PCR, indicating high false-negative results of the RIDT. Quantitative RT-PCR results demonstrated that false-negative RIDT results were owing to low quantity of virus present in the sample. IDSA recommends that follow-up testing with RT-PCR or other molecular assays should be performed to confirm negative RIDT results [2]. Our study suggests that additional sample collection is not necessarily required for a following molecular assay because the suspension remained after use of the immunochromatographic assay could be used for RT-PCR.

It should be noted that antiviral treatment decisions should not be made based on RIDT results. If clinically indicated, antiviral treatment should not be withheld from patients with suspected influenza, even if RIDT results are negative [4]. In other words, antiviral treatment decisions are primarily based on patients' signs and symptoms. RIDTs can assist in making clinical decision but can mislead clinicians if negative results are misinterpreted.

2.2 *Molecular Assays*

A number of molecular assays are available for clinical use. They can detect influenza viral RNA with high sensitivity and specificity. Some platforms are rapid enough to yield results within 30 min and/or portable enough to test at the point of care. The amplification method, turnaround time, and size of instruments vary by platforms. Some instruments enable to detect multiple pathogens including influenza virus by a single test. Sensitivities of molecular assays are higher than those of RIDTs, suggesting that false-negative results of molecular assays are less likely. IDSA recommends use of molecular assays. Some molecular assays are as easy as RIDTs. Furthermore, molecular assays can identify specific influenza viral subtypes. Taking together, rapid molecular assays will replace RIDTs in the future.

It is important to note that antiviral treatment should not be delayed while awaiting testing results. Antiviral treatment should be started as soon as possible because the greatest clinical benefit is when treatment is initiated as close to illness onset as possible, especially for hospitalized patients and outpatients at high risk of serious complications [5].

2.2.1 Rapid Molecular Assays

Cobas Liat is a portable real-time polymerase chain reaction (PCR) instrument manufactured by Roche molecular diagnostics [6–8]. It is easy, simple, and small enough to be used in a physician's office. Cobas Influenza A/B & RSV can identify influenza and RS viruses within 20 min after loading samples in the instrument [9].

Another molecular assay based on loop-medicated isothermal amplification (LAMP) is available for diagnostic use in Japan. The LAMP technology was developed and applied to detect pathogens by Eiken Chemical. It detects a single target by a single test. Therefore, it cannot detect multiple targets by a single test. However, it enables highly efficient amplification with high specificity without the need of a thermal cycler. LAMP products can be detected visually or by measuring the turbidity of the reaction mixture caused by pyrophosphate produced in the process of amplification. Influenza virus A and its subtype can be identified within 3 h [10].

ID NOW, formerly Alere i, is another molecular POCT instrument provided by Abbott [8, 11, 12]. The ID NOW technology is based on isothermal amplification and following detection of fluorescently labeled products. It enables detecting influenza A and B by a single test and providing results within a half hour. Its sensitivity is not as good as that of other molecular assays [7, 8, 13].

2.2.2 Multiplex Molecular Assays

FilmArray, Verigene, GenMark Dx, GeneXpert, and BD Max instruments allow to identify multiple respiratory pathogens including influenza virus [7, 8, 12, 13]. They are easy to operate and provide results within 2 h. FilmArray, Verigene, and GenMark Dx systems can detect multiple respiratory viruses including influenza A and B in a single respiratory panel assay, whereas GeneXpert and BD Max platforms detect multiple pathogens by using multiple single tests. When using GeneXpert or BD Max instrument, clinicians choose single tests for suspected pathogens and can test for them simultaneously. All platforms allow to detect many respiratory pathogens and help make a differential diagnosis of influenza-like respiratory illnesses.

2.3 Viral Culture

Viral culture is not recommended in the IDSA guideline [2]. It does not provide timely results and therefore does not help in diagnosis. However, viral culture is important to characterize the virus and help in developing vaccine.

2.4 Serology

Serologic tests detect antibodies produced against influenza viral antigens in blood. Centers for disease control and prevention (CDC) and ISDA do not recommend serologic testing, because it does not help in timely diagnosis. The presence of antibodies does not readily indicate acute infection. Clinicians should measure the antibodies again when the patient is recovering. Diagnosis of acute infection is generally made when the antibody titer of the initial serum is four times higher than that collected after 2–3 weeks.

3 How to Use Influenza Diagnostic Tests in Clinical Practice

3.1 Which Patients Should Clinicians Test for Influenza?

Influenza testing is not needed to decide use of antivirals. Clinicians should consider antiviral treatment regardless of testing when patients' signs and symptoms are compatible with influenza infection. However, influenza testing helps in clinical management in the following cases.

3.1.1 Outbreaks

When an outbreak of a respiratory illness occurs in closed settings such as nursing home and hospitals, influenza diagnostic tests are useful to identify the cause of the outbreak.

3.1.2 Outpatients at High Risk

Influenza testing is not always needed for outpatients. During an influenza outbreak, diagnosis of influenza infection can be made clinically without testing in outpatients who are not at risk, because influenza is typically self-limited infection in otherwise healthy outpatients. However, influenza infection is associated with increased morbidity and mortality in high-risk populations. Therefore, influenza testing is recommended in immunocompromised hosts and high-risk outpatients with pneumonia or nonspecific respiratory illness (Table 7.1).

Table 7.1 How to use influenza testing

Whom to test	What test	Why
Outpatients not at high risk	Not needed	During an influenza outbreak, acute febrile respiratory illnesses in patients who are not at high risk for influenza complications and who do not require hospital admission can be diagnosed as influenza with a high likelihood by clinical criteria alone [14]
Outpatients at high risk [15] • Children <5 years, but especially <2 years • Adults ≥65 years of age • Women who are pregnant or up to 2 weeks postpartum • Residents of nursing homes and long-term care facilities • Native Americans, including Alaska natives • People with medical conditions including: – Asthma – Neurologic and neurodevelopmental conditions – Chronic lung disease – Heart disease – Blood disorders – Endocrine disorders – Kidney disorders – Liver disorders – Metabolic disorders – Weakened immune system due to disease or medication – Children <19 years of age who are receiving long-term aspirin therapy – People with extreme obesity	Rapid molecular assays	Test results are anticipated to influence management decisions (initiating antiviral and/or antibacterial therapy, performing other diagnostic tests, and/or implementing infection control measures)
Hospitalized patients	Molecular assays	

3.1.3 Hospitalized Patients

Clinicians should test for influenza on admission in all patients requiring hospitalization with an acute respiratory illness. Antiviral treatment should not be withheld while awaiting the test results. CDC emphasizes that antiviral treatment should be started as soon as possible because antiviral treatment is clinically most beneficial when started as close to illness onset as possible [5].

3.2 What Test Should Clinicians Use?

IDSA recommends use of rapid molecular assays over RIDTs for outpatients. Conventional RT-PCR or other molecular assays are recommended for all hospitalized patients. IDSA recommends that clinicians should use rapid molecular tests and should NOT use RIDTs for hospitalized patients except when molecular assays are not available [2]. The availability of molecular assays varies in countries, regions, and institutions. Use of molecular assays is currently limited in Japan, because molecular assays are not necessarily approved for clinical use.

3.3 How to Interpret the Testing Results?

It is important to interpret test results properly, because misinterpretation can lead to improper clinical management.

3.3.1 Interpretation of Negative Results

When RIDTs are used, careful interpretation is needed especially for negative results. The question is whether negative results are true-negative or false-negative. When clinicians obtain a negative result, they should take disease prevalence into consideration, because disease prevalence in the population being tested affects the negative predictive value (NPV). The NPV is the proportion of true-negative results in negative results. The NPV indicates, in this case, the proportion of patients without influenza infection in patients who test negative. If negative results are totally true-negative, NPV is 100%. Suppose a clinician use a RIDT that detect influenza virus with 70% sensitivity and 95% specificity and obtain a negative result (Fig. 7.2a). The NPV decreases when influenza prevalence is high. This means that

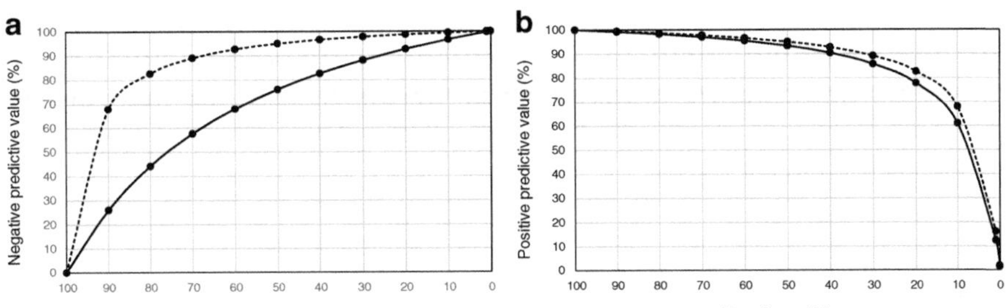

Fig. 7.2 Negative and positive predictive values using a test with 95% specificity and the indicated sensitivity. (**a**) Negative predictive values (NPVs) using a test with 70% (solid line) and 95% (dot line) sensitivity are shown. NPVs decrease when disease prevalence is high especially when the test sensitivity is low. (**b**) Positive predictive values (PPVs) using a test with 70% (solid line) and 95% (dot line) sensitivity are shown. PPVs decrease when disease prevalence is low, but the test sensitivity has little effect on PPVs

the negative result is likely a false-negative result if influenza is circulating in the community (high prevalence) but likely a true-negative result when influenza is not circulating in the community (low prevalence). The NPV can increase if clinicians use other tests with higher sensitivity. FDA requires at least 80% sensitivity for all RIDTs to reduce as much false-negative results as possible. However, even if clinicians use molecular assays with 95% sensitivity, they should consider the potential of a false-negative result, because the NPVs are not perfect and decrease when influenza prevalence is very high (Fig. 7.2a).

3.3.2 Interpretation of Positive Results

When clinicians obtain positive results, the results are likely a true-positive result especially during periods of high influenza activity in the population being tested. There is the possibility of a false-positive result. However, the false-positive result is unlikely when influenza prevalence of the tested population is high. Suppose a clinician use a RIDT that detects influenza virus with 70% sensitivity and 95% specificity and obtain a positive result (Fig. 7.2b). The difference in sensitivity of tests has little effect on the positive predictive value, which is the proportion of true-positive results in positive results. Specificities of most influenza diagnostic tests including RIDTs are as high as 95%. Therefore, the positive result of the influenza diagnostic tests including RIDTs is likely a true-positive result particularly during periods of high influenza activity in the tested population. However, the potential for a false-positive result should be taken into consideration when influenza is not circulating the community.

4 Conclusion

Influenza testing is not needed for outpatients who are not at high risk during periods of high influenza activity in the population being tested but needed for outpatients at high risk for influenza complications and all hospitalized patients. When testing for influenza, molecular assays are recommended over RIDTS to minimize false-negative results. Clinicians should be aware of false-negative RIDT results especially when influenza is circulating in the community. Antiviral treatment should not be decided based on RIDT results and should not be delayed while awaiting molecular testing results.

References

1. Chartrand C, Leeflang MM, Minion J, Brewer T, Pai M. Accuracy of rapid influenza diagnostic tests: a meta-analysis. Ann Intern Med. 2012;156(7):500–11.
2. Uyeki TM, Bernstein HH, Bradley JS, Englund JA, File TM, Fry AM, et al. Clinical practice guidelines by the Infectious Diseases Society of America: 2018 update on diagnosis, treat-

ment, chemoprophylaxis, and institutional outbreak management of seasonal influenza. Clin Infect Dis. 2019;68(6):895–902.

3. Tsushima Y, Uno N, Sasaki D, Morinaga Y, Hasegawa H, Yanagihara K. Quantitative RT-PCR evaluation of a rapid influenza antigen test for efficient diagnosis of influenza virus infection. J Virol Methods. 2015;212:76–9.
4. Centers for Disease Control and Prevention. Rapid influenza diagnostic tests. https://www.cdc.gov/flu/professionals/diagnosis/clinician_guidance_ridt.htm. Accessed 20 Feb 2020.
5. Centers for Disease Control and Prevention. Information on rapid molecular assays, RT-PCR, and other molecular assays for diagnosis of influenza virus infection. https://www.cdc.gov/flu/professionals/diagnosis/molecular-assays.htm. Accessed 20 Feb 2020.
6. Gibson J, Schechter-Perkins EM, Mitchell P, Mace S, Tian Y, Williams K, et al. Multi-center evaluation of the cobas((R)) Liat((R)) influenza A/B & RSV assay for rapid point of care diagnosis. J Clin Virol. 2017;95:5–9.
7. Young S, Illescas P, Nicasio J, Sickler JJ. Diagnostic accuracy of the real-time PCR cobas((R)) Liat((R)) influenza A/B assay and the Alere i influenza A&B NEAR isothermal nucleic acid amplification assay for the detection of influenza using adult nasopharyngeal specimens. J Clin Virol. 2017;94:86–90.
8. Nolte FS, Gauld L, Barrett SB. Direct comparison of Alere i and cobas Liat influenza A and B tests for rapid detection of influenza virus infection. J Clin Microbiol. 2016;54(11):2763–6.
9. Binnicker MJ, Espy MJ, Irish CL, Vetter EA. Direct detection of influenza A and B viruses in less than 20 minutes using a commercially available rapid PCR assay. J Clin Microbiol. 2015;53(7):2353–4.
10. Ito M, Watanabe M, Nakagawa N, Ihara T, Okuno Y. Rapid detection and typing of influenza A and B by loop-mediated isothermal amplification: comparison with immunochromatography and virus isolation. J Virol Methods. 2006;135(2):272–5.
11. Bell J, Bonner A, Cohen DM, Birkhahn R, Yogev R, Triner W, et al. Multicenter clinical evaluation of the novel Alere i influenza A&B isothermal nucleic acid amplification test. J Clin Virol. 2014;61(1):81–6.
12. Chen JH, Lam HY, Yip CC, Cheng VC, Chan JF, Leung TH, et al. Evaluation of the molecular Xpert Xpress flu/RSV assay vs. Alere i influenza A & B assay for rapid detection of influenza viruses. Diagn Microbiol Infect Dis. 2018;90(3):177–80.
13. Nie S, Roth RB, Stiles J, Mikhlina A, Lu X, Tang YW, et al. Evaluation of Alere i influenza A&B for rapid detection of influenza viruses A and B. J Clin Microbiol. 2014;52(9):3339–44.
14. Dolin R. Diagnosis of seasonal influenza in adults. UpToDate. https://www.uptodate.com/contents/diagnosis-of-seasonal-influenza-in-adults/print?search=influenza%20virus&source=search_result&selectedTitle=6~150&usage_type=default&display_rank=6. Accessed 20 Feb 2020.
15. Centers for Disease Control and Prevention. People at high risk for flu complications. https://www.cdc.gov/flu/highrisk/index.htm. Accessed 20 Feb 2020.

Chapter 8
Differential Diagnosis Between Influenza and Other Respiratory Viral Infections: What Are the Differential Diagnoses?

Takeshi Kinjo and Jiro Fujita

Abstract Respiratory viruses causing seasonal epidemics in the community are called community-acquired respiratory viruses (CARVs). CARVs include RNA viruses such as human rhinovirus, human respiratory syncytial virus, human parainfluenza virus, human coronavirus, human metapneumovirus, human enterovirus, human parechovirus, and DNA viruses such as human adenovirus and human bocavirus. Needless to say, influenza-like illness (ILI) is caused not only by influenza virus but also by other CARVs. Epidemiological studies targeting ILI patients revealed that CARVs other than influenza are universally detected, predominantly the rhinovirus. However, the viral etiology of ILI is affected by many factors such as the study population, season, setting (community or outpatient or inpatient), and regions. Previous studies investigated the utility of fever and cough as clinical diagnosis markers of influenza, nonetheless the sensitivity and specificity were modest. Since CARVs fairly cause respiratory and general symptoms including fever, cough, coryza, sore throat, headache, myalgia, and chills, predicting the causative virus by clinical symptoms is further difficult in most cases, except for diseases presenting with unique features such as laryngotracheobronchitis (croup), herpangina, and hand-foot-and-mouth disease. Consequently, clinical manifestations are not reliable enough for the differential diagnosis between influenza and other CARVs infection, therefore a rapid antigen test or molecular assay is critical to confirm the causative virus.

Keywords Community-acquired respiratory virus · Influenza-like illness
Taxonomy · Etiology

T. Kinjo (✉) · J. Fujita
Department of Infectious, Respiratory, and Digestive Medicine,
Graduate School of Medicine, University of the Ryukyus,
Okinawa, Japan

J. Fujita (ed.), *Influenza*, Respiratory Disease Series: Diagnostic Tools and Disease Managements, https://doi.org/10.1007/978-981-15-9109-9_8

1 Introduction

Respiratory viruses causing seasonal epidemics in the community are called community-acquired respiratory viruses (CARVs). Besides influenza virus, CARVs include human rhinovirus (HRV), human respiratory syncytial virus (RSV), human parainfluenza virus (HPIV), human adenovirus (HAdV), human coronavirus (HCoV), human metapneumovirus (HMPV), human bocavirus (HBoV), human enterovirus (HEV), and human parechovirus (HPeV). CARVs usually cause temporally upper respiratory tract infections in immunocompetent individuals; however, they can also cause severe lower respiratory tract infections (LRTIs) in susceptible individuals such as infants, elders, and immunocompromised patients. Although a vaccine and antiviral treatment have been established only against the influenza virus, knowledge about each CARV is also important from the perspective of clinical practice and infection control. This chapter focuses on CARVs other than influenza virus. Each CARV is briefly overviewed at the beginning, and then clinical aspects, emphasizing on the differential diagnosis between influenza and other respiratory viral infections, are discussed.

2 Brief Summary of CARVs

In this section, basic information for each CARV is briefly described. The taxonomy for CARVs is summarized in Table 8.1.

Table 8.1 Brief description of CARVs taxonomy

Genome	Family	Genus	Species	Envelope
RNA	*Picornaviridae*	*Enterovirus*	Human rhinovirus A, B, C	
			Human enterovirus A, B, C, D	(−)
			Human parechovirus 1, 2, 3, 4, 5, 6	
	Coronaviridae	*Alphacoronavirus*	Human coronavirus NL63, 229E	
		Betacoronavirus	Human coronavirus OC43, HKU1, SARS-CoV-1/2, MERS-CoV	(+)
	Pneumoviridae	*Metapneumovirus*	Human metapneumovirus A, B	
		Orthopneumovirus	Human respiratory syncytial virus A, B	(+)
	Paramyxoviridae	*Respirovirus*	Human parainfluenza virus 1, 3	
		Rubulavirus	Human parainfluenza virus 2, 4	(+)
	Orthomyxoviridae	*Alphainfluenzavirus*	Influenza A virus	
		Betainfluenzavirus	Influenza B virus	(+)
		Gammainfluenzavirus	Influenza C virus	
DNA	*Adenoviridae*	*Mastadenovirus*	Human adenovirus A, B, C, D, E, F, G	(−)
	Parvoviridae	*Bocavirus*	Human bocavirus 1, 2, 3, 4	(−)

2.1 Human Rhinovirus (HRV)

HRV, first reported in 1956 [1], is a single-stranded, positive-sense RNA virus that belongs to the family *Picornaviridae*. The name originally derived from "rhinos" in Greek, meaning "of the nose." HRV consists of more than 160 serotypes and is classified into three genotypes (A, B, and C) [2]. Although previous studies indicated that HRV-C was more virulent than other genotypes, being associated with asthma exacerbation and LRTIs, recent studies showed that specific genotypes are not linked to illness severity [3].

HRV is known as the most common virus causing mild self-limiting upper respiratory tract infections across all age groups; however, HRV can also cause severe LRTIs in immunocompromised patients [4]. Seo et al. reported that the mortality of transplant recipients with HRV present in the lower respiratory tract was as high as the rates of other viral pneumonias caused by RSV, HPIV, and influenza virus [5]. Respiratory viral infections often cause asthma exacerbation and chronic obstructive pulmonary disease (COPD), and HRV is known as the most detected virus in such vulnerable patients [6, 7]. Moreover, experimental inoculation studies revealed that HRV infection induced asthma exacerbations and COPD in human subjects [8–10].

2.2 Human Respiratory Syncytial Virus (RSV)

RSV, reclassified into the family *Pneumoviridae* in 2016 (previously *Paramyxoviridae*), is a single-stranded, negative-sense RNA virus. This virus was firstly isolated from chimpanzees in 1955, and shortly thereafter detected in infants with respiratory symptoms [11]. There are two genotypes (RSV-A and RSV-B) and no difference in virulence was shown in previous studies between genotypes [12, 13]. Approximately 60% of infants under 1-year-old experience a RSV infection and almost all children become infected with this virus at least once by the age of 2 or 3 years old [14]. RSV is the most common virus causing bronchiolitis and pneumonia in infants. A multicenter study targeting 5067 children revealed that RSV was detected in 18% of all children with acute respiratory infections, and that 61% of these patients required hospitalization. Additionally, 2–3% of children younger than 12 months were hospitalized annually due to RSV infections in the United States [15]. RSV also causes LRTIs and exacerbations of underlying diseases in adults, especially in the elderly and in immunocompromised patients [16].

2.3 Human Parainfluenza Virus (HPIV)

HPIV, first isolated from infants with croup in 1956 [17], is a single-stranded, negative-sense RNA virus belonging to the family *Paramyxoviridae*. There are four serotypes (1, 2, 3, and 4); HPIV-1 and HPIV-3 are classified in the genus *Respirovirus*, while HPIV-2 and HPIV-4 belong to the genus *Rubulavirus*. Clinically, HPIV-1 and HPIV-2 are the leading cause of laryngotracheobronchitis (croup) in children, accounting for 60–75% of croup illnesses [18]. HPIV-3 is the most commonly detected serotype in all age groups and it often causes pneumonia and outbreaks in long-term care facilities [19]. The epidemiology of HPIV-4 infections is not well understood because the detection is relatively difficult and its symptoms often present as subclinical [18].

2.4 Human Adenovirus (HAdV)

HAdV was firstly isolated from surgically resected adenoid tissue of children and initially reported as a "cytopathogenic agent" in 1953 [20]. HAdV is a double-stranded DNA virus categorized into the *Adenoviridae* family. HAdV is further classified into seven species (HAdV-A through HAdV-G) containing 67 immunologically distinct serotypes [21]. HAdV infects the mucosal tissue and each serotype presents with tissue/organ tropism, therefore, HAdV causes a variety of illnesses including respiratory infections, keratoconjunctivitis, and gastroenteritis (Table 8.2). Among these serotypes, 1–5, 7, 21, and 41 are most commonly associated with human disease [22]. Serotypes 4, 7, 14, and 55 were reported to cause severe pneumonia in immunocompetent adults, and of note, the former two (HAdV-4, 7) are known as a common cause of respiratory illness among military recruits in the United States [22–24]. Although temporarily suspended, an oral live nonattenuated vaccine against both HAdV-4 and HAdV-7 is administered to military recruits in the United States [25]. It is also clinically important to consider that gastrointestinal symptoms are sometimes intercurrent in patients (especially in children) having a HAdV respiratory illness [22].

Table 8.2 Disease types and associated serotypes of HAdV

Disease type	Patient population	Common serotypes
Pharyngitis	All age groups	1–7
Pharyngoconjunctival fever	Children	3, 4, 7
Pneumonia	Younger children	1–7
Pneumonia	Adults	3, 4, 7, 14, 21, 55
Epidemic keratoconjunctivitis	All age groups	8, 19, 37, 53, 54, 56
Gastroenteritis	Younger children	40, 41
Hemorrhagic cystitis	HSCT, SOT recipients	3, 7, 11, 21, 34, 35
CNS infections	Children, immunocompromised host	1–3, 6, 7, 12, 32
Myocarditis	Children, adults	1, 2, 5–7, 21
Disseminated disease	Children, immunocompromised host	1–3, 5, 7

CNS central nervous system, *HSCT* hematopoietic stem cell transplant, *SOT* solid organ transplant

2.5 Human Coronavirus (HCoV)

HCoV is a single-stranded, positive-sense RNA virus and belongs to the family *Coronaviridae*. The term of "corona" derives from the crown-like appearance of virions, meaning crown in Latin, by electron microscopy. CoV is further classified into four genera: alpha-, beta-, gamma-, and delta-coronavirus. HCoV was first isolated from the nasal discharge of common cold patients in 1965 [26]. To date, there are seven HCoVs including two alpha-CoVs (HCoV-NL63, HCoV-229E) and five beta-CoVs (HCoV-OC43, HCoV-HKU1, severe acute respiratory syndrome-CoV (SARS-CoV)-1, SARS-CoV-2, and Middle East respiratory syndrome-CoV (MERS-CoV)) [27, 28]. HCoVs were initially considered as a mere pathogen causing common cold-like symptoms; however, emergence of SARS-CoV in 2002 [29], MERS-CoV in 2012 [30], and SARS-CoV-2 in 2019 [28] has reminded us of its significant impact on human public health.

2.6 Human Metapneumovirus (HMPV)

HMPV was first identified from nasopharyngeal samples in children with respiratory symptoms in 2001 [31]. HMPV is a single-stranded, negative-sense RNA virus, and currently reclassified into the family *Pneumoviridae*, which also includes RSV. A seroprevalence study revealed that most children experience HMPV infection at least once by 5 years of age and re-infection occurs throughout the life [32]. HMPV preferentially infects respiratory ciliated epithelial cells and causes a variety of respiratory symptoms. A study investigating the clinical features of HMPV pneumonia in long-term care facilities in Japan showed that HMPV pneumonia patients experienced wheezing more frequently compared to non-pneumonia HMPV infected patients (43% vs. 9%; $p < 0.0001$). Additionally, the authors suggested that proximal bronchial wall thickenings radiating outward from the hilum on chest X-ray is a common finding in HMPV induced pneumonia [33].

2.7 Human Bocavirus (HBoV)

HBoV was first isolated from the respiratory samples of infants as an unknown human parvovirus in 2005 [34]. HBoV is a single-stranded DNA virus belonging to the family *Parvoviridae* and further classified into four subtypes (HBoV-1, -2, -3, and -4). HBoV-1 causes respiratory illness especially in young children, while HBoV-2, -3, and -4 are associated with gastroenteritis [35].

2.8 *Human Enterovirus (HEV) and Parechovirus (HPeV)*

HEV and HPeV are positive-sense, single-stranded RNA virus and belong to the family *Picornaviridae*. HEV is classified into four species (HEV-A, -B, -C, and -D) and traditional viral names such as coxsackievirus, echovirus, and poliovirus are still retained for individual serotypes [36]. HEV causes a variety of diseases involving not only respiratory organs, but also the skin, eyes, heart, and central nervous system (Table 8.3). Acute flaccid paralysis/myelitis caused by wild-type poliovirus has been eradicated from most countries including Japan. Based on genetic analysis, echovirus 22 and 23 were reclassified into a new genus *Parechovirus* and renamed HPeV-1 and -2, respectively, in 1999. Currently, 16 different parechovirus genotypes are identified and HPeV 1-6 cause infectious diseases in human. Among these genotypes, HPeV-1, -3, and -6 are associated with respiratory infections, and HPeV-3 is known as a cause of sepsis-like illness in neonates [37].

3 Viral Etiology in Patients with Influenza-Like Illness

World Health Organization defines influenza-like illness (ILI) as "an acute respiratory illness with a measured temperature of ≥38 °C and cough; with onset within the past 10 days" [38]. It is well known that CARVs other than influenza can cause ILI. A prospective, multinational, active community surveillance study involving 17 centers in eight countries was conducted from February 2010 to August 2011 [39].

Table 8.3 Disease types and associated serotypes of HEV

Disease type	Patient population	Common species/serotypes
Common cold	All age groups	Not specified
Herpangina	Children (mostly 1–7 years old)	Group A coxsackieviruses
HFMD	Children	Enterovirus 71, coxsackievirus A6, A16
Acute hemorrhagic conjunctivitis	All age groups	Enterovirus 70, coxsackievirus A24
Bronchitis, pneumonia	All age groups	Enterovirus D68
Acute flaccid paralysis/myelitis	Children	Poliovirus 1, 2, 3, enterovirus A71, D68
Aseptic meningitis	Infants (mostly <1-year-old)	Group B coxsackieviruses, echoviruses
Maculopapular eruptions	Children	Echoviruses
Petechiae/purpuric rash	All age groups	Echovirus 9, coxsackievirus A9
Epidemic Pleurodynia	Adolescents, younger adults	Group B coxsackieviruses
Myopericarditis	Adults	Group B coxsackieviruses

HFMD hand-foot-and-mouth disease

In this study, upper respiratory specimens were collected from 2421 children aged 6 months to 10 years (3717 ILI episodes) and tested by multiplex PCR. As a result, CARVs were detected in 2958 of 3717 episodes (79.6%) and the most commonly detected virus was HRV/HEV (41.5%), followed by influenza (15.8%), HAdV (9.8%), HPIV and RSV (both 9.7%), HCoV (5.6%), HMPV (5.5%), and HBoV (2.0%). The assay used in the study was unable to distinguish between HRV and HEV. Another study enrolling 1023 children with ILI revealed HRV as the most detected virus (49.4%), followed by HPIV-3 (19.5%), HMPV (16.5%), and influenza (5.4%) [40]. Table 8.4 summarizes representative large-scale studies investigating viral etiology in adult patients with ILI [41–47]. Most studies revealed that HRV, as well as influenza virus, were the leading cause of ILI. Needless to say, the viral etiology of ILI varies by many factors such as the study sample (e.g., age, influenza vaccination history), season, setting (e.g., community or outpatient or inpatient), and regions. However, the important thing is that CARVs other than influenza virus are commonly detected even during influenza epidemics [39, 48].

4 Are Specific Symptoms Useful in Distinguishing Between Influenza and Other CARVs?

Before discussing symptoms, the most important factor in clinically diagnosing influenza is whether the patient presenting with ILI visits a clinic during an influenza epidemic. Some studies investigated the utility of fever and cough symptoms to predict the likelihood of influenza [49–51]. Michiels et al. reported that the likelihood of influenza was quite low in patients without fever and cough during influenza non-epidemic periods [49]. On the other hand, the presence of "previous flu-like contacts," cough, "expectoration on the first day of illness," and fever higher than 37.8 °C during an influenza epidemic increased the likelihood of influenza threefold. Ebell et al. reviewed five studies examining the diagnostic accuracy based on the "fever and cough rule" during the influenza season [51]. The sensitivity and specificity of the rule for influenza diagnosis was 30–78% and 55–94%, respectively, and the authors concluded that the rule had a modest accuracy. We should keep in mind that ILI symptoms sometimes lack in some population types such as the elderly, for example. Therefore, clinical diagnosis of influenza should be carefully made by taking a comprehensive decision based on several factors such as the epidemic situation around the region and patient background.

Predicting causative CARV by clinical symptoms is further difficult, except for diseases presenting unique features such as bronchiolitis in children (mostly caused by RSV [52]), laryngotracheobronchitis, known as croup (mostly caused by HPIV [53]), hand-foot-and-mouth disease and herpangina (both caused by HEV). Bellei et al. compared the clinical manifestations (fever, cough, coryza, sore throat, headache myalgia, and chills) of seven CARVs (influenza, HRV, HMPV, HAdV, RSV, HCoV, and HEV) in adult patients with acute respiratory symptoms [46]. Although

Table 8.4 Viral etiology in adult ILI patients

			Number of samples		Percentage of each virus[b]							
Authors [References]	Country	Period	Total	Positives[a] (%)	Flu	HRV	RSV	HAdV	HCoV	HMPV	HPIV	Others
Al-Romaihi et al. [41]	Qatar	2012–2017	43.597	20,278 (47%)	49	18	5	5	9	5	5	3
Tan et al. [42]	Singapore	2009–2012	7.733	3794 (49%)	36	15	NT	17	9	4	3	22
Noh et al. [43]	Korea	2011–2012	1.983	1100 (55%)	77	8	3	0.6	3	6	3	NT
Todd et al. [44]	Vietnam	2013–2015	1.152	651 (57%)	70	9	2	3	2	1	8	4
Falsey et al. [45]	Multinational	2008–2010	556	340 (61%)	35	24	12	0.3	9	9	0.4	NT
Bellei et al. [46]	Brasil	2001–2003	420	274 (65%)	32	38	4	6	7	9	1	3
Louie et al. [47]	USA	2002	266	147 (55%)	35	16	8	0.7	1	3	0.7	9

Flu influenza virus, *HRV* human rhinovirus, *RSV* human respiratory syncytial virus, *HAdV* human adenovirus, *HCoV* human coronavirus, *HMPV* human metapneumovirus, *HPIV* human parainfluenza virus, *NT* not tested

[a]Number of samples positive for at least one virus

[b]Number of positives for each virus/number of positive of any virus

the frequency of fever was relatively higher in patients with influenza (91%) compared to other viruses (51–60%), there was no virus-specific symptom overall. To identify the causative CARVs in patients with respiratory infections, rapid antigen tests using immunochromatography or molecular assays including nucleic acid amplification tests are useful [54].

5 Conclusions

In this chapter, basic information regarding viral and clinical aspects of CARVs other than influenza is briefly summarized. From an epidemiological point, CARVs other than influenza virus are commonly detected even during influenza epidemics, thus a differential diagnosis between influenza and other CARVs infections is important. Additionally, identification of CARVs is sometimes critical especially when managing severe pneumonia patients or in an outbreak setting. Since the usefulness of clinical manifestations for differential diagnosis between influenza and other CARVs infection is limited in most cases, rapid antigen tests or molecular assays are needed to confirm a causative virus.

References

1. Price WH. The isolation of a new virus associated with respiratory clinical disease in humans. Proc Natl Acad Sci U S A. 1956;42(12):892–6.
2. Bochkov YA, Grindle K, Vang F, Evans MD, Gern JE. Improved molecular typing assay for rhinovirus species A, B, and C. J Clin Microbiol. 2014;52:2461–71. https://doi.org/10.1128/JCM.00075-14.
3. Ljubin-Sternak S, Mestrovic T, Ivkovic-Jurekovic I, Kolaric B, Slovic A, Forcic D, et al. The emerging role of rhinoviruses in lower respiratory tract infections in children - clinical and molecular epidemiological study from Croatia, 2017-2019. Front Microbiol. 2019;10:2737. https://doi.org/10.3389/fmicb.2019.02737.
4. Gutman JA, Peck AJ, Kuypers J, Boeckh M. Rhinovirus as a cause of fatal lower respiratory tract infection in adult stem cell transplantation patients: a report of two cases. Bone Marrow Transplant. 2007;40(8):809–11. https://doi.org/10.1038/sj.bmt.1705827.
5. Seo S, Waghmare A, Scott EM, Xie H, Kuypers JM, Hackman RC, et al. Human rhinovirus detection in the lower respiratory tract of hematopoietic cell transplant recipients: association with mortality. Haematologica. 2017;102(6):1120–30. https://doi.org/10.3324/haematol.2016.153767.
6. Dougherty RH, Fahy JV. Acute exacerbations of asthma: epidemiology, biology and the exacerbation-prone phenotype. Clin Exp Allergy. 2009;39(2):193–202. https://doi.org/10.1111/j.1365-2222.2008.03157.x.
7. Hewitt R, Farne H, Ritchie A, Luke E, Johnston SL, Mallia P. The role of viral infections in exacerbations of chronic obstructive pulmonary disease and asthma. Ther Adv Respir Dis. 2016;10(2):158–74. https://doi.org/10.1177/1753465815618113.
8. Jackson DJ, Makrinioti H, Rana BM, Shamji BW, Trujillo-Torralbo MB, Footitt J, et al. IL-33-dependent type 2 inflammation during rhinovirus-induced asthma exacerbations in vivo. Am J Respir Crit Care Med. 2014;190(12):1373–82. https://doi.org/10.1164/rccm.201406-1039OC.

9. Message SD, Laza-Stanca V, Mallia P, Parker HL, Zhu J, Kebadze T, et al. Rhinovirus-induced lower respiratory illness is increased in asthma and related to virus load and Th1/2 cytokine and IL-10 production. Proc Natl Acad Sci U S A. 2008;105(36):13562–7. https://doi.org/10.1073/pnas.0804181105.
10. Mallia P, Message SD, Gielen V, Contoli M, Gray K, Kebadze T, et al. Experimental rhinovirus infection as a human model of chronic obstructive pulmonary disease exacerbation. Am J Respir Crit Care Med. 2011;183(6):734–42. https://doi.org/10.1164/rccm.201006-0833OC.
11. Chanock R, Roizman B, Myers R. Recovery from infants with respiratory illness of a virus related to chimpanzee coryza agent (CCA). I. Isolation, properties and characterization. Am J Hyg. 1957;66(3):281–90. https://doi.org/10.1093/oxfordjournals.aje.a119901.
12. Martinello RA, Chen MD, Weibel C, Kahn JS. Correlation between respiratory syncytial virus genotype and severity of illness. J Infect Dis. 2002;186(6):839–42. https://doi.org/10.1086/342414.
13. Espinosa Y, San Martin C, Torres AA, Farfan MJ, Torres JP, Avadhanula V, et al. Genomic loads and genotypes of respiratory syncytial virus: viral factors during lower respiratory tract infection in Chilean hospitalized infants. Int J Mol Sci. 2017;18(3):654. https://doi.org/10.3390/ijms18030654.
14. Glezen WP, Taber LH, Frank A, Kasel J. Risk of primary infection and reinfection with respiratory syncytial virus. Am J Dis Child. 1986;40:543–6.
15. Hall CB, Weinberg GA, Iwane MK, Blumkin AK, Edwards KM, Staat MA, et al. The burden of respiratory syncytial virus infection in young children. N Engl J Med. 2009;360(6):588–98. https://doi.org/10.1056/NEJMoa0804877.
16. Nam HH, Ison MG. Respiratory syncytial virus infection in adults. BMJ. 2019;366:–l5021.
17. Chanock RM. Association of a new type of cytopathogenic myxovirus with infantile croup. J Exp Med. 1956;104:555–76.
18. Branche AR, Falsey AR. Parainfluenza virus infection. Semin Respir Crit Care. 2016;37(4):538–54. https://doi.org/10.1055/s-0036-1584798.
19. Russell E, Ison MG. Parainfluenza virus in the hospitalized adult. Clin Infect Dis. 2017;65(9):1570–6. https://doi.org/10.1093/cid/cix528.
20. Rowe WP, Huebner RJ, Gilmore LK. Isolation of a cytopathogenic agent from human adenoids undergoing spontaneous degeneration in tissue culture. Proc Soc Exp Biol Med. 1953;84(3):570–3. https://doi.org/10.3181/00379727-84-20714.
21. Ison MG, Hayden RT. Adenovirus. Microbiol Spectr. 2016; https://doi.org/10.1128/microbiolspec.DMIH2-0020-2015.
22. Lynch JP III, Kajon AE. Adenovirus: epidemiology, global spread of novel serotypes, and advances in treatment and prevention. Semin Respir Crit Care Med. 2016;37(4):586–602. https://doi.org/10.1055/s-0036-1584923.
23. Low SY, Tan TT, Lee CH, Loo CM, Chew HC. Severe adenovirus pneumonia requiring extracorporeal membrane oxygenation support--serotype 7 revisited. Respir Med. 2013;107(11):1810–3. https://doi.org/10.1016/j.rmed.2013.09.008.
24. Sun B, He H, Wang Z, Qu J, Li X, Ban C, et al. Emergent severe acute respiratory distress syndrome caused by adenovirus type 55 in immunocompetent adults in 2013: a prospective observational study. Crit Care. 2014;18(4):456. https://doi.org/10.1186/s13054-014-0456-6.
25. Kuschner RA, Russell KL, Abuja M, Bauer KM, Faix DJ, Hait H, et al. A phase 3, randomized, double-blind, placebo-controlled study of the safety and efficacy of the live, oral adenovirus type 4 and type 7 vaccine, in U.S. military recruits. Vaccine. 2013;31(28):2963–71. https://doi.org/10.1016/j.vaccine.2013.04.035.
26. Tyrrell DA, Bynoe ML. Cultivation of a novel type of common-cold virus in organ cultures. Br Med J. 1965;1(5448):1467–70. https://doi.org/10.1136/bmj.1.5448.1467.
27. Cui J, Li F, Shi ZL. Origin and evolution of pathogenic coronaviruses. Nat Rev Microbiol. 2019;17(3):181–92. https://doi.org/10.1038/s41579-018-0118-9.

28. Zhu N, Zhang D, Wang W, Li X, Yang B, Song J, et al. A novel coronavirus from patients with pneumonia in China, 2019. N Engl J Med. 2020;382(8):727–33. https://doi.org/10.1056/NEJMoa2001017.
29. Ksiazek TG, Erdman D, Goldsmith CS, Zaki SR, Peret T, Emery S, et al. A novel coronavirus associated with severe acute respiratory syndrome. N Engl J Med. 2003;348(20):1953–66. https://doi.org/10.1056/NEJMoa030781.
30. Zaki AM, van Boheemen S, Besterbroer TN, Osterhaus AD, Fouchier RA. Isolation of a novel coronavirus from a man with pneumonia in Saudi Arabia. N Engl J Med. 2012;367(19):1814–20. https://doi.org/10.1056/NEJMoa1211721.
31. van den Hoogen BG, de Jong JC, Groen J, Kuiken T, de Groot R, Fouchier RAM, et al. A newly discovered human pneumovirus isolated from young children with respiratory tract disease. Nat Med. 2001;7(6):719–24. https://doi.org/10.1038/89098.
32. Williams JV, Harris PA, Tollefson SJ, Halburnt-Rush LL, Pingsterhaus JM, Edwards KM, et al. Human metapneumovirus and lower respiratory tract disease in otherwise healthy infants and children. N Engl J Med. 2004;350(5):443–50. https://doi.org/10.1056/NEJMoa025472.
33. Karimata Y, Kinjo T, Parrott G, Uehara A, Nabeya D, Haranaga S, et al. Clinical features of human metapneumovirus pneumonia in non-immunocompromised patients: an investigation of three long-term care facility outbreaks. J Infect Dis. 2018;218(6):868–75. https://doi.org/10.1093/infdis/jiy261.
34. Allander T, Tammi MT, Eriksson M, Bjerkner A, Tiveljung-Lindell A, Andersson B. Cloning of a human parvovirus by molecular screening of respiratory tract samples. Proc Natl Acad Sci U S A. 2005;102(36):12891–6. https://doi.org/10.1073/pnas.0504666102.
35. Broccolo F, Falcone V, Esposito S, Toniolo A. Human bocaviruses: possible etiologic role in respiratory infection. J Clin Virol. 2015;72:75–81. https://doi.org/10.1016/j.jcv.2015.09.008.
36. Dunn JJ. Enteroviruses and parechoviruses. Microbiol Spectr. 2016; https://doi.org/10.1128/microbiolspec.DMIH2-0006-2015.
37. Olijve L, Jennings L, Walls T. Human parechovirus: an increasingly recognized cause of sepsis-like illness in young infants. Clin Microbiol Rev. 2017;31(1):e00047–17. https://doi.org/10.1128/CMR.00047-17.
38. Fitzner J, Qasmieh S, Mounts AW, Alexander B, Besselaar T, Briand S, et al. Revision of clinical case definitions: influenza-like illness and severe acute respiratory infection. Bull World Health Organ. 2018;96(2):122–8. https://doi.org/10.2471/BLT.17.194514.
39. Taylor S, Lopez P, Weckx L, Borja-Tabora C, Ulloa-Gutierrez R, Lazcano-Ponce E, et al. Respiratory viruses and influenza-like illness: epidemiology and outcomes in children aged 6 months to 10 years in a multi-country population sample. J Infect. 2017;74(1):29–41. https://doi.org/10.1016/j.jinf.2016.09.003.
40. Chang ML, Jordan-Villegas A, Evans A, Bhore R, Brock E, Mejias A, et al. Respiratory viruses identified in an urban children's hospital emergency department during the 2009 influenza a(H1N1) pandemic. Pediatr Emerg Care. 2012;28(10):990–7. https://doi.org/10.1097/PEC.0b013e31826ca980.
41. Al-Romaihi HE, Smatti MK, Ganesan N, Nadeem S, Farag E, Coyle PV, et al. Epidemiology of respiratory infections among adults in Qatar (2012-2017). PLoS One. 2019;14(6):e0218097. https://doi.org/10.1371/journal.pone.0218097.
42. Tan XQ, Zhao X, Lee VJ, Loh JP, Tan BH, Koh WHV, et al. Respiratory viral pathogens among Singapore military servicemen 2009-2012: epidemiology and clinical characteristics. BMC Infect Dis. 2014;14:204. https://doi.org/10.1186/1471-2334-14-204.
43. Noh JY, Song JY, Cheong HJ, Choi WS, Lee J, Lee JS, et al. Laboratory surveillance of influenza-like illness in seven teaching hospitals, South Korea: 2011-2012 season. PLoS One. 2013;8(5):e64295. https://doi.org/10.1371/journal.pone.0064295.
44. Todd S, Huong NTC, Thanh NTL, Vy NHT, Hung NT, Thao TTN, et al. Primary care influenza-like illness surveillance in Ho Chi Minh City, Vietnam 2013-2015. Influenza Other Respir Viruses. 2018;12(5):623–31. https://doi.org/10.1111/irv.12574.

45. Falsey AR, McElhaney JE, Beran J, van Essen GA, Duval X, Esen M, et al. Respiratory syncytial virus and other respiratory viral infections in older adults with moderate to severe influenza-like illness. J Infect Dis. 2014;209(12):1873–81. https://doi.org/10.1093/infdis/jit839.
46. Bellei N, Carraro E, Perosa A, Watanabe A, Arruda E, Granato C. Acute respiratory infection and influenza-like illness viral etiologies in Brazilian adults. J Med Virol. 2008;80(10):1824–7. https://doi.org/10.1002/jmv.21295.
47. Louie JK, Hacker JK, Gonzales R, Mark J, Maselli JH, Yagi S, Drew WL. Characterization of viral agents causing acute respiratory infection in a San Francisco university medical center clinic during the influenza season. Clin Infect Dis. 2005;41(6):822–8. https://doi.org/10.1086/432800.
48. Jain A, Prakash S, Jain B. Contribution of non- influenza respiratory viruses in causation of influenza like illness (ILI) during influenza epidemic: a laboratory based study. Clin Epidemiol Glob Health. 2017; https://doi.org/10.1016/j.cegh.2017.06.001.
49. Michiels B, Thomas I, Van Royen P, Coenen S. Clinical prediction rules combining signs, symptoms and epidemiological context to distinguish influenza from influenza-like illnesses in primary care: a cross sectional study. BMC Fam Pract. 2011;12:4. https://doi.org/10.1186/1471-2296-12-4.
50. Eskin B, Levy R. Evidence-based emergency medicine/rational clinical examination abstract. Does this patient have influenza? Ann Emerg Med. 2007;49(1):103–5. https://doi.org/10.1016/j.annemergmed.2006.08.016.
51. Ebell MH, Afonso A. A systematic review of clinical decision rules for the diagnosis of influenza. Ann Fam Med. 2011;9(1):69–77. https://doi.org/10.1370/afm.1192.
52. Meissner HC. Viral bronchiolitis in children. N Engl J Med. 2016;374(1):62–72. https://doi.org/10.1056/NEJMra1413456.
53. Smith DK, McDermott AJ, Sullivan JF. Croup: diagnosis and management. Am Fam Physician. 2018;97:575–80.
54. Zhang N, Wang L, Deng X, Liang R, Su M, He C, et al. Recent advances in the detection of respiratory virus infection in humans. J Med Virol. 2020;92(4):408–17. https://doi.org/10.1002/jmv.25674.

Chapter 9
Radiologic Findings of Influenza Pneumonia: What Are the Recent Radiological Findings?

Takeshi Johkoh

Abstract Classically, influenza pneumonia commonly shows focal, multifocal, or diffuse ground-glass opacity (GGO) and areas of consolidation along bronchovascular bundles on CT. HiN1/H7N9 influenza pneumonia depicts the parenchymal opacities of ground-glass opacity and consolidation have a predominant peribronchovascular and subpleural distribution on CT, resembling organizing pneumonia. If influenza pneumonia shows bronchopneumonia and/or bronchiolitis on CT, it is not difficult to differentiate it from COVID-19 pneumonia. Although they share peripheral predominant GGO and/or consolidation on CT, which looks like cryptogenic organizing pneumonia, differentiation of both diseases is often impossible by using CT.

Keywords Chest radiography · CT · H1N1 influenza pneumonia · COVID-19 pneumonia

1 General

The radiologic findings of viral pneumonia are diverse and may be affected by the immune status of the host and the underlying pathophysiology of the viral pathogen. Although not all cases demonstrate typical imaging patterns, most viral pneumonia patterns exhibit similarity on the basis of viridae [1]. CT pattern of viral pneumonias (Fig. 9.1) are as follows: (a) Pneumonia due to varicella-zoster virus shows multifocal 1–10-mm well-defined or ill-defined nodular opacity (arrows) with a surrounding halo or patchy ground-glass opacity (GGO) (arrowheads) in both lungs, (b) Pneumonia due to cytomegalovirus shows diffuse ill-defined patchy GGO with

T. Johkoh (✉)
Department of Radiology, Kansai Rosai Hospital, Amagasaki, Hyogo, Japan

J. Fujita (ed.), *Influenza*, Respiratory Disease Series: Diagnostic Tools and Disease Managements, https://doi.org/10.1007/978-981-15-9109-9_9

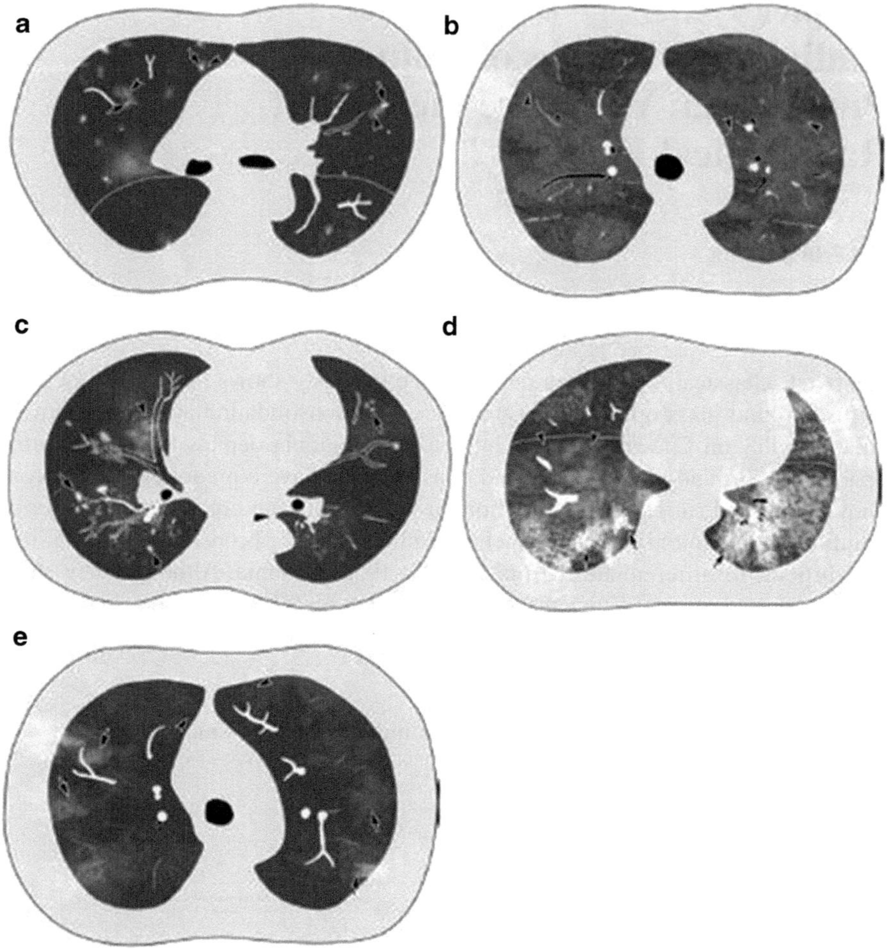

Fig. 9.1 Schematic illustrations of typical CT patterns of viral pneumonia. In general, CT findings of viral pneumonia are classified into these five patterns [1]

interlobular septal thickening (arrowheads) in both lungs, (c) Pneumonia due to human metapneumovirus shows multiple ill-defined nodules (arrows) or GGO (arrowhead) along the bronchovascular bundles in both lungs. These findings are similar to those of human parainfluenza virus pneumonia, which belongs to the same viridae, (d) Pneumonia due to influenza A virus shows multiple irregular areas of consolidation (arrows) along the bronchovascular bundles and diffuse GGO (arrowheads) with interlobular septal thickening in both lungs, and (e) Pneumonia due to rhinovirus shows multiple ill-defined patchy areas of GGO (arrows) with interlobular septal thickening (arrowheads) in both lungs [1]. These CT patterns are not always specific for each viral pneumonia, generally shared with each other, and often found altogether in one case.

2 Classical Imaging Findings of Influenza Pneumonia

Classically, chest radiographs in patients with influenza pneumonia show bilateral reticulonodular areas of opacity with or without focal areas of consolidation, usually in the lower lobes. On CT, focal, multifocal, or diffuse GGO and areas of consolidation are commonly seen. Centrilobular nodules, pseudocavitation, pneumatocele formation, and lymphadenopathy also are seen often [1, 2] (Fig. 9.2). Fujita et al. reported that in six patients with influenza pneumonia, four had no pleural effusion and two patients had pleural effusion. In these six patients, ground-glass opacities were the predominant finding; in five of the six, the opacities were bilateral and the opacities were unilateral in one patient. The ground-glass opacities showed upper lobe predominance in all six patients [2]

3 H1N1 Influenza Pneumonia

Influenza A (H1N1) virus infection is reported an outbreak in Mexico in April 2009 [3]. Since then it has spread rapidly worldwide. This pandemic influenza caused increased morbidity and mortality in a young population who were not generally at risk for severe illness with the usual seasonal influenza [3]. Although the majority of H1N1 influenza cases have been mild influenza-like illness, the most common

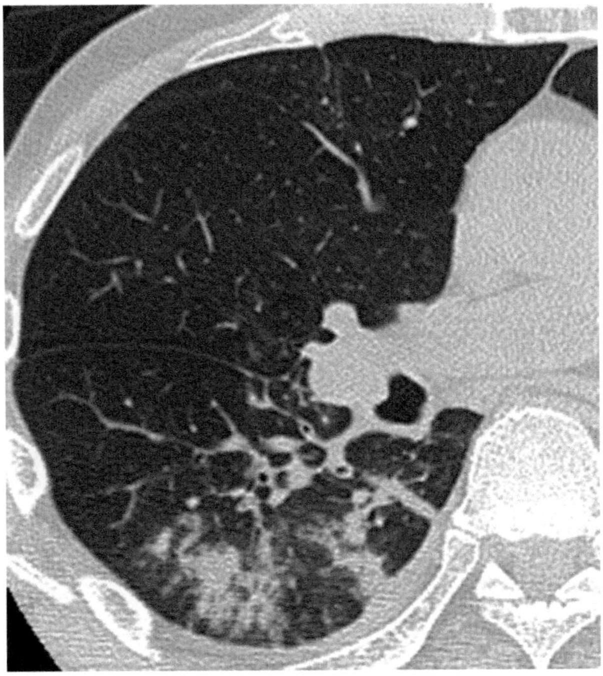

Fig. 9.2 Bronchopneumonia and bronchiolitis due to influenza A virus. Patchy shadow, lobular consolidation, and centrilobular branching structures are segmentally distributed in apical segment of right lower lobe

causes of death due to H1N1 infection are pneumonia and acute respiratory distress syndrome [4]. The main pathological finding in patients with H1N1 infection was reported to be exudative diffuse alveolar damage (DAD) with variable degrees of pulmonary hemorrhage and necrotizing bronchiolitis [5, 6]. There are also few case reports describing pathological findings of organizing pneumonia (OP) associated with influenza A (H1N1) virus infection [3, 7]. Moreover, Cornejo et al. suggested that the clinical symptoms of severe respiratory failure observed in these patients do not seem to resemble those of OP due to other causes [7].

Chest radiograph with a mild and self-limited clinical course of infection is often normal, but it may demonstrate prominent peribronchial markings with hyperinflation. Bilateral symmetric and multifocal areas of consolidation, often associated with ground-glass opacities, are the predominant radiographic findings in patients with a severe clinical course of infection [8–11]. Chest radiologic findings are most commonly seen in lower and central lung zones [11].

On CT, the parenchymal opacities of ground-glass opacity and consolidation have a predominant peribronchovascular and subpleural distribution, resembling organizing pneumonia [8] (Fig. 9.3). Several small ground-glass opacity may also be seen (Fig. 9.4). However, Shim et al. described that involvement of central lung parenchyma was more common than a mixed peripheral and central pattern or a subpleural pattern [12]. Li et al. reported that the predominant CT findings in the patients at presentation were unilateral or bilateral multifocal asymmetric ground-glass opacities alone with unilateral or bilateral consolidation which had peribronchovascular and subpleural predominance [13]. Namely, some cases with H1N1 influenza pneumonia look like cryptogenic organizing pneumonia and others show bronchiolitis-bronchopneumonia pattern (Fig. 9.3). Extensive involvement of both lungs, evidenced by the presence of multizonal and bilateral peripheral opacities, is associated with a required ICU admission, mechanical ventilation [11], and diverse prognosis [13–15]. In some cases, ground-glass opacities and/or consolidation on initial CT tend to resolve to fibrosis, which then resolve completely or display substantially reduced residual disease [16].

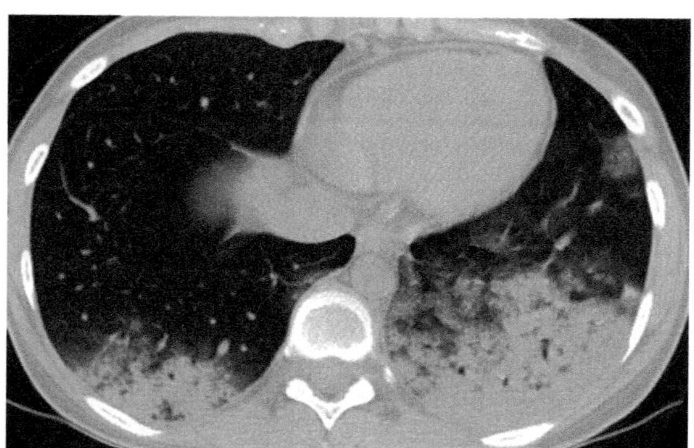

Fig. 9.3 H1N1 influenza pneumonia. Areas of ground-glass attenuation and consolidation are non-segmentally distributed in the subpleural lung zone of bilateral basal segments

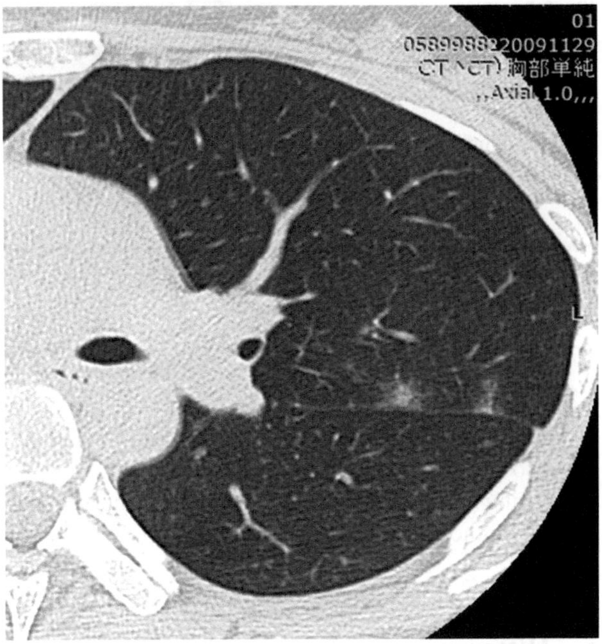

Fig. 9.4 H1N1 influenza pneumonia. Small ground-glass opacities surrounded areas with ground-glass opacity (halo sign) are seen in the left upper segment

4 H7N9 Influenza Pneumonia

Human infection with avian influenza A H7N9 virus firstly emerged in Anhui Province and Shanghai City, P.R. China in February, 2013 [17]. The condition of patients with H7N9 infection can deteriorate rapidly, with acute respiratory distress syndrome (ARDS) in 5–7 days, multiorgan failure, and even death.

Wang et al. reported imaging findings of 12 cases with H7N9 influenza pneumonia [18]. CT findings included ground-glass opacities (GGOs) (in 12 of 12 patients), consolidations (in 11 patients), air bronchograms (in 11patients), interlobular septal thickening (in 11 patients), centrilobular nodules (in 7 patients), reticulations (in 7 patients), cystic changes (in 4 patients), bronchial dilatation (in 3 patients), and subpleural linear opacities (in 3 patients). The lung lesions involved three or more lobes in all cases and were mostly detected in the right lower lobe (in 11 patients). Qi et al. described CT findings of six cases with H7N9 influenza pneumonia [19]. In the early stage, the right lung was more commonly affected (particularly in the right upper and middle lobes). The lesions rapidly expanded to the entire lungs and were characterized primarily by ground-glass opacities (GGOs) combined with consolidation. Diffuse GGO was observed in all six cases (1 was symmetric, and 5 were non-symmetric) (Fig. 9.5) [19]. Rapidly progressive GGOs and consolidations with air bronchograms and interlobular septal thickening, with right lobe predominance, are the main imaging findings in H7N9 pneumonia. GGO and consolidation often shows segmental or lobar distribution [21].

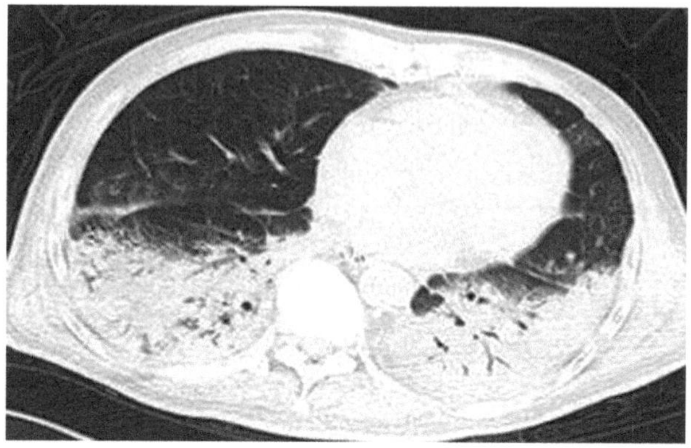

Fig. 9.5 H7N9 influenza pneumonia. Areas of consolidation are non-segmentally distributed in the subpleural lung zone of bilateral basal segments [20]

Extent of abnormalities on initial CT is associated with not only disease severity but also prognosis in patients with avian influenza H7N9 pneumonia [21, 22]. In recovering stage, fibrosis and traction bronchiectasis are seen on CT [20, 21]. Patients sometimes recover remaining fibrosis.

5 Differentiation from COVID-19 Pneumonia

On March 11, 2020 the World Health Organization (WHO) officially characterized the rapid global spread of coronavirus disease 2019 (COVID-19) as a pandemic and called for urgent international action in four key areas: to prepare and be ready; detect, protect, and treat; reduce transmission; and innovate and learn [23]. At the time of writing (May 27, 2020), the first pandemic is coming to an end in the world. However, the second and the third pandemics are sure to happen. If the future pandemic begins in the winter season, the differentiation of influenza pneumonia from COVID-19 pneumonia will be critical in the daily clinical practice.

Characteristic CT findings of COVID-19 infection on imaging were bilateral and peripheral ground-glass opacity and consolidation (Fig. 9.6) [24, 25]. With a longer time after the onset of symptoms, CT findings were more frequent, including consolidation, bilateral and peripheral disease, greater total lung involvement, linear opacities, "crazy-paving" pattern, and the "reverse halo" sign.

Bay et al. compared CT findings of 424 patients with COVID-19 pneumonia with those of 205 patients with other viral infection including influenza pneumonia [26]. Compared to non-COVID-19 pneumonia, COVID-19 pneumonia was more likely to have a peripheral distribution (80% vs. 57%, $p < 0.001$), ground-glass opacity (91% vs. 68%, $p < 0.001$), fine reticular opacity (56% vs. 22%, $p < 0.001$), and *vascular thickening* (59% vs. 22%, $p < 0.001$), but less likely to have a central + peripheral distribution (14.% vs. 35%, $p < 0.001$), pleural effusion (4.1% vs. 39%, $p < 0.001$), and lymphadenopathy (2.7% vs. 10.2%, $p < 0.001$). Wan et al.

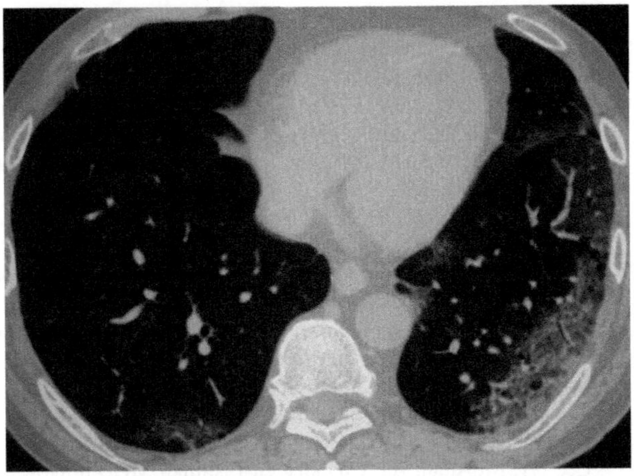

Fig. 9.6 COVID-19 pneumonia. Areas of ground-glass attenuation and consolidation are non-segmentally distributed in the subpleural lung zone of bilateral basal segments

described the comparison of CT findings of 13 patients with COVID-19 pneumonia to those of 92 patients with influenza pneumonia [27]. Peripheral and non-specific distributions in COVID-19 showed a markedly higher frequency compared with the influenza group ($p < 0.05$). Most lesions in COVID-19 showed balanced lobe localization, while in influenza pneumonia they were predominantly located in the inferior lobe ($p < 0.05$). COVID-19 presented a clear lesion margin and a shrinking contour compared with influenza pneumonia ($p < 0.05$).

COVID-19 had a patchy or combination of GGO and consolidation opacities, while a cluster-like pattern and bronchial wall thickening were more frequently seen in influenza pneumonia ($p < 0.05$). The lesion number and attenuation, air bronchogram, tree-in-bud sign, interlobular septal thickening, and intralobular septal thickening were not significantly different between the two groups (all $p > 0.05$).

If influenza pneumonia shows bronchopneumonia and/or bronchiolitis on CT, it is not difficult to differentiate it from COVID-19 pneumonia. Although they share peripheral predominant GGO and/or consolidation on CT, which looks like cryptogenic organizing pneumonia, differentiation of both diseases is often impossible by using CT.

References

1. Koo HY, Lim S, Choe J, Choi SH, Sung H, Do KY. Radiographic and CT features of viral pneumonia. Radiographics. 2018;38:719–39.
2. Fujita J, Bandoh S, Yamaguchi M, et al. Chest CT findings of influenza virus-associated pneumonia in 12 adult patients. Influenza Other Respir Viruses. 2008;1(5–6):183–7.
3. Perez-Padilla R, de la Rosa-Zamboni D, Ponce de Leon S, Hernandez M, Quiñones-Falconi F, Bautista E, et al. Pneumonia and respiratory failure from swine-origin influenza A (H1N1) in Mexico. N Engl J Med [Internet]. 2009 [cited 2018 Jun 9];361(7):680–9. Available from: http://www.ncbi.nlm.nih.gov/pubmed/19564631.

4. Torrego A, Pajares V, Mola A, Lerma E, Franquet T. Influenza A (H1N1) organising pneumonia. Case Rep [Internet]. 2010 [cited 2017 Aug 11]:bcr1220092531. Available from: http://www.ncbi.nlm.nih.gov/pubmed/22736390.
5. Mauad T, Hajjar LA, Callegari GD, da Silva LFF, Schout D, Galas FRBG, et al. Lung pathology in fatal novel human influenza A (H1N1) infection. Am J Respir Crit Care Med [Internet]. 2010 [cited 2018 Jun 9];181(1):72–9. Available from: http://www.ncbi.nlm.nih.gov/pubmed/19875682.
6. Nin N, Sánchez-Rodríguez C, Ver LS, Cardinal P, Ferruelo A, Soto L, et al. Lung histopathological findings in fatal pandemic influenza A (H1N1). Med Intensiva [Internet]. 2012 [cited 2018 Nov 4];36(1):24–31. Available from: http://www.ncbi.nlm.nih.gov/pubmed/22154847
7. Cornejo R, Llanos O, Fernandez C, Carlos Diaz J, Cardemil G, Salguero J, et al. Organizing pneumonia in patients with severe respiratory failure due to novel A (H1N1) influenza. BMJ Case Rep [Internet]. 2010 [cited 2017 Aug 11];2010(Jul 16 2). https://doi.org/10.1136/bcr.02.2010.2708. Available from: http://www.ncbi.nlm.nih.gov/pubmed/22767562.
8. Ajlan AM, Quiney B, Nicolaou S, Muller NL. Swine-origin influenza A (H1N1) viral infection: radiographic and CT findings. AJR Am J Roentgenol. 2009;193:1494–9.
9. Lee EY, McAdam AJ, Chaudry G, Fishman MP, Zurakowski D, Boiselle PM. Swine-origin influenza A (H1N1) viral infection in children: initial chest radiographic findings. Radiology. 2010;254:934–41.
10. Bai L, Li Gu L, Cao B, et al. Clinical features of pneumonia caused by 2009 Influenza A(H1N1) virus in Beijing, China. Chest. 2011;139(5):1156–64.
11. Agarwa PP, Cinti S, Kazerooni EA. Chest radiographic and CT findings in novel swine-origin influenza A (H1N1) virus (S-OIV) infection. AJR. 2009;193:1488–93.
12. Shim SS, Kim Y, Ryu JY. Novel influenza A (H1N1) infection: chest CT findings from 21 cases in Seoul, Korea. Clin Radiol. 2011;66(2):118–24.
13. Li P, Dong-Ju Sub D-J, Ji-Feng Zhanga J-F, et al. Pneumonia in novel swine-origin influenza A (H1N1) virus infection: high-resolution CT findings. Eur J Radiol. 2011;80:e146–52.
14. Aviram G, Bar-Shai A, Sosna J, et al. H1N1 influenza: initial chest radiographic findings in helping predict patient outcome. Radiology. 2010;255:252–9.
15. Grieser C, Goldmann A, Steffen IG, et al. Computed tomography findings from patients with ARDS due to Influenza A (H1N1) virus-associated Pneumonia. Eur J Radiol. 2012;81:389–94.
16. Li P, Zhang JF, Xia X-D. Serial evaluation of high-resolution CT findings in patients with pneumonia in novel swine-origin influenza A (H1N1) virus infection. Br J Radiol. 2012;85:729–35.
17. Gao RB, Cao B, Hu YW, et al. Human infection with a novel avian-origin influenza A (H7N9) virus. N Engl J Med. 2013;368:1888–97.
18. Wang Q, Zhang Z, Shi Y. JiangY emerging H7N9 Influenza A (Novel Reassortant avian-Origin) Pneumonia: radiologic findings. Radiology. 2013;268:882–9.
19. Lin ZQ, Xu XQ, Zhang KP, et al. Chest X-ray and CT findings of early H7N9 avian Influenza cases. Acta Radiol. 2015;56(5):552–6. https://doi.org/10.1177/0284185114535209.
20. Chen C, Chen J, Huang J-A. Persistence of lymphocytopenia with CT abnormalities among patients with critical H7N9 swine-origin influenza A virus infection. Jpn J Radiol. 2015;33:657–62.
21. Wang X-M, Hu S, Hu C-H, et al. Chest imaging of H7N9 subtype of human avian influenza. Radiol Infect Dis. 2015;1:51e56.
22. Feng F, Jiang Y, Yuan M, et al. Association of Radiologic Findings with mortality in patients with avian influenza H7N9 pneumonia. PLoS One. 2014;9(4):e93885. https://doi.org/10.1371/journal.pone.0093885.
23. World Health Organization: Director-General's opening remarks at the media briefing on COVID-19. 2020. Available from: https://www.who.int/dg/speeches/detail/who-director-general-s-opening-remarks-at-the-media-briefing-on-covid-19%2D%2D-11-march-2020. Updated 11 March 2020. Accessed 1 April 2020.
24. Song F, Shi N, Shan F, et al. Emerging 2019 novel coronavirus (2019-nCoV) pneumonia. Radiology. 2020;295:210–7.

25. Bernheim A, Mei X, Mingqian Huang M, et al. Chest CT findings in coronavirus disease-19 (COVID-19): relationship to duration of Infection. Radiology. 2020;295:200463. https://doi.org/10.1148/radiol.2020200463.
26. Bai XH, Hsieh B, Zeng Xiong Z, et al. Performance of radiologists in differentiating COVID-19 from viral pneumonia on chest CT. Radiology. 2020;20:200463. https://doi.org/10.1148/radiol.2020200463.
27. Wang H, Wei R, Rao G, Zhu J, Song B. Characteristic CT findings distinguishing 2019 novel coronavirus disease (COVID-19) from influenza pneumonia. Eur Radiol. 2020;30:4910–7. https://doi.org/10.1007/s00330-020-06880-z.

Chapter 10
Oral Findings of Influenza Viral Infection: What Are the Characteristic Pharyngeal Findings of Influenza?

Yuichiro Tamaki

The pharyngeal findings in influenza infection were first discovered by Miyamoto and Watanabe [1] and reported as influenza follicles. Influenza follicles, which can be detected in early phase of fever, are more sensitive than rapid influenza diagnostic tests, and therefore one of the physical findings useful for early diagnosis (Figs. 10.1 and 10.2).

The best light source to use is an LED light, but use of multi-LED lights or orange light, which often modify the shadow and color of follicles, may affect observation of follicles.

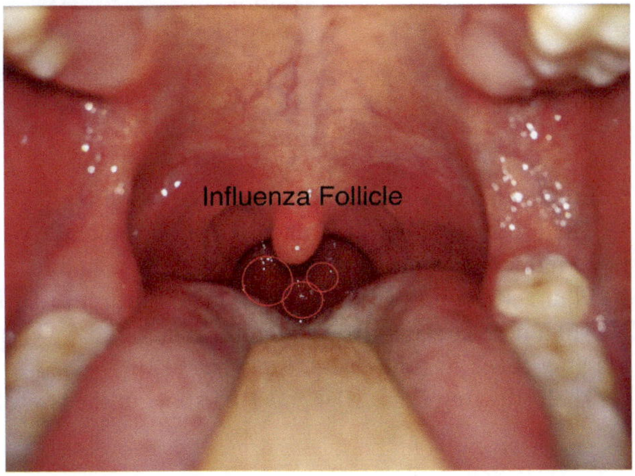

Fig. 10.1 16-year-old female, influenza type B, outpatient consultation within 12 h after fever

Y. Tamaki (✉)
Division of Emergency and Critical Care, University of the Ryukyus Hospital, Nishihara, Nakagami District, Okinawa, Japan
e-mail: doris@med.u-ryukyu.ac.jp

J. Fujita (ed.), *Influenza*, Respiratory Disease Series: Diagnostic Tools and Disease Managements, https://doi.org/10.1007/978-981-15-9109-9_10

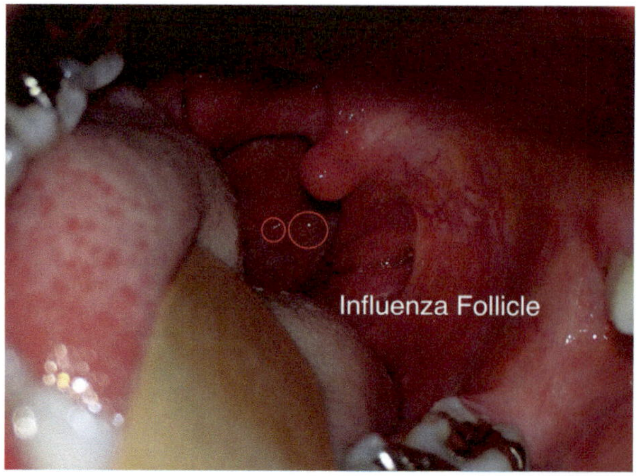

Fig. 10.2 19-year-old female, influenza type A, outpatient consultation within 12 h after fever

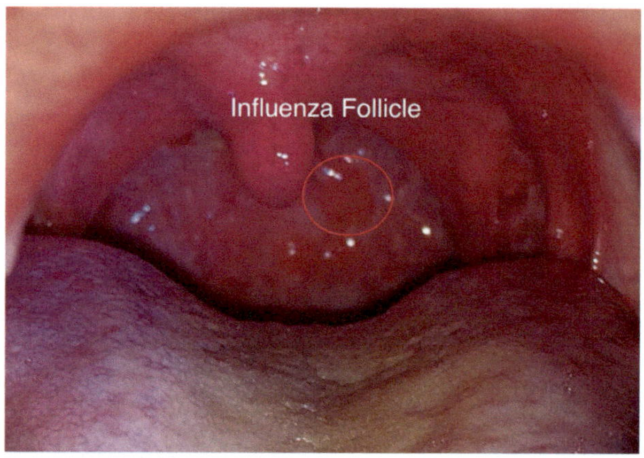

Fig. 10.3 39-year-old female, influenza negative, outpatient consultation over 12 h after fever

Influenza pharyngeal findings are shown below.

The following Figs. 10.3 and 10.4 show the cases with type A negative by initial rapid influenza test followed by positive the next day.

Figure 10.4 shows the case with the use of multi-LED light source.

Miyamoto et al. named small influenza follicles, which were observed as early as 1 h after fever, as influenza follicle buds [2].

The following Figs. 10.4 and 10.5 show influenza follicle buds.

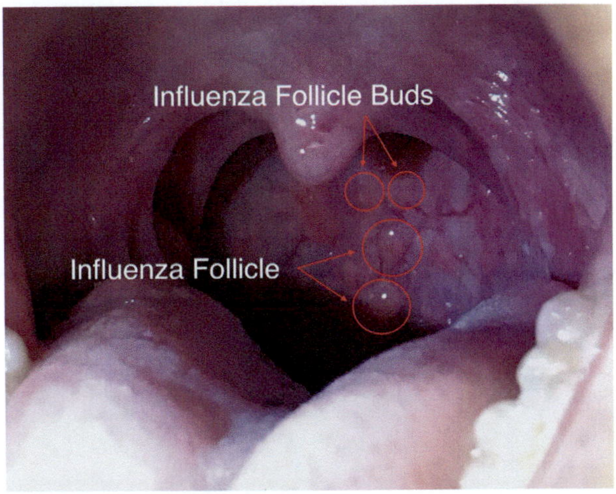

Fig. 10.4 21-year-old female, influenza negative, outpatient consultation within about 2 h after fever

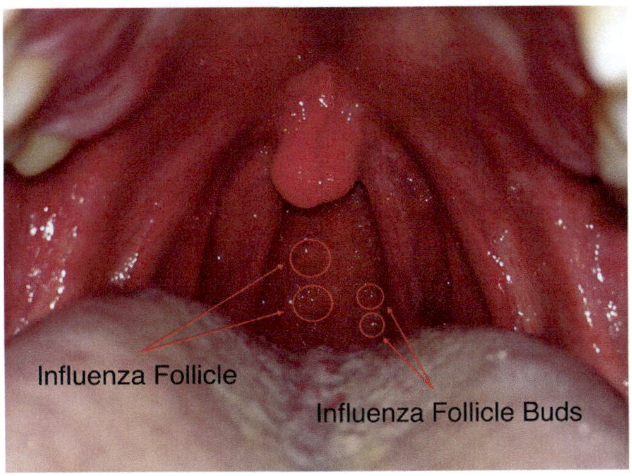

Fig. 10.5 24-year-old male, influenza type A, outpatient consultation within 1 h after fever

References

1. Miyamoto A, Watanabe S. Posterior pharyngeal wall follicles as diagnostic marker for seasonal and novel influenza. Gen Med. 2011;12:51–60.
2. Miyamoto A, Watanabe S. Influenza follicles and their buds as early diagnostic marker of influenza:typical images. Postgrad Med J. 2016;92(1091):560–1.

Part IV
Complication

Chapter 11
Classification of Pneumonia Complicated with Influenza Viral Infection: What Are the Patterns of Pneumonia?

Yuji Fujikura

Abstract Pulmonary complications associated with influenza, particularly pneumonia, are well recognized and are referred to as influenza (associated) pneumonia. Influenza-associated pneumonia can be classified into several subtypes, including viral pneumonia and superimposed or sequential bacterial pneumonia. Pure influenza viral pneumonia manifests in widespread diffuse lung inflammation, resulting in severe respiratory conditions. Secondary bacterial pneumonia is often seen as a post-influenza complication arising as a consequence of epithelial damage during viral infection. Viral and bacterial pneumonia can co-occur and each can promote the other. Because influenza pneumonia comprises several distinct subtypes with different clinical courses and pathophysiology, it is difficult to uniformly assess pneumonia severity. However, mortality may be slightly higher than expected, based on conventional severity indicators of community-acquired pneumonia.

Keywords Influenza pneumonia · Pure influenza viral pneumonia · Secondary bacterial pneumonia · Mixed viral and bacterial pneumonia

1 Introduction

Pulmonary complications associated with influenza, particularly pneumonia, are well recognized, and were described in the historical literature as "perineumony," [1] even in the era before imaging modalities or stethoscopes. Numerous cases of pneumonia following influenza were reported during the Spanish influenza

Y. Fujikura (✉)
Division of Infectious Diseases and Respiratory Medicine, Department of Internal Medicine, National Defense Medical College, Tokorozawa, Saitama, Japan
e-mail: fujikura@ndmc.ac.jp

J. Fujita (ed.), *Influenza*, Respiratory Disease Series: Diagnostic Tools and Disease Managements, https://doi.org/10.1007/978-981-15-9109-9_11

pandemic of 1918. Pneumonia during or post-influenza virus infection is referred to as "influenza(-associated) pneumonia," which can sometimes result in serious outcomes.

2 Severity of Influenza Pneumonia

Influenza may be accompanied by pneumonia either during or after illness, which can be fatal. There are no clear statistical data on the incidence of influenza pneumonia or influenza-related deaths during each season of influenza epidemics. At present, influenza-related death rates are estimated by the concept of excess mortality [2]. Thousands of extra deaths are recorded in Japan each season, which may include deaths from influenza pneumonia.

Influenza pneumonia comprises several distinct subtypes, each with different clinical courses and pathophysiology. Therefore, it is difficult to assess the severity of pneumonia uniformly, with no established evaluation method at present. Assessing the severity of influenza pneumonia is important for patient management. Various mortality prediction models such as the Pneumonia Severity Index [3], CURB-65 [4], and A-DROP [5] were verified during the 2009 pandemic; however, no definitive model has been established [6]. Among these three prediction models, the A-DROP system had the strongest discrimination power for point of mortality during the influenza pandemic of 2009 [7]. However, observed mortality tended to be higher than expected mortality predicted from any of these indicators (Fig. 11.1). Influenza pneumonia is not necessarily categorized as community-acquired pneumonia. In general, patients with underlying conditions are at risk of pulmonary complications from influenza and may contribute to this increased mortality. A recent multicenter cohort study reported that mortality was higher among immunocompromised patients in the 2009 influenza pandemic than during seasonal influenza [8]. From these findings, it is possible that mortality may be slightly higher than expected based on conventional indicators.

3 Classification of Influenza Pneumonia

A detailed analysis of influenza pneumonia was first documented during the Asian flu of 1957–1958. Louria classified pulmonary complications associated with influenza into four distinct syndromes on the basis of clinical history, chest X-ray, and viral and bacterial analysis [9]. Three of these syndromes are considered pneumonia, while the fourth is a syndrome comprising physical signs of lower respiratory tract involvement with no infiltrate on X-ray imaging. This classification distinguishes pneumonia due to influenza from cases caused by secondary or

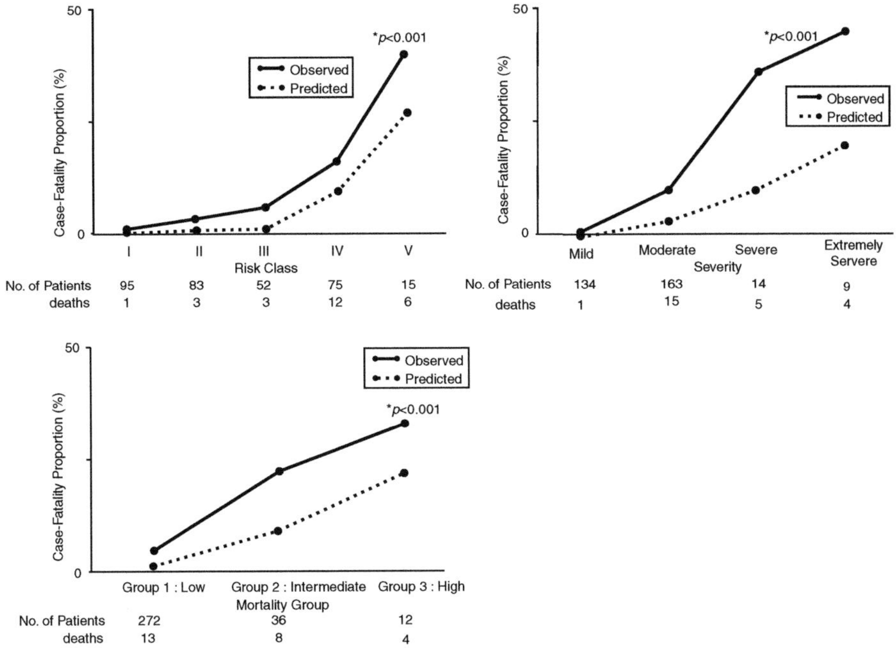

Fig. 11.1 Comparison of observed and predicted mortality according to (**a**) pneumonia severity index (PSI), (**b**) CURB-65 (confusion, urea, respiratory rate, blood pressure, and age $\geq$ 65 years), and (**c**) A-DROP (age, dehydration, respiration, disorientation, and blood pressure) [7]

Fig. 11.2 Pure influenza viral pneumonia: CT scan showing diffuse infiltration resembling heart failure

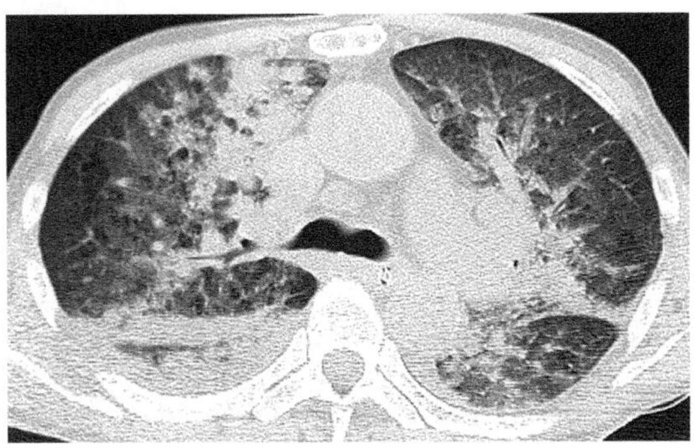

simultaneous bacterial infection. This concept is important when considering the pathophysiology of influenza pneumonia. Pure influenza pneumonia is caused by viral infection alone, described by Louria as a serious pneumonia represented by diffuse infiltrate similar to heart failure with rapid progression (Fig. 11.2). Such cases occur in relatively young individuals, and bloody sputum is often observed in clinical course. Although pure influenza viral pneumonia is considered common during pandemics, it is also observed during seasonal influenza [10]. Bacterial pneumonia is often experienced during or after influenza virus infection. Bacterial pneumonia is mainly composed of either secondary bacterial pneumonia (Fig. 11.3) or mixed influenza viral and bacterial pneumonia.

Influenza pneumonia presents various radiological findings depending on the pathophysiology described above. Direct viral infection of the lung parenchyma tends to show diffuse ground-glass opacity or consolidation [11], while secondary bacterial pneumonia is generally recognized as a localized consolidation which is observed easily in typical bacterial pneumonia. However, it is not always easy to discriminate whether pneumonia is being caused by virus alone or includes a bacterial contribution.

Comparative characteristics of these types of influenza pneumonia are shown in Table 11.1.

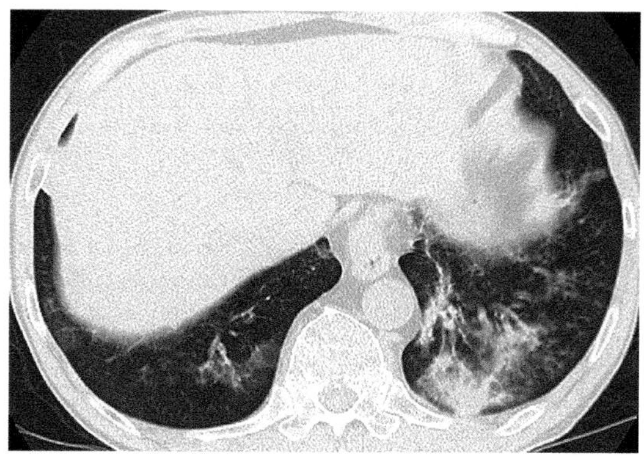

Fig. 11.3 Secondary bacterial pneumonia: CT scan showing local consolidation in lower left lung; *Haemophilus influenzae* was isolated from sputum culture

Table 11.1 Classification and comparative features of influenza pneumonia

	Pure influenza viral pneumonia	Secondary bacterial pneumonia	Mixed viral and bacterial pneumonia
Background	Younger individual or cardiovascular disease Observed more frequently during influenza pandemic	Older individual or underlying diseases	Variable
Clinical course	Rapid progress of respiratory symptoms such as dyspnea and distressing cough, resulting in respiratory failure. Occasionally, bloody sputum is observed.	Reappearance of lower respiratory tract symptoms after relief of typical influenza symptoms	Variable
Chest imaging	Bilateral diffuse infiltration mimicking pulmonary edema	Diffuse pulmonary involvement was not observed, but lobar involvement was seen.	Features of both viral and bacterial pneumonia
Mortality	High	Low	Variable

4 Pathophysiology of Influenza Pneumonia

4.1 Primary Influenza Viral Pneumonia

Sialic acid (SA), an important binding factor facilitating hemagglutinin binding of the human influenza virus, is expressed on human tracheal epithelium [12]. SA at the end of the receptor is linked to galactose (Gal) in two ways: via an α2,3 and α2,6 linkage. The influenza virus recognizes mainly host cell receptors bearing SAα2,6-Gal sequences [13], which are found on the surface of ciliated tracheal epithelium. Human receptors containing SAα2,6-Gal are widely distributed in the upper respiratory tract [14] and are associated with efficient viral infection and propagation.

In contrast, receptors containing SAα2,3-Gal sequences are found only in part of the respiratory bronchioles and alveoli. If the antigenicity of an influenza virus changes drastically, as seen in pandemic viruses (through antigenic shift), they can develop greater affinity for receptors with α2,3 binding. This subsequently results in efficient virus replication in the respiratory bronchioles and alveoli. Infection of the lung parenchyma causes inflammation with cytotoxicity of the vascular endothelium and alveolar epithelium. Depending on the immune response of the host, this may be clinically diffuse and cause rapid lung deterioration. In autopsy findings, diffuse alveolar damage in lung tissue, including microvascular thrombi and inflammatory cell infiltration and edema of interstitial structures, alveolar hemorrhage and formation of a hyaline membrane, is clinically suggestive of acute respiratory distress syndrome (ARDS) [15, 16]. This appears to be a severe form of primary influenza virus pneumonia and is considered a relatively common phenomenon during a pandemic [17]. Affinity for human airway epithelium receptor through antigenic shift and subsequent excessive host response are one explanation for pure influenza viral pneumonia.

4.2 Secondary Bacterial Pneumonia

During influenza virus infection, multifocal destruction and desquamation of the tracheal and bronchial mucosal epithelia are observed in the acute phase. Submucosal infiltration of inflammatory cells as well as edema and congestion are also observed at this time [16]. This damage leads to a decrease in bacterial clearance due to ciliary immobility and leukocyte and macrophage malfunction. Additionally, increased neuraminidase activity promotes pneumococcal adhesion to airway epithelial cells [18]. *Streptococcus pneumoniae* and *Staphylococcus aureus* are considered the most common pneumonia-associated bacteria. In Japan, the same results were obtained for both the 2009 pandemic [19] (Table 11.2) and seasonal influenza [20].

Table 11.2 Causative pathogens of influenza pneumonia during the 2009 pandemic

Causative pathogen	*n* (%)
Streptococcus pneumoniae	67 (34.2)
Haemophilus influenzae	10 (5.1)
Methicillin-sensitive *Staphylococcus aureus*	7 (3.6)
Mycoplasma pneumoniae	4 (2.0)
Moraxella catarrhalis	4 (2.0)
Pseudomonas aeruginosa	4 (2.0)
Klebsiella pneumoniae	3 (1.5)
Streptococcus viridans	2 (1.0)
Enterobacter cloacae	1 (0.5)
Enterococcus faecalis	1 (0.5)
Leuconostoc spp.	1 (0.5)
	($n = 198$)

4.3 Mixed Viral and Bacterial Pneumonia

Although there are no clear descriptions of mixed pneumonia in previous reports, viral and bacterial pneumonia can exist simultaneously and even promote one another. As described above, influenza can damage the airway epithelium, facilitating bacterial infection. It has also been demonstrated that some *Staphylococcus* and *Streptococcus* strains may promote viral replication and pathogenicity [21]. Although lesions compatible with uncomplicated viral pneumonia have been widely described, premortem and postmortem findings from lung specimens also suggest a combined role for both bacterial and viral pathogens. In fact, postmortem findings from lung specimens of those who succumbed to Spanish influenza, the largest influenza pandemic of the twentieth century, suggest a predominant role for bacterial pneumonia [22].

5 Conclusion

Influenza pneumonia is classified into several subtypes, viral pneumonia and superimposed or sequential bacterial pneumonia. In particular, pure influenza viral pneumonia is known to progress rapidly, often with fatal complications. It is therefore important to understand the pathophysiology to provide appropriate disease management.

References

1. Thompson T, Todd RB. Annals of influenza, or, epidemic catarrhal fever in Great Britain from 1510 to 1837. London: Sydenham Society; 1852.
2. Assaad F, Cockburn WC, Sundaresan TK. Use of excess mortality from respiratory diseases in the study of influenza. Bull World Health Organ. 1973;49(3):219–33.
3. Fine MJ, Auble TE, Yealy DM, Hanusa BH, Weissfeld LA, Singer DE, et al. A prediction rule to identify low-risk patients with community-acquired pneumonia. N Engl J Med. 1997;336(4):243–50.
4. Lim WS, van der Eerden MM, Laing R, Boersma WG, Karalus N, Town GI, et al. Defining community acquired pneumonia severity on presentation to hospital: an international derivation and validation study. Thorax. 2003;58(5):377–82.
5. The Committee for the Japanese Respiratory Society Guidelines in the Management of Respiratory Infections. Guidelines for the management of community acquired pneumonia in adults, revised edition. Respirology. 2006;11(Suppl 3):S79–133.
6. Bjarnason A, Thorleifsdottir G, Love A, Gudnason JF, Asgeirsson H, Hallgrimsson KL, et al. Severity of influenza A 2009 (H1N1) pneumonia is underestimated by routine prediction rules. Results from a prospective, population-based study. PLoS One. 2012;7(10):e46816.
7. Fujikura Y, Kawano S, Kouzaki Y, Shinoda M, Hara Y, Shinkai M, et al. Mortality and severity evaluation by routine pneumonia prediction models among Japanese patients with 2009 pandemic influenza A (H1N1) pneumonia. Respir Investig. 2014;52(5):280–7.
8. Garnacho-Montero J, Leon-Moya C, Gutierrez-Pizarraya A, Arenzana-Seisdedos A, Vidaur L, Guerrero JE, et al. Clinical characteristics, evolution, and treatment-related risk factors for mortality among immunosuppressed patients with influenza A (H1N1) virus admitted to the intensive care unit. J Crit Care. 2018;48:172–7.
9. Louria DB, Blumenfeld HL, Ellis JT, Kilbourne ED, Rogers DE. Studies on influenza in the pandemic of 1957-1958. II. Pulmonary complications of influenza. J Clin Invest. 1959;38(1 Part 2):213–65.
10. Jain S, Williams DJ, Arnold SR, Ampofo K, Bramley AM, Reed C, et al. Community-acquired pneumonia requiring hospitalization among U.S. children. N Engl J Med. 2015;372(9):835–45.
11. Agarwal PP, Cinti S, Kazerooni EA. Chest radiographic and CT findings in novel swine-origin influenza A (H1N1) virus (S-OIV) infection. AJR Am J Roentgenol. 2009;193(6):1488–93.
12. Couceiro JN, Paulson JC, Baum LG. Influenza virus strains selectively recognize sialyloligosaccharides on human respiratory epithelium; the role of the host cell in selection of hemagglutinin receptor specificity. Virus Res. 1993;29(2):155–65.
13. Rogers GN, Paulson JC. Receptor determinants of human and animal influenza virus isolates: differences in receptor specificity of the H3 hemagglutinin based on species of origin. Virology. 1983;127(2):361–73.
14. Shinya K, Ebina M, Yamada S, Ono M, Kasai N, Kawaoka Y. Avian flu: influenza virus receptors in the human airway. Nature. 2006;440(7083):435–6.
15. Winternits MC, Wason IM, McNamara FP. The pathology of influenza. New Haven: Yale University Press; 1920.
16. Taubenberger JK, Morens DM. The pathology of influenza virus infections. Annu Rev Pathol. 2008;3:499–522.
17. Rothberg MB, Haessler SD. Complications of seasonal and pandemic influenza. Crit Care Med. 2010;38(4 Suppl):e91–7.
18. Peltola VT, Murti KG, McCullers JA. Influenza virus neuraminidase contributes to secondary bacterial pneumonia. J Infect Dis. 2005;192(2):249–57.
19. Fujikura Y, Kawano S, Kouzaki Y, Shinoda M, Hara Y, Shinkai M, et al. The (H1N1) 2009 pandemic influenza pneumonia among adult patients in Japan. Jpn J Infect Dis. 2014;67:100–4.
20. Maruyama T, Fujisawa T, Suga S, Nakamura H, Nagao M, Taniguchi K, et al. Outcomes and prognostic features of patients with influenza requiring hospitalization and receiving early antiviral therapy: a prospective multicenter-cohort study. Chest. 2016;149(2):526–34.

21. Scheiblauer H, Reinacher M, Tashiro M, Rott R. Interactions between bacteria and influenza A virus in the development of influenza pneumonia. J Infect Dis. 1992;166(4):783–91.
22. Morens DM, Taubenberger JK, Fauci AS. Predominant role of bacterial pneumonia as a cause of death in pandemic influenza: implications for pandemic influenza preparedness. J Infect Dis. 2008;198(7):962–70.

Chapter 12
Influenza Encephalopathy: What Is Encephalopathy?

Mitsuru Tsuge, Masato Yashiro, Naoki Ohno, and Hirokazu Tsukahara

Abstract Influenza encephalopathy is defined as an acute onset of consciousness disorders secondary to an influenza virus infection and shows neurological symptoms such as impaired consciousness, convulsions, and abnormal behavior. It commonly affects younger children, but an increasing number of cases have recently been reported in adults. The fatality related to influenza encephalopathy has decreased to 7%; however, the rate of neurologic sequelae is still high. Influenza encephalopathy cannot be detected in the brain and can cause diffuse brain edema without infiltrating the inflammatory cells. The levels of several inflammatory cytokines increase in the serum and cerebrospinal fluid, particularly in severe cases, which can contribute to the pathogenesis of influenza encephalopathy. Diagnosis is based on the development of neurological symptoms such as consciousness disturbance or convulsions, as well as the findings in electroencephalograms or brain imaging. Influenza encephalopathy is classified into several types based on its pathogenesis, and characteristic clinical courses and brain imaging findings were found to be different in each type of the classification. Treatment of influenza encephalopathy includes specific treatments such as methylprednisolone pulse therapy, in addition to supportive care that stabilizes the general condition of the patient. Epidemiologic analysis of compiled cases, development of biomarkers for the diagnosis or classification of influenza encephalopathy, and research into the effectiveness of specific treatment methods are now expected.

Keywords Influenza · Encephalopathy · Convulsion · Cytokine · Brain edema

---

M. Tsuge (✉) · M. Yashiro · H. Tsukahara
Department of Pediatrics, Okayama University Graduate School of Medicine, Dentistry, and Pharmaceutical Sciences, Okayama, Japan
e-mail: tsugemitsuru@okayama-u.ac.jp

N. Ohno
Department of Pediatrics, Kawasaki Medical School, Kurashiki, Okayama, Japan

J. Fujita (ed.), *Influenza*, Respiratory Disease Series: Diagnostic Tools and Disease Managements, https://doi.org/10.1007/978-981-15-9109-9_12

1 Introduction

Influenza encephalopathy is a syndrome defined as an acute onset of consciousness disorders secondary to infection by the influenza virus. It develops rapidly, demonstrating neurological symptoms such as impaired consciousness, convulsions, and abnormal behavior. Poor prognosis has been reported despite appropriate treatment being followed. Significant progress on its classification, understanding its pathogenesis, and the development of treatment have been made in recent years.

2 Epidemiology

Cases of influenza encephalopathy have previously been reported in East Asia. In Japan, a number of cases of influenza encephalopathy were reported in 1997/1998 [1]. A nationwide survey in Japan reported that the fatality rate caused by influenza encephalopathy was 30%; however, fatality has markedly declined to approximately 7% after the development of specific treatment, such as methylprednisolone pulse therapy [2, 3]. A new strain of the influenza virus (A/H1N1pdm09) that originated in Mexico in 2009 spread globally, thus increasing the number of reported cases of influenza encephalopathy [4–7] (Fig. 12.1). A nationwide survey in Japan revealed that the incidence of encephalopathy caused by a pandemic influenza virus was higher in older children than that of encephalopathy caused by seasonal influenza [8]. Cases of influenza encephalopathy in adults have been identified (Fig. 12.2), and recent nationwide survey in Japan reported lower incidence of influenza encephalopathy in adults (0.19 cases per million), fewer seizures (35%), and a higher rate of fatality (13.7%) compared with children [9].

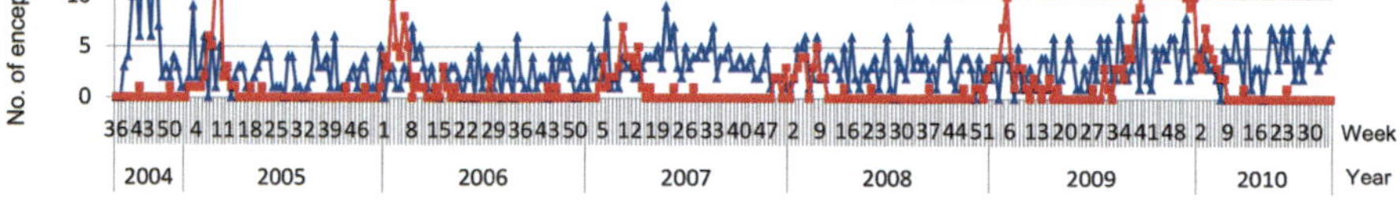

Fig. 12.1 Number of cases of influenza encephalopathy during 2004–2010 seasons in Japan [4]

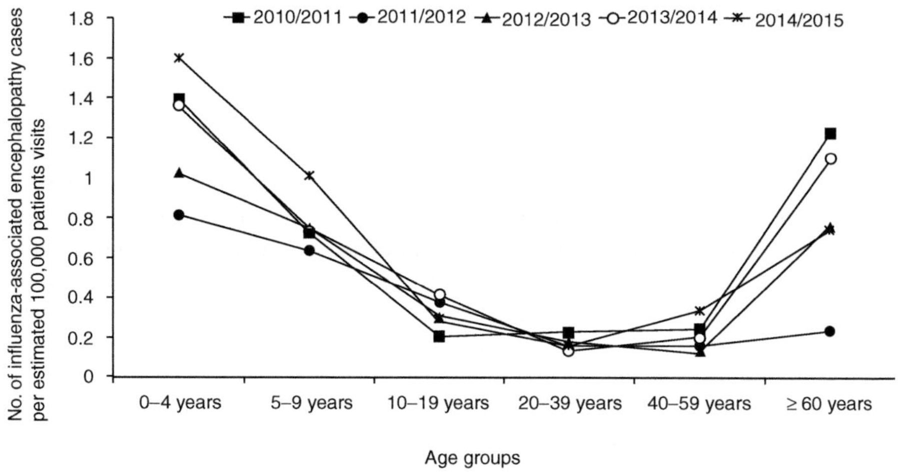

Fig. 12.2 Age distribution of influenza encephalopathy during 2010–2014 seasons in Japan [9]

3 Pathogenesis

Autopsies results showed non-inflammatory pathological changes such as brain edema without the infiltration of inflammatory cells, vasogenic edema with plasma extravasation, microhemorrhage, and necrosis of the brain parenchyma. The levels of inflammatory cytokines such as inteleukin-6, tumor necrosis factor-α, and interleukin-10 were elevated in the serum and cerebrospinal fluid in patients with influenza encephalopathy [10]. Further investigation revealed increased serum levels of nitrite/nitrate [11], matrix metalloproteinases-9 (MMP-9) [12], brain-derived neurotrophic factor (BDNF) [13], and high mobility group box-1 (HMGB-1) [14]. These observations suggest that influenza encephalopathy occurred due to the elevated levels of inflammatory cytokines in the blood (hypercytokinemia), caused by an activated host immune response triggered by an infection in the respiratory tract. Excessive production of inflammatory cytokines in the blood impairs the cerebrovascular endothelium, increasing the permeability of the blood-brain barrier, resulting in brain edema [15]. The use of non-steroidal anti-inflammatory drugs (NSAIDs) such as diclofenac and mefenamic acid exacerbates the overproduction of inflammatory cytokines. In addition, several gene mutations or polymorphisms, such as carnitine palmitoyl transferase II (CPT II) [16], adenosine A2a receptor (ADORA2A) [17], sodium voltage-gated channel alpha subunit 1 (SCN1A) [18], ran binding protein 2 (RANBP2) [19], and toll-like receptor 3 (TLR3) [20], have also been reported to be associated with influenza encephalopathy. These genetic backgrounds can contribute to the pathogenesis of influenza encephalopathy.

4 Diagnosis

Diagnosis of influenza encephalopathy is obtained based on a combination of the degree and duration of neurological symptoms, blood test, electroencephalography (EEG), and brain imaging. The diagnosis also needs to be distinguished from other neurological diseases such as bacterial meningitis, viral encephalitis, diabetic coma, hypocalcemia, congenital metabolism disorder, poisoning, child abuse, and heatstroke. The difference between mild influenza encephalopathy and complicated febrile seizures or delirium is not always clear. The neurological symptoms of influenza encephalopathy include consciousness disturbance, convulsions, and abnormal behavior. The duration between onset of fever and the onset of neurological symptoms is within 48 h in more than 70% of all cases [1]. Consciousness disturbance is the most significant clinical manifestation, and persistent consciousness disturbance (Glasgow coma scale <13) for more than 12 h suggests the onset of influenza encephalopathy. The diagnosis is confirmed with consciousness disturbance (Glasgow coma scale <10–11) for more than 24 h or the deterioration of consciousness disturbance during the course of disease. The difficulty in evaluating mild consciousness disturbance, particularly in children, after using anticonvulsants for prolonged seizures should be taken into consideration. The extent of convulsions can vary from few minutes to an intussusception state lasting $\geq$15 min. Abnormal behaviors such as delirium, stupor, visual hallucinations, anger, fear, and emotional incontinence are often observed in the early stage of influenza encephalopathy, which needs to be distinguished from benign febrile delirium. Blood tests can reveal thrombocytopenia, elevated transaminase, elevated creatine kinase, abnormal blood glucose, abnormal coagulopathy, elevated urea nitrogen and creatinine, and hyperammonemia. These findings suggest hypercytokinemia and are factors that show poor prognosis in influenza encephalopathy [21]. EEG findings in influenza encephalopathy present various findings such as generalized high-amplitude slow waves, low-amplitude fast waves. Multifocal, diffuse spikes and slow wave bursts, and periodic lateralized epileptiform discharge may also be observed. A computed tomography (CT) scan of the head can show diffuse low-absorption areas, blurring of the corticomedullary junction, narrowing of the subarachnoid space and ventricles of the brain, localized low-absorption areas, and brain stem edema. Diffusion weighted imaging (DWI) of magnetic resonance (MR) imaging scans of the head can detect abnormal high signal lesions at an early stage; therefore, it is particularly useful for diagnosis. MR imaging can also be used to classify influenza encephalopathy by identifying characteristic abnormalities (Fig. 12.3) [22].

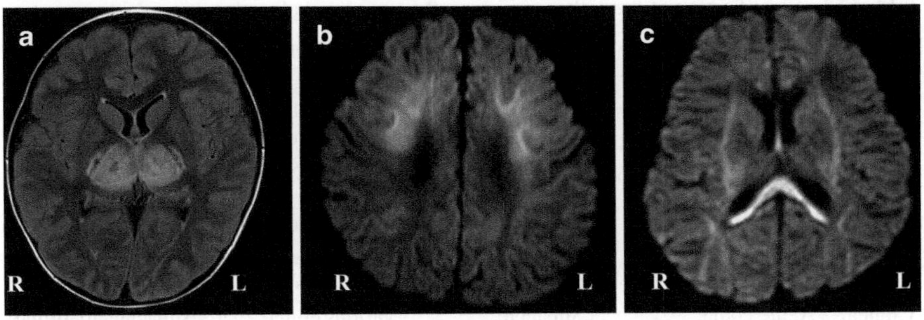

Fig. 12.3 MR imaging findings in influenza encephalopathy. (**a**) Local high intensity in bilateral thalamus (ANE, T2/FLAIR), (**b**) bright tree appearance in bilateral frontal and occipital subcortical white matter (AESD, DWI), (**c**) high intensity area in the corpus callosum (MERS, DWI), *MR* magnetic resonance, *FLAIR* fluid-attenuated inversion recovery, *ANE* acute necrotizing encephalopathy, *DWI* diffusion weighted image, *AESD* acute encephalopathy with biphasic seizures and late reduced diffusion, *MERS* clinically mild encephalitis/encephalopathy with a reversible splenial lesion

5 Classification

Influenza encephalopathy is classified according to its pathophysiology into "hypercytokinemia type," "excitotoxicity type," and "metabolic disorder type." In addition to these three groups, clinically mild encephalitis/encephalopathy with a reversible splenial lesion (MERS) is also significant (Table 12.1).

5.1 Hypercytokinemia Type

Hypercytokinemia type includes acute necrotizing encephalopathy (ANE) and hemorrhagic shock and encephalopathy (HSE). ANE primarily affects children aged 1–5 years and is characterized by the development of high fever, rapid disturbance of consciousness, and convulsions. It is complicated with disseminated intravascular coagulation (DIC), hemophagocytic syndrome, and multiple organ failure (MOF). Blood tests show thrombocytopenia, liver dysfunction, renal dysfunction, and acute coagulopathy. CT and MR imaging scans of the head show edematous necrotic lesions in the bilateral thalamus, basal ganglia, periventricular white matter of the lateral ventricle, dentate nucleus of the cerebellum, and pontomesencephalic tegmentum. The prognosis is often poor, accounting for 28% fatality rate and 61% sequelae rate in ANE cases [2]. Cases with severe sequelae show severe

Table 12.1 Classification of the pathogenesis in influenza encephalopathy

Type	Hypercytokinemia type	Excitotoxic type	Metabolic disorder type	MERS
Disease	ANE HSES	AESD	Congenital metabolic disease Classical Reye syndrome	MERS
Risk factor	NSAIDs	Theophylline	Salicylic acid	Unknown
Age	1–5 years old	0–1 years old	6–12 years old	3–8 years old
Clinical course	Acute coma, convulsion, diarrhea, shock, DIC, MOF	Subacute, biphasic (onset) febrile convulsion (3–7 days later) Afebrile convulsion, Impaired consciousness	Various coma, convulsion	Subacute abnormal behavior, mild impaired consciousness
Blood test	Elevation of serum Aminotransferases No hyperammonemia	Non-specific	Metabolic acidosis Hyperammonemia Hypoglycemia	Hyponatremia
Brain imaging	Diffuse cerebral edema Bilaterally symmetric Necrotic lesions (ANE) Cerebral hemorrhage	Localized cerebral edema High signal intensity in subcortical white matter	Diffuse cerebral edema	High signal intensity lesion in the splenium of corpus callosum
Fatality	30–50%	<5%	10%	0%

ANE acute necrotizing encephalopathy, *HSES* hemorrhagic shock and encephalopathy syndrome, *NSAIDs* non-steroidal anti-inflammatory drugs, *DIC* disseminated intravascular coagulation, *MOF* multiple organ failure, *AESD* acute encephalopathy with biphasic seizures and late reduced diffusion, *MERS* clinically mild encephalitis/encephalopathy with a reversible splenial lesion

intellectual disability, quadriplegia, and epilepsy. HSE primarily affects infants and is characterized by the development of high fever, impaired consciousness, convulsions, diarrhea, and bleeding from the lungs and intestines. Blood tests show severe anemia, thrombocytopenia, liver dysfunction, renal dysfunction, and acute coagulopathy. CT scans of the head show edematous lesions of the entire cerebrum, and MR imaging scans show high signal intensity lesions in the bilateral symmetrical frontal and parietal temporal lobes on DWI. EEG tests show multifocal spike-waves, generalized high-amplitude slow waves, and low-amplitude waves. The prognosis is also poor, accounting for 55% fatality rate and 30% sequelae rate in HSE cases [2].

5.2 Excitotoxicity Type

Excitotoxicity type involves acute encephalopathy with biphasic seizures and late reduced diffusion (AESD). AESD causes selective and delayed neuronal damage due to excessive release of glutamate, associated with prolonged convulsions [23]. AESD mainly affects infants aged <2 years, and febrile convulsions develop within 24 h of fever onset. Neurological symptoms are relatively mild after the onset of febrile convulsions; however, afebrile convulsions present 3–7 days after the onset of the disease, with progressive deterioration of the consciousness disturbance. Thereafter, cerebral cortical dysfunctions, including speech disorders, gradually become apparent. Blood tests and CT and MR imaging scans of the head do not show apparent unusual findings on the onset of febrile convulsions; however, several days after, CT scans of the head reveal lobar cerebral edema, and MR imaging scans on DWI show high signal lesion in the subcortical white matter of frontal lobe or frontal parietal lobe (bright tree appearance) [24]. AESD shows lower fatality rates (1%) and a high sequelae rate (66%) accompanied by brain atrophy, decreased cerebral blood flow, and neurological sequelae such as intellectual disability, motor paralysis, and epilepsy [2, 25].

5.3 Metabolic Disorder Type

Metabolic disorder type includes congenital metabolic disorders such as organic acid or fatty acid metabolism disorders and classical Reye syndrome. Patients with congenital metabolic disorders often suffer from rapid consciousness disturbance with severe ketosis, hypoglycemia, hyperammonemia, metabolic acidosis, coagulopathy, and abnormal liver function accompanied by the influenza infection [26]. Congenital metabolic disorders are present in approximately 5% of cases with influenza encephalopathy. Classical Reye syndrome leads to uncharacteristic liver mitochondrial morphology and function due to influenza infection with the usage of aspirin, causing neurological symptoms with brain edema, hepatic dysfunction, hypoglycemia, hyperlactatemia, and hyperammonemia.

5.4 Clinically Mild Encephalitis/Encephalopathy with a Reversible Splenial Lesion (MERS)

MERS is characterized by neurological symptoms such as delirium, stupor, and convulsions, but its pathogenesis has not been elucidated. Visual hallucinations, emotional changes, and inconsistent conversations are also observed. These symptoms appear within 1 week in the febrile phase but dissipate within 10 days in many cases [27]. MERS is most frequently seen in children aged 3–8 years. Hyponatremia is frequently observed, and EEG tests show high-amplitude slow waves in approximately half of the cases. MR imaging scans on DWI show a high signal in the cerebral corpus callosum at the early stages of onset, and this signal often disappears within 1 week, leaving no atrophy. The rates of death and sequelae were 0% and 7%, respectively.

6 Management

Influenza encephalopathy is managed by supportive treatment to maintain the general condition and specific treatment for hypercytokinemia or excitotoxicity. Since the progression of influenza encephalopathy is often rapid, it is important to carry out sufficient systemic management before a definite diagnosis. When the diagnosis is suspected or confirmed, specific treatment should be performed without delay. General conditions, vital signs, and neurological symptoms should be observed using techniques such as EEG or brain imaging tests during treatment. After the treatment, neurological sequelae such as paralysis, epilepsy, and mental retardation should be evaluated for the necessity of rehabilitation.

6.1 Supportive Treatment

It is important to immediately evaluate consciousness, airway, respiration, and circulation upon onset of the disease and to provide appropriate supportive care for respiratory circulation, convulsions, intracranial pressure, body temperature, electrolytes, blood sugar, and body fluid content. Airway intubation and artificial respiration should be considered in cases of impaired consciousness; hypercapnia should be avoided because it increases intracranial pressure. Intravenous fluids should be administered to maintain the body water content sufficiently. Hypotonic infusions may cause hyponatremia and should not be used. Rapid consciousness deterioration, loss of light reflex, pupil irregularity, and bradycardia are signs of imminent cerebral hernia. D-mannitol can be administered intravenously to control intracranial hypertension. Cooling and acetaminophen administration should be performed; however, aspirin, diclofenac, and mefenamic acid should not be used in influenza encephalopathy. Administration of midazolam or thiopental can be considered for the treatment of prolonged severe convulsions. Continuous monitoring using amplitude-integrated EEG is useful for understanding anti-convulsant effects, changes in brain function, and unexpected subclinical seizures [28].

6.2 Specific Treatment

Specific treatment such as the administration of an anti-influenza agent, methylprednisolone pulse therapy, high-dose immunoglobulin therapy, cerebral hypothermia, blood purification therapy, and free radical scavengers may be performed (Fig. 12.4). However, evidence to support their therapeutic effects are insufficient. Anti-influenza drugs are often used in cases of influenza encephalopathy to suppress viral replication in the bronchus. Peramivir, a neuraminidase inhibitor, is predominantly used because it can be administered intravenously. Methylprednisolone pulse therapy is effective in suppressing excessive immune response and cytokine production in the blood and brain, thus alleviating cerebral edema, which has been associated with improved prognosis in influenza encephalopathy [8]. High-dose immunoglobulin therapy is also thought to have an effect on hypercytokinemia. Blood purification therapy can remove cytokines or harmful metabolites in the blood to prevent the progression of tissue damage. Early initiation of cerebral

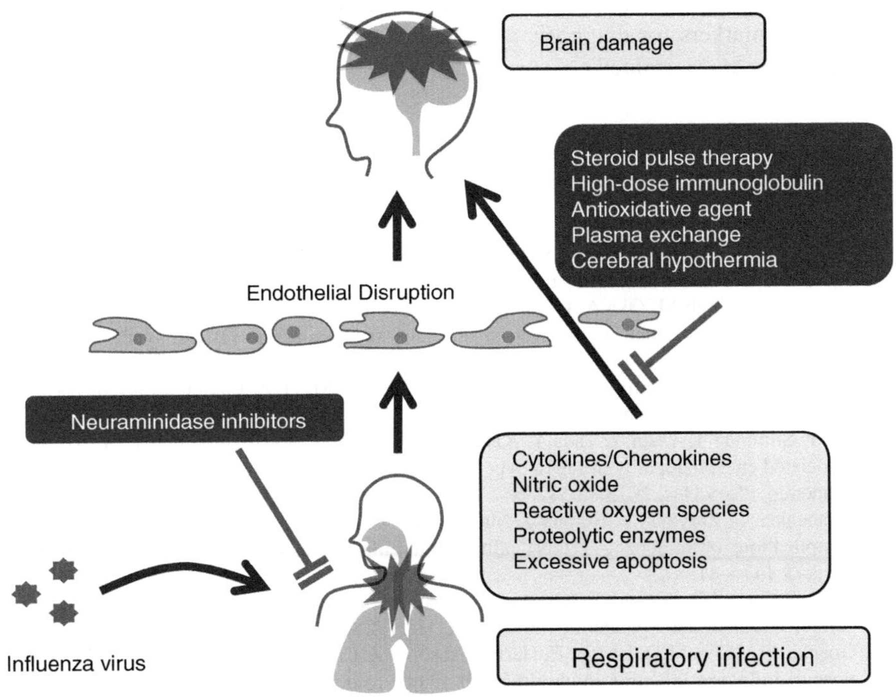

Fig. 12.4 Specific treatment for influenza encephalopathy to suppress the progression of cerebrovascular endothelial disruption and brain damage

hypothermia therapy using intracranial pressure monitoring can improve the neurological outcome [29]. Induced normothermia therapy has also been reported to be therapeutically efficacious [30]. Thrombomodulin α is used because it is expected to have anti-inflammatory and protective effects on the vascular endothelium in addition to improving disseminated intravascular coagulation by anti-thrombin effect and activation of protein C. Edaravone is used in influenza encephalopathy to reduce the oxidative damage caused in the brain. Although continuous intravenous injection of cyclosporine is expected to suppress apoptosis associated with hypercytokinemia and prevent the progression of cell and tissue damage [31].

7 Conclusion

Influenza encephalopathy has been recognized to cause a high neurologic sequelae rate, although the fatality rate is on the decline. Rapid diagnosis of influenza encephalopathy and adequate treatment for its individual pathogenesis are required to improve the neurological outcome. Further epidemiologic analysis, development of specific biomarkers for diagnosis and classification, and research for novel therapeutic agents are warranted.

References

1. Morishima T, Togashi T, Yokota S, Okuno Y, Miyazaki C, Tashiro M, et al. Encephalitis and encephalopathy associated with an influenza epidemic in Japan. Clin Infect Dis. 2002;35:512–7.
2. Hoshino A, Saitoh M, Oka A, Okumura A, Kubota M, Saito Y, et al. Epidemiology of acute encephalopathy in Japan, with emphasis on the association of viruses and syndromes. Brain Dev. 2012;34:337–43.
3. Goto S, Nosaka N, Yorifuji T, Wada T, Fujii Y, Yashiro M, et al. Epidemiology of pediatric acute encephalitis/encephalopathy in Japan. Acta Med Okayama. 2018;72:351–7.
4. Gu Y, Shimada T, Yasui Y, Tada Y, Kaku M, Okabe N. National surveillance of influenza-associated encephalopathy in Japan over six years, before and during the 2009-2010 influenza pandemic. PLoS One. 2013;8:e54786.
5. Khandaker G, Zurynski Y, Buttery J, Marshall H, Richmond PC, Dale RC, et al. Neurologic complications of influenza A (H1N1)pdm09: surveillance in 6 pediatric hospitals. Neurology. 2012;79:1474–81.
6. Kedia S, Stroud B, Parsons J, Schreiner T, Curtis DJ, Bagdure D, et al. Pediatric neurological complications of 2009 pandemic influenza A (H1N1). Arch Neurol. 2011;68:455–62.
7. Goenka A, Michael BD, Ledger E, Hart IJ, Absoud M, Chow G, et al. Neurological manifestations of influenza infection in children and adults: results of a National British Surveillance Study. Clin Infect Dis. 2014;58:775–84.
8. Kawashima H, Morichi S, Okumara A, Nakagawa S, Morishima T. National survey of pandemic influenza A (H1N1) 2009-associated encephalopathy in Japanese children. J Med Virol. 2012;84:1151–6.
9. Okuno H, Yahata Y, Tanaka-Taya K, Arai S, Satoh H, Morino S, et al. Characteristics and outcomes of influenza-associated encephalopathy cases among children and adults in Japan, 2010-2015. Clin Infect Dis. 2018;66:1831–7.

10. Ichiyama T, Isumi H, Ozawa H, Matsubara T, Morishima T, Furukawa S. Cerebrospinal fluid and serum levels of cytokines and soluble tumor necrosis factor receptor in influenza virus-associated encephalopathy. Scand J Infect Dis. 2003;35:59–61.
11. Kawashima H, Watanabe Y, Morishima T, Togashi T, Yamada N, Kashiwagi Y, et al. NOx (nitrite/nitrate) in cerebral spinal fluids obtained from patients with influenza-associated encephalopathy. Neuropediatrics. 2003;34:137–40.
12. Ichiyama T, Morishima T, Kajimoto M, Matsushige T, Matsubara T, Furukawa S. Matrix metalloproteinase-9 and tissue inhibitors of metalloproteinases 1 in influenza-associated encephalopathy. Pediatr Infect Dis J. 2007;26:542–4.
13. Morichi S, Yamanaka G, Ishida Y, Oana S, Kashiwagi Y, Kawashima H. Brain-derived neurotrophic factor and interleukin-6 levels in the serum and cerebrospinal fluid of children with viral infection-induced encephalopathy. Neurochem Res. 2014;39:2143–9.
14. Momonaka H, Hasegawa S, Matsushige T, Inoue H, Kajimoto M, Okada S, et al. High mobility group box 1 in patients with 2009 pandemic H1N1 influenza-associated encephalopathy. Brain Dev. 2014;36:484–8.
15. Tsuge M, Yasui K, Ichiyawa T, Saito Y, Nagaoka Y, Yashiro M, et al. Increase of tumor necrosis factor-alpha in the blood induces early activation of matrix metalloproteinase-9 in the brain. Microbiol Immunol. 2010;54:417–24.
16. Chen Y, Mizuguchi H, Yao D, Ide M, Kuroda Y, Shigematsu Y, et al. Thermolabile phenotype of carnitine palmitoyltransferase II variations as a predisposing factor for influenza-associated encephalopathy. FEBS Lett. 2005;579:2040–4.
17. Shinohara M, Saitoh M, Nishizawa D, Ikeda K, Hirose S, Takanashi J, et al. ADORA2A polymorphism predisposes children to encephalopathy with febrile status epilepticus. Neurology. 2013;80:1571–6.
18. Saitoh M, Shinohara M, Hoshino H, Kubota M, Amemiya K, Takanashi JL, et al. Mutations of the SCN1A gene in acute encephalopathy. Epilepsia. 2012;53:558–64.
19. Neilson DE, Adams MD, Orr CM, Schelling DK, Eiben RM, Kerr DS, et al. Infection-triggered familial or recurrent cases of acute necrotizing encephalopathy caused by mutations in a component of the nuclear pore, RANBP2. Am J Hum Genet. 2009;84:44–51.
20. Hidaka F, Matsuo S, Muta T, Takeshige K, Mizukami T, Nunoi H. A missense mutation of the Toll-like receptor 3 gene in a patient with influenza-associated encephalopathy. Clin Immunol. 2006;119:188–94.
21. Nagao T, Morishima T, Kimura H, Yokota S, Yamashita N, Ichiyama T, et al. Prognostic factors in influenza-associated encephalopathy. Pediatr Infect Dis J. 2008;27:384–9.
22. Mizuguchi M, Yamanouchi H, Ichiyama T, Shiomi M. Acute encephalopathy associated with influenza and other viral infections. Acta Neurol Scand. 2007;115:45–56.
23. Fujita Y, Takanashi J, Takei H, Ota S, Fujii K, Sakuma H, et al. Activated microglia in acute encephalopathy with biphasic seizures and late reduced diffusion. J Neurol Sci. 2016;366:91–3.
24. Takanashi J, Mizuguchi M, Terai M, Barkovich AJ. Disrupted glutamate-glutamine cycle in acute encephalopathy with biphasic seizures and late reduced diffusion. Neuroradiology. 2015;57:1163–8.
25. Ito Y, Natsume J, Kidokoro H, Ishihara N, Azuma Y, Tsuji T, et al. Seizure characteristics of epilepsy in childhood after acute encephalopathy with biphasic seizures and late reduced diffusion. Epilepsia. 2015;56:1286–93.
26. Purevsuren J, Hasegawa Y, Kobayashi H, Endo M, Yamaguchi S. Urinary organic metabolite screening of children with influenza-associated encephalopathy for inborn errors of metabolism using GC/MS. Brain Dev. 2008;30:520–6.
27. Iwata A, Matsubara K, Nigami H, Kamimura K, Fukaya T. Reversible splenial lesion associated with novel influenza A (H1N1) viral infection. Pediatr Neurol. 2010;42:447–50.
28. Okumura A, Komatsu M, Abe S, Kitamura T, Matsui K, Ikeno M, et al. Amplitude-integrated electroencephalography in patients with acute encephalopathy with refractory, repetitive partial seizures. Brain Dev. 2011;33:77–82.

29. Kawano G, Iwata O, Iwata S, Kawano K, Obu K, Kuki I, et al. Determinants of outcomes following acute child encephalopathy and encephalitis: pivotal effect of early and delayed cooling. Arch Dis Child. 2011;96:936–41.
30. Murata S, Kashiwagi M, Tanabe T, Oba C, Shigehara S, Yamazaki S, et al. Targeted temperature management for acute encephalopathy in a Japanese secondary emergency medical care hospital. Brain Dev. 2016;38(3):317–23.
31. Watanabe Y1, Motoi H, Oyama Y, Ichikawa K, Takeshita S, Mori M, et al. Cyclosporine for acute encephalopathy with biphasic seizures and late reduced diffusion. Pediatr Int. 2014;56:577–82.

Part V
Management

Chapter 13
Treatment Guidelines for Influenza Virus Infection: What Does the Recent Guideline State?

Tadashi Ishida

Abstract The efficacy of anti-influenza drugs (neuraminidase inhibitor—NAI) has been examined before and after the 2009 H1N1 pandemic. Recent studies indicated that NAI administration reduced risk of lower respiratory tract complications, and admittance to hospital, moreover, shortened the duration of fever and viral RNA shedding. NAI administration was also associated with reduced ICU length of stay and mortality.

The clinical practice guidelines were released from the Infectious Diseases Society of America in 2018. In the treatment section of the guidelines, antivirals should be administered as soon as possible to those who are hospitalized, with severely ill or progressed disease, or at high risk for complications from influenza. Antiviral treatment can be done to those who are not at high risk of influenza complications if onset is within 48 h. Other causes including influenza NAI resistance should be investigated in influenza patients who fail to improve or deteriorate despite antiviral treatment. Adjunctive therapy such as corticosteroid or immunoglobulins is not recommended. Baloxavir marboxil was a newly released drug after the finalization of the guidelines. Thus, the guidelines did not refer to recommendations of this drug.

Keywords Anti-influenza drugs · The guidelines of the Infectious Diseases Society of America · Neuraminidase inhibitor · Antiviral resistant virus · Baloxavir marboxil

---

T. Ishida (✉)
Department of Respiratory Medicine, Ohara Memorial Kurashiki Medical Foundation, Kurashiki Central Hospital, Kurashiki, Okayama, Japan
e-mail: ishidat@kchnet.or.jp

J. Fujita (ed.), *Influenza*, Respiratory Disease Series: Diagnostic Tools and Disease Managements, https://doi.org/10.1007/978-981-15-9109-9_13

1 Introduction

Influenza causes epidemics worldwide every winter and is associated with mortality and morbidity. Influenza-related deaths are estimated to be 3000–10,000 every year in Japan, and especially excess death in the elderly is a serious problem [1].

Influenza presents a wide range of clinical findings from self-limited upper respiratory tract infection to life-threatening illness which includes respiratory failure, encephalopathy, and so on.

Many studies of neuraminidase inhibitor (NAI) have been done during and after the 2009 H1N1 pandemic. Most of them proved the efficacy of NAI. On the other hand, NAI treatment in generally healthy outpatients is controversial. Furthermore, a novel anti-influenza drug which has a different mechanism as cap-dependent endonuclease inhibitor, "baloxavir marboxil," was released on March, 2018. However, the evaluation of this drug is not decided due to lack of evidence.

Several guidelines for influenza treatment have been published. Among them, the clinical practice guidelines by the Infectious Diseases Society of America in 2018 [2] will be taken up mainly in this article, and explained in summary.

2 Essential Way of Thinking for Antiviral Treatment

The efficacy of NAI has been examined after the 2009 H1N1 pandemic. A Chinese observational study reported that oseltamivir administration restrained development to pneumonia and shortened the duration of fever and viral RNA shedding [3]. A prospective, observational study of a cohort of ICU patients with confirmed 2009 H1N1 infection reported that early oseltamivir administration was associated with reduced ICU length of stay and mortality [4].

The World Health Organization (WHO) revised the guidelines for influenza treatment in February 2010 which recommended the use of antivirals as soon as possible to those who were at high risk for complications or who had severe or progressive clinical presentation [5]. On the other hand, the WHO stated that antiviral treatment with NAI within 48 h is reasonable in otherwise healthy patients with uncomplicated illness in another review article [6].

In 2014, Jefferson and colleagues analyzed randomized, placebo-controlled trials (RCTs) on healthy adults and children and concluded that oseltamivir and zanamivir had small, non-specific effects on reducing the time to alleviation of influenza symptoms [7]. They also stated that NAI treatment had limited efficacy, and caused adverse effects in another paper [8]. In response to these results, the WHO excluded oseltamivir from essential medicine, and recommended to place it as the only listed option for "critically ill" hospitalized patients and for pandemic influenza preparedness [9].

However, the reports of Jefferson et al. were analysis of intention to treat (ITT) cases, thus diseases other than influenza might be included. On the other hand,

Dobson and colleagues analyzed the same RCTs as Jefferson's and showed that oseltamivir accelerated time to clinical symptom alleviation, reduced risk of lower respiratory tract complications, and hospital admittance [10]. The point that should be mentioned specially is that this paper analyzed only intention to treat infection (ITTI) cases who were proven to have influenza infection through laboratory examinations.

After that, it was reported that NAI treatment significantly reduced the likelihood of requiring hospital admission in outpatients with confirmed or suspected A(H1N1) pdm09 and at high risk of hospitalization [11]. A systematic review published in 2017 reported that NAI treatment was effective at reducing mortality among hospitalized patients, and symptom duration, by up to 1 day in the general population [12]. This review also showed that oseltamivir or zanamivir prophylaxis was effective at reducing secondary symptomatic influenza transmission.

3 The Guidelines of the Infection Disease Society of America 2018

The Infection Diseases Society of America published the guidelines for seasonal influenza in 2018 [2]. These clinical guidelines are an update of the guidelines in 2009 which is prior to the 2009 H1N1 influenza pandemic. They referred to diagnosis, treatment, chemoprophylaxis, and institutional outbreak management of seasonal influenza.

In the treatment part, some clinical questions were raised, and recommendations to those were described.

CQ1 Which patients with suspected or confirmed influenza should be treated with antivirals?

Antiviral treatment as soon as possible is recommended for adults and children with documented or suspected influenza irrespective of influenza vaccination history, who meet the criteria listed in Table 13.1.

Clinicians can consider antiviral treatment for adults and children who are not at high risk of influenza complications, with documented or suspected influenza, irrespective of influenza vaccination history listed in Table 13.2.

Table 13.1 Those who require antiviral treatment as soon as possible

1. Persons of any age who are hospitalized with influenza, regardless of illness duration prior to hospitalization.
2. Outpatients of any age with severe or progressive illness, regardless of illness duration.
3. Outpatients who are at high risk of complications from influenza, including those with chronic medical conditions and immunocompromised patients.
4. Children younger than 2 years and adults ≧65 years.
5. Pregnant women and those within 2 weeks postpartum.

Table 13.2 Those who may receive antiviral treatment

1. Outpatients with illness onset within 2 days before presentation.
2. Symptomatic outpatients who are household contacts of persons who are at high risk of developing complications from influenza, particularly those who are severely immunocompromised.
3. Symptomatic healthcare providers who care for patients who are at high risk of developing complications from influenza, particularly those who are severely immunocompromised.

Table 13.3 Persons who are at high risk of complications from influenza

1. Children aged <5 years, and especially aged <2 years
2. Adults aged ≧65 years
3. Persons with chronic pulmonary (including asthma), cardiovascular (except hypertension alone), renal, hepatic, hematologic (including sickle cell disease), or metabolic disorders (including diabetes mellitus), or neurologic and neurodevelopment conditions (including disorders of the brain, spinal cord, peripheral nerve, and muscle such as cerebral palsy, epilepsy [seizure disorders], stroke, intellectual disability [mental retardation], moderate to severe developmental delay, muscular dystrophy, or spinal cord injury)
4. Persons with immunosuppression, including that caused by medications or by HIV infection
5. Women who are pregnant or postmortem (within 2 weeks after delivery)
6. Children and adolescents through 18 years who are receiving aspirin- or salicylate-containing medications and who might be at risk for experiencing Reye syndrome after influenza virus infection
7. American Indian/Alaska Native people
8. Persons with extreme obesity, i.e., body mass index ≧40 kg/m^2
9. Residents of nursing homes and other chronic care facilities

Those who are at high risk of complication from influenza are defined as listed in Table 13.3, which is adapted from the report of the advisory committee on immunization practices of the Center of Disease Control and Prevention [13].

CQ2 For patients who are recommended to receive antiviral treatment for suspected or confirmed influenza, which antiviral should be prescribed, at what dosing, for what duration?

In the guidelines, a single neuraminidase inhibitor (NAI) oseltamivir, zanamivir, or peramivir is recommended for antiviral treatment. Laninamivir can be used only in Japan, because it is still under clinical evaluation in other countries.

The doses of antivirals should be according to the US Food and Drug Administration-approved ones. The duration of treatment is 5 days with oseltamivir or zanamivir, or a single dose of intravenous peramivir in otherwise healthy patients. Longer duration can be considered for patients with immunocompromising conditions or requiring hospitalization for severe lower respiratory tract disease such as pneumonia or acute respiratory distress syndrome (ARDS).

CQ3 In a patient with suspected or confirmed influenza, when should bacterial coinfection of the upper or lower respiratory tract be considered, investigated, and treated?

It is recommended to investigate and empirically treat bacterial coinfection in patients who present initially with severe disease (extensive pneumonia, respiratory failure, hypotension, and fever), patients who deteriorate after initial improvement, particularly those who undergo antiviral treatment, or patients who fail to improve after 3–5 days of antiviral treatment.

CQ4 If a patient with influenza does not demonstrate clinical improvement with antiviral treatment or demonstrates clinical deterioration during or after treatment, what additional testing and therapy should be considered?

Clinicians should investigate other causes besides influenza virus infection in influenza patients who fail to improve or deteriorate despite antiviral treatment.

CQ5 When should testing be done for infection with an antiviral-resistant influenza virus?

Influenza NAI resistance testing can be considered for

- Patients who develop laboratory-confirmed influenza while or immediately after NAI chemoprophylaxis.
- Patients with an immunocompromising condition and evidence of persistent-influenza viral replication (after days, demonstrate by persistently positive RT-PCR or viral culture results) and remain ill during or after NAI treatment.
- Patients with laboratory-confirmed influenza who inadvertently received sub-therapeutic NAI dosing.
- Patients with severe influenza who do not improve with NAI treatment and have evidence of persistent-influenza viral replication.

CQ6 Should adjunctive therapy be administered to patients with suspected or confirmed influenza?

One systemic review and meta-analysis suggested that corticosteroid therapy for presumed influenza-associated complications is associated with increased mortality despite the limitation of the included studies [14]. Another meta-analysis of published observational studies showed that corticosteroid treatment was significantly associated with mortality. Moreover, nosocomial infection, duration of mechanical ventilation and ICU stay were both markedly longer in the corticosteroid treatment group than in the control group [15].

Taking these results into consideration, the guidelines do not recommend corticosteroid adjunctive therapy for the treatment of adults or children with suspected or confirmed influenza, influenza-associated pneumonia, respiratory failure, or ARDS, unless clinically indicated for other reasons.

A randomized, double-blind, phase 3 trial was done to assess the efficacy of high-titer anti-influenza plasma (hemagglutination inhibition antibody titer $\geq$1:80) compared with low-titer plasma ($\leq$1:10) [16]. High-titer anti-influenza plasma conferred no significant benefit over non-immune plasma. The guidelines do not recommend to routinely administer immunoglobulin for treatment of adults or children with suspected or confirmed seasonal influenza.

4 Baloxavir Marboxil

Baloxavir marboxil was approved by the FDA in the USA after the finalization of the IDSA guidelines. Thus, the guidelines did not make recommendation on the use of baloxavir. In a phase 3 randomized control trial of baloxavir performed in the USA and Japan, baloxavir significantly shortened the median time for alleviation of symptoms compared with placebo and the median duration of infectious virus detection in upper respiratory tract specimens, which was significantly shorter for baloxavir compared with oseltamivir [17].

However, PAI38X amino acid substitution was detected after initiation of the trial in 9.7% of baloxavir recipients [17]. Similar amino acid substitution was recognized in a clinical case who was not given baloxavir, that consequently human to human transmission of the virus exhibiting reduced baloxavir susceptibility was suggested [18].

The emergence of viruses with PAI38X substitutions following baloxavir treatment was associated with low baseline neutralizing virus antibody titer [19]. For that reason, those who are at risk of variant virus emergence are thought to be young children, seriously ill patients, hospitalized patients, or immunocompromised ones.

The influenza committee of the Japanese Association for Infectious Diseases released the statement about the usage of anti-influenza drugs in October 2019 [20]. Recommendations for a single use of baloxavir are as follows.

1. For adolescents from 12 to 19 years old and adults; the committee cannot recommend or discourage baloxavir because of lack of evidence.
2. For children under 12 years old; clinicians should examine the administration of baloxavir considering that the emergence of viruses with reduced baloxavir susceptibility will increase in this population.
3. For immunocompromised patients and severely ill patients; the committee does not recommend administration of a single use of baloxavir.

5 Conclusion

The essential way of thinking for anti-influenza medications and the concept of the IDSA guidelines in 2018 were summarized. The guidelines recommend positive administration of antiviral drugs to hospitalized patients, severely ill patients, or patients who are at high risk of complications from influenza. Outpatients who are not at high risk of complications might be administered antiviral drugs within 48 h from the onset. The Centers of Disease Control and Prevention released a similar recommendation like the IDSA guidelines [21]. Clinical evidence of baloxavir is insufficient at present. Future guidelines will include recommendation for the usage of baloxavir.

References

1. National Institute of Infectious Diseases. Infectious agents surveillance report. IASR. 2019;40(11).
2. Uyeki TM, Bernstein HH, Bladley JS, Englund JA, File TM, Fry AM, et al. Clinical practice guidelines by the Infectious Diseases Society of America: 2018 update on diagnosis, treatment, chemoprophylaxis, and institutional outbreak management of seasonal influenza. Clin Infect Dis. 2019;68:895–902.
3. Yu H, Liao Q, Yuan Y, Zhou L, Xiang N, Huai Y, et al. Effectiveness of oseltamivir on disease progression and viral RNA shedding in patients with mild pandemic 2009 influenza A H1N1: opportunistic retrospective study of medical charts in China. BMJ. 2010;341:c4779.
4. Rodriguez A, Diaz E, Martin-Loches I, Canadell L, Díaz JJ, Figueira JC, et al. Impact of early oseltamivir treatment on outcome in critically ill patients with 2009 pandemic influenza A. J Antimicrob Chemother. 2011;66:1140–9.
5. World Health Organization. WHO guidelines for pharmacological management of pandemic (H1N1) 2009 influenza and other influenza viruses. Part I: recommendations. 2010. http://www.who.int/csr/resources/publications/swineflu/h1n1_guidelines_pharmaceutical_mngt.pdf?ua=1.
6. Writing Committee of the WHO Consultation on Clinical Aspects of Pandemic (H1N1) 2009 Influenza. Clinical aspects of pandemic 2009 influenza A (H1N1) virus infection. N Engl J Med. 2010;362:1708–19.
7. Jefferson T, Jones MA, Doshi P, Del Mar CB, Hama R, Thompson MJ, et al. Neuraminidase inhibitors for preventing and treating influenza in healthy adults and children. Cochrane Database Syst Rev. 2014;(4):CD008965.
8. Jefferson T, Jones MA, Doshi P, Elizabeth AS, Igho O, Carl JH. Oseltamivir for influenza in adults and children: systematic review of clinical study reports and summary of regulatory comments. BMJ. 2014;348:g2545.
9. World Health Organization. Executive summary: the selection and use of essential medicines. 2017. http://www.who.int/medicines/publications/essentialmedicines/EML_2017_EC21_Unedited_Full_Report.pdf.
10. Dobson J, Whitley RJ, Pocock S, Monto AS. Oseltamivir treatment for influenza in adults: a meta-analysis of randomized controlled trials. Lancet. 2015;385:1729–37.
11. Venkatesan S, Myles PR, Leonardi-Bee J, Muthuri SG, Al Masri M, Andrews N, et al. Impact of outpatient neuraminidase inhibitor treatment in patients infected with influenza A(H1N1) pdm09 at high risk of hospitalization: an individual participant data meta-analysis. Clin Infect Dis. 2017;64:1328–34.
12. Doll MK, Winters N, Boikos C, Kraicer-Melamed H, Gore G, Quach C. Safety and effectiveness of neuraminidase inhibitors for influenza treatment, prophylaxis, and outbreak control: a systematic review of systematic reviews and/or meta-analyses. J Antimicrob Chemother. 2017;72:2990–3007.
13. Grohskopf LA, Alyanak E, Broder KR, Walter EB, Fry AM, Jernigan DB. Prevention and control of seasonal influenza with vaccines: recommendations of the Advisory Committee on Immunization Practices—United States, 2019-20 influenza season. MMWR Recomm Rep. 2019;68:1–21.
14. Rodrigo C, Leonardi-Bee J, Nguyen-Van-Tam JS, Lim WS. Effect of corticosteroid therapy on influenza-related mortality: a systematic review and meta-analysis. J Infect Dis. 2015;212:183–94.
15. Yang JW, Fan LC, Miao XY, Mao B, Li MH, Lub HW, et al. Corticosteroids for the treatment of human infection with influenza virus: a systematic review and meta-analysis. Clin Microbiol Infect. 2015;21:956–63.
16. Beigel JH, Aga E, Elie-Turenne MC, Cho J, Tebas P, Clark CL, et al. Anti-influenza immune plasma for the treatment of patients with severe influenza A: a randomised, double-blind, phase 3 trial. Lancet Respir Med. 2019;7:941–50.

17. Hayden FG, Sugaya N, Hirotsu N, Lee N, de Jong MD, Hurt AC, et al. Baloxavir marboxil for uncomplicated influenza in adults and adolescents. N Engl J Med. 2018;379:913–23.
18. Takashita E, Ichikawa M, Morita H, Ogawa R, Fujisaki S, Shirakura M, et al. Human-to-human transmission of influenza A(H3N2) virus with reduced susceptibility to baloxavir, Japan February 2019. Emerg Infect Dis. 2019;25:2108–11.
19. Uehara T, Hayden FG, Kawaguchi K, Omoto S, Hurt AC, De Jong D, et al. Treatment-emergent influenza variant viruses with reduced baloxavir susceptibility: impact on clinical and virologic outcomes in uncomplicated influenza. J Infect Dis. 2019;221:346–55.
20. The influenza committee of the Japanese Association for Infectious Diseases the statement: about anti-influenza medications. http://www.kansensho.or.jp/uploads/files/guidelines/191024_teigen.pdf.
21. The Centers of Disease Control and Prevention. Influenza antiviral medications: summary for clinicians. https://www.cdc.gov/flu/professionals/antivirals/summary-clinicians.htm.

Chapter 14
Treatment Strategy for Influenza Viral Infection in Adolescent: What Is the Current Adolescent Treatment?

Yosuke Aoki

Abstract The influenza virus infection poses a life-threatening impact even in adolescents and working adults. Careful attention should be particularly paid in pandemic flu, during which health care burden in this relatively young population is prominent.

While (When) seeing patients with fever and systemic condition, physicians must bear in mind a differential list of influenza-like illnesses, including systemic infection by herpesviridae, human immunodeficiency virus infection, streptococcal infection that rapidly deteriorates, and other sexually transmitted infection that are frequently encountered in this age group of patients.

Although prudent use of antimicrobial agents is a clinical rule, it must always be weighed against disease severity of patients, the evaluation of which should reflect upon the age, chronic health condition, immune status, and coexisting bacterial infections.

Among the anti-influenza agents clinically available, suitable ambulatory preparation (oral, inhalational, or intravenous) is to be chosen on the basis of compliance, upper gastrointestinal function, and patients' preference as well.

Although the emergence of drug-insensitivity virus is of concern, significant mutation of the target molecule that renders antiviral agents ineffective has been observed on very few occasions.

While appropriately observing droplet and contact precautions for infection prevention, vigorous attempts to identify severe complications should be made not to delay in putting patients on the right track of multidisciplinary treatment.

Keywords Adolescent · Differential diagnosis · Severity · Complications

---

The original version of this chapter was revised. The correction to this chapter can be found at https://doi.org/10.1007/978-981-15-9109-9_23

Y. Aoki (✉)
Division of Infectious Disease, Department of International Medicine, Faculty of Medicine, Saga University, Saga, Japan
e-mail: aokiy3@cc.saga-u.ac.jp

J. Fujita (ed.), *Influenza*, Respiratory Disease Series: Diagnostic Tools and Disease Managements, https://doi.org/10.1007/978-981-15-9109-9_14

1 Introduction

Influenza virus has been circulating the globe all around the year causing human being (and mammals) a significant health care burden in the vast majority of the countries and regions. Although influenza virus infection basically behaves as a self-limiting communicable disease even among elderly and young children, close attention should be paid and vigorous treatment strategies must be provided in a timely fashion to those patients with chronic disease of the heart, lung, liver, and kidney, and immunocompromising disease or on immunosuppressive therapy in order to avoid exacerbation of the systemic condition that requires intensive care, heavy medical expenditure, let alone death.

This remains the same after the devastating pandemic "Spanish flu" in 1918, even though the world has witnessed development of socio-economic improvement and advancement of health care services encompassing public hygiene and preventive medicine.

It has been reported that in pandemic influenza the number of working adults hospitalized by influenza virus infection was larger than that of the elderly [1, 2].

In this chapter, basic strategy for the treatment of influenza viral infection in adolescents and working adults is reviewed and discussed.

2 Epidemiology of Influenza in Adolescents and Adults

Influenza virus poses a continuous threat to human health, afflicting all generations with 600,000–700,000 deaths every year [3]. In influenza pandemic accompanying antigenic shift/drift of the virus, much can't be hoped for influenza vaccine to prevent developing acute viral respiratory disease. Younger children, who are too young to mount a protective immunological response against virus, as well as elderly population with senescent immune response, are at high risk of contracting severe influenza virus infection. It is generally accepted that these subgroups of patients are subject to hospitalization or significant morbidity during the annual epidemic influenza virus infection.

Previous studies, however, have observed that adolescents and previously healthy working adults have an increased chance of hospitalization in pandemic influenza compared to the endemic seasonal influenza [4, 5].

As with 2009 influenza pandemic caused by pdm A (H1N1), Perez-Padilla et al. reported from Mexico city that 10 out of 18 PCR-positive patients (Age; 9 months to 61 years, mean 38 years) had no underlying diseases, and none of them including 7 fatal cases had received anti-influenza drug prior to hospitalization: they were all started on therapy with antiviral agents on the average of 8 days after the onset of the illness [6]. By utilizing a population-based surveillance, Reed et al. also have found that adults hospitalized with pdm A (H1N1) 2009 (median age 47 years;

$n = 4962$) were younger than those with seasonal influenza (median age 68 years; $n = 5270$) ($p < 0.01$) [7].

This is considered due partly to the insufficient cummulative immunity against influenza virus in the adolescent population. By and large, the majority of this age group is expected to restore their usual health without complication. On the other hand, some patients may develop very severe systemic disease via what is called cytokine storm, an uncontrollable proinflammatory response triggered via interaction between host and influenza virus. Additionally, it should be reminded that this age group of patients is not an exception to develop systemic life-threatening complications such as severe bacterial pneumonia, sepsis, or neurologic complications [7]. In one cohort study, 50% (19/38 cases with median age of 52 years old) of those who contracted severe influenza had no significant problems in their chronic health; 11 (29%) had a simultaneous or secondary bacterial pneumonia, 24 (63%) required intensive care unit admission for a median of 11 days, and 17 (45%) died [8].

These findings clearly indicate that even working adults should also be paid as close attention to their systemic condition following influenza infection as that given to the vulnerable age group with either immature or senescent immune function.

3 Differential Diagnosis in Primary Care Setting

Before touching on the treatment strategy, essential tips in differential diagnosis of influenza-like illness (ILI) in a primary care setting are briefly mentioned for the sake of appropriate use of antiviral agents.

Upper respiratory symptom, including nasal discharge, sore throat, or cough, accompanied with subjective fever is a leading cause of seeking medical attention in primary care setting. A differential list of pharyngitis-like symptom is shown in Table 14.1 [9] .

Rhinovirus, coronavirus, and adenovirus are predominant agents in viral respiratory infection, in which category influenza virus is included. They all manifest clinically as common cold except that adenovirus sometimes manifest pharyngo-conjunctival infection or encephalitis in rare cases. Clinical presentation of influenza can be far more salient especially in non-immunized individuals than these respiratory virus infection in that the disease onset is acute, highly feverish, with prominent general exhaustion, although the degree of disease severity varies among patients depending on chronic health or previous vaccination status.

Herpesviruses have historically been known to cause systemic illness presenting pharyngitis-like symptoms. Infections caused by Epstein–Barr virus, cytomegalovirus, and herpes simplex virus present as febrile mononucleosis with or without anicteric hepatitis. HHV-6 is a well-known cause of exanthema subitum (Roseola infantum or Sixth disease).

Table 14.1 Infectious agents and clinical manifestation of pharyngitis-like symptoms

Pathogen	Affected age group	Clinical features, complication
Respiratory viral infection		
• Rhinovirus • Coronavirus • Adenovirus • *Influenza virus*	All	Common cold[a] Common cold, SARS[b] (SARS-CoV, MERS-CoV, SARS-CoV-2) Pharyngo-conjunctival fever, encephalitis High fever, general malaise, myalgia, encepalopathy
Systemic viral infection		
• Epstein–Barr virus • Cytomegalovirus • Herpes simplex virus • Human herpesvirus 6 • HIV[d]	Adolescents and adults Adolescent and adults Children ~adolescent Adolescent and adults	Classical infectious mononucleosis [9] Mononucleosis, anicteric hepatitis Gingivostomatitis, painful vesicules, shallow ulceration, STI[c] Exanthema subitum Acute HIV infection (mononucleosis-like syndrome)
Bacterial infection		
• GA/GC/GG Streptococcus and *M. pneumoniae* • *N. gonorrhea*, *T. pallidum*, and *C. trachomatis*[e]	School-age children, adolescent, young adults Adolescents and adults	Fever, severe pharyngeal pain, tender lymph nodes (Stereptococci) Sore throat, bronchitis, pneumonia, extrapulmonary manifestations Gonorrhea: supprative urethritis, oligo-polyarthritis, tenosynovitis, skin lesions (DGI)[f], genital ulcers, scaly rash in palm sole (syphilis), non-supprative urethritis, pelvic inflammatory disease (*C. trachomatis*)

[a]Chillness, throat dryness, sore throat, rhinorrhea, nasal obstruction, cough, hoarseness, running nose, general fatigue, etc.
[b]Severe acute respiratory syndrome
[c]Sexually transmitted infection
[d]Human immunodeficiency virus
[e]*Neisseria gonorrhea, Treponema pallidum, Chamydophila trachomatis*
[f]*DGI* disseminated gonococcal infection

Of prime importance is to consider acute HIV infection with high index of suspicion in every adolescent patient presenting as pharyngitis-like illness or mononucleosis mimicking influenza. Although it is never easy to detect a single case of acute HIV infection among many ILI outpatients particularly in high influenza season, physicians should be cautious not to be predisposed to make an at-a-glance diagnosis of influenza, or an unanticipated HIV-infected patient will be left undiagnosed and untreated.

Pharyngitis caused by streptococci, a classical pathogen of sore throat, should also be paid alertness so that proper antibiotic treatment that help prevent cardiac or renal complications can be initiated without delay.

Sexually transmitted pharyngitis such as those caused by gonorrhea, syphilis, or chlamydial infection must also be considered in adolescent and adult patients.

4 Treatment Strategy

The morbidity and mortality from seasonal influenza is assumed to be getting milder than those once observed in preceding pandemia namely due to the development of worldwide strategies for disease control and prevention. However, emphasis on the use of antiviral agents should not be lifted for the adolescent and adult patients in order to prevent severe illness or death, reduce the need for hospitalization rate as well as the duration of hospital stays.

Treatment strategy of influenza is divided into two categories: (1) Treatment of influenza virus infection with specific anti-influenza agents and (2) Treatment of secondary bacterial infection with antibiotics. Multidisciplinary treatment including intensive care or infection prevention and control are not within the scope of this chapter.

4.1 Anti-influenza Agents (AIAs) (Table 14.2)

Although physicians may differ in to what degree they encourage the use of AIAs in otherwise healthy patients, the best clinical outcome can be achieved, regardless of the utility, with early administration of this class of drug that is highly active against influenza viruses.

There have been four classes of government-approved AIAs so far, each of which differ in the mechanism of action: ion channel inhibitor, neuraminidase inhibitor, (RNA) polymerase inhibitor, and cap-dependent endonuclease inhibitor.

One-hundred percent of clinical strain of influenza A (both H1N1 and H3N2) subjected to the in vitro analyses have shown resistance to the ion channel (M2 protein) inhibitor for now. Inconsistent clinical efficacy and potential teratogenicity have restricted clinical application of RNA polymerase inhibitor to the seasonal influenza. Thus, neuraminidase inhibitor and cap-dependent endonuclease inhibitor have been clinically utilized.

4.1.1 Neuraminidase Inhibitor

It has been over two decades since the development of neuraminidase inhibitor. A systemic review regarding oseltamivir and zanamivir has documented their clinical efficacy (reduction of the median duration of symptoms and median time to return to normal activity) and utility verified on the basis of economic evaluation [10, 11]. Any neuraminidase inhibitor treatment had a survival benefit in observational studies of patients including pregnant women hospitalized with 2009 H1N1 virus infection [12, 13].

Table 14.2 Anti-influenza agents: indications and mutations of drug target

	Neuraminidase inhibitor				Endonuclease inhibitor	RNA polymerase inhibitor
	Oseltamivir	Zanamivir	Lanimamivir	Peramivir	Baloxavir-marboxyl	Favipiravir
Newborn (<1 year old)	Applicable	Not recommended		Good indication when oral administration is impossible or upon poor inhalational performance.	Applicable: BW ≧10 kg 10 mg/day BW ≧20 kg 20 mg/day BW ≧40 kg 40 mg/day BW ≧80 kg 80 mg/day	Approved for HPAI or human influenza viruses insensitive to the currently approved drug. Off-label or compassionate use for infections due to Ebola virus, SFTS, or SARS-CoV-2.
Toddler (1 to 4 years old)	Applicable	Not applicable due to poor inhalational performance				
Young children (5–15 years old)	Applicable	May be used with good inhalational performance				
Adolescent ~Adult	Applicable	Applicable				
Patients with underlying lung disease		Use with caution (due to inducible bronchoconstriction)				
Mutation in amino-acid sequence of the target molecule	1–1.5% in A (H1N1), 0% in A (H3N2), and B	0%		1–1.5% in A (H1N1), 0% in A (H3N2), and B	0.14% in A (H1N1), 0% in A (H3N2), and B	

Prevalence data of drug insensitivities derives from National Institute of Infectious Diseases (https://www.niid.go.jp/niid/ja/influ-resist/9592-flu-r20200430.html): last-updated 2020 April 30

HPAI highly pathogenic avian influenza, *SFTS* severe fever with thrombocytopenia syndrome, *SARS* severe acute respiratory syndrome

Zanamivir

Zanamivir is the first neuraminidase inhibitor manufactured in 1993 based on the analyses of crystallographic structure of sialidase, a synonym of neuraminidase [14]. Zanamivir was later found to be capable of inhibiting neuraminidase activity in all antigenic subtypes of Influenza A and Influenza B virus [15], as well as Influenza A (H5N1) [16]. The bioavailability of this drug, however, was estimated to be 2% when orally administered so that it was developed as an inhalational preparation [16].

Oseltamivir

Li et al. [17] successfully developed an ethyl-ester prodrug (Oseltamivir) with good bioavailability that is capable of strongly inhibiting neuraminidase, acting against Influenza virus A and B. Since then, no doubt that oseltamivir has demonstrated apparent clinical benefit as a leading AIA worldwide [10, 11]. There once had been a concern in terms of safety, however, with the use of this drug: In Japan, since 2004, sporadic cases of transient neuropsychiatric behavioral abnormality (self-injury, agitation, delirium, etc.) that developed after oseltamivir use among young patients had been observed post-marketing such that Japanese government issued an emergency safety information in patients with influenza in adolescents and young adults [18]. Although no causal connection between oseltamivir and abnormal behavior has been confirmed [19], careful 2-day attention by caregivers is encouraged.

Peramivir

Peramivir is the only AIA available as an intravenous preparation. Long serum half-life and high binding affinity to viral neuraminidase have made once-daily dosing possible [16, 20]. Patients with vomiting or upper gastrointestinal malfunction that may interfere with drug absorption or those who can't be orally medicated for any reason should benefit from peramivir.

Laninamivir

Laninamivir, a lipophilic derivative, is another inhalational AIA for once-daily dosing. Inhibitory concentration is a little higher for Influenza A (H3N2) and B than that of oseltamivir, but it is capable of inhibiting replication of Influenza A (H5N1) as well as oseltamivir-insensitive virus in vitro [21].

4.1.2 RNA Polymerase Inhibitor

Favipiravir

Favipiravir, developed and approved in Japan in 2014, is known to act against PB1 of influenza virus as a purine analogue and has been shown to exert antiviral effect, as seen in IC50, that was 30-times potent as that of another purine analogue ribavirin without causing any damage to DNA and RNA synthesis of the host [22]. Unfortunately, clinical application of this drug has been suspended by the time being due to (1) inconsistent therapeutic efficacy with variable dosing regimen observed in clinical study enrolling those with uncomplicated influenza and (2) possible toxicity for reproduction and development of the fetus [23]. On the other hand, broad application of this drug to the infections caused by other RNA viruses, such as Ebola virus or SARS-CoV-2 has been under investigation.

4.1.3 Cap-Dependent Endonuclease Inhibitor

Baloxir Marboxil

Influenza viruses snatch the first 10–20 residues of a host cell RNA (cap structure), thereby enabling its genetic replication within the host cells via cap-dependent endonuclease (CEN) activity intrinsic to RNA polymerase PA protein [24].

Baloxavir, a CEN inhibitor, is the newest anti-influenza agent, the clinical efficacy of which has been demonstrated in otherwise healthy adult patients [25], those who are at high risk of developing complication [26], and children under 12 years old [27].

This single-dosing regimen drug has received a lot of interest and also concern in terms of the treatment-emergent variant viruses [28]. The current nation-wide surveillance of the emergence of this low-sensitivity virus, however, has been much lower than initially anticipated.

4.2 Treatment of Secondary Bacterial Infection (Table 14.3)

It has become even a clinical axiom that secondary bacterial infection frequently develops as a complication of influenza, which significantly affects the prognosis of patients. *Streptococcus pneumonia* is among the most prevalent and virulent pathogen regardless of the drug sensitivity that quickly deteriorates patients' condition. Including *Staphylococcus aureus*, and *Streptococcus pyogenes*, these 3S have been reported to be found in 50% of fatal cases in pandemic influenza [29]. When encountering with an influenza patient, physicians should consider every relevant clinical

Table 14.3 Secondary bacterial infection and antimicrobial therapy

Pathogens	Common, severe clinical features	Specific clinical features	Antimicrobial therapy
Streptococcus pneumoniae	Bacteremia ~ Sepsis Fever, Hypothermia Tachypnea, Tachycardia, Hypotension Thrombocytopenia, Purpura Renal failure Metabolic acidosis	Lobar pneumonia Multifocal bronchopneumonia (without cavity formation) Meningitis, infective endocarditis	High-dose PenicillinG Ceftriaxone and Vancomycin (meningitis caused by penicillin-resistant strain)
Staphylococcus aureus		Infective endocarditis Bronchopneumonia (may form cavity) Bronchitis	Ceftriaxone Vancomycin, Daptomycin (not approved for pneumonia), Linezolid
Streptococcus pyogenes		Pharyngitis Bronchitis, Bronchopneumonia Necrotizing fasciitis	Penicillin G Pen allergy: Erythromycin, Azithromycin, Clindamycin, Cefazolin, Cefotaxime, Vancomycin

Besides rapid influenza diagnostic test, complete blood count, blood chemistry, and two sets of blood culture must be ordered
Severe streptococcal infections tend to rapidly progress in the pace of "hours", whereas staphylococcal infections in "days"

detail to make sure that severe complications such as infective endocarditis or bacterial meningitis due to these classical pathogen are not overlooked in the presence of overwhelming respiratory distress from severe pneumonia. Additionally, bactericidal antimicrobial agents against these 3S pathogen must immediately be administered intravenously (Table 14.3).

5 Conclusion

Wide range of population is afflicted by influenza virus infection every year. Adolescent and young adults are not the exception, who also needs immediate antiviral treatment.

Differential list of influenza must be retrieved when seeing young adult with pharyngitis-like symptoms, particularly in high season of influenza infection.

There is no strict difference in which AIAs should be selected. Oral or inhalational medications are convenient for outpatient treatment, while parenteral preparation should be given in patients with severe systemic condition who should be hospitalized.

Physicians should always be alert in identifying coexisting bacterial infection such that bactericidal antibiotics can be administered without delay.

References

1. Viboud C, Simonsen L, Fuentes R, Flores J, Miller MA, Chowell G. Global mortality impact of the 1957–1959 influenza pandemic. J Infect Dis. 2016;213:738–45.
2. Shrestha SS, Swerdlow DL, Borse RH, Prabhu VS, Finelli L, Atkins CY, et al. Estimating the burden of 2009 pandemic influenza A (H1N1) in the United States (April 2009–April 2010). Clin Infect Dis. 2011;52(S1):S75–82.
3. Thompson WW, Weintraub E, Dhankhar P, Cheng PY, Brammer L, Meltzer MI, et al. Estimates of US influenza-associated deaths made using four different methods. Influenza Other Respir Viruses. 2009;3:37–49.
4. Yang L, Wong CS, Chiu SSS, Cowling BJ, Oeiris JSM. Estimation of excess moratlity and hospitalization associated with 2009 pandemic influenza. Hong Kong Med J. 2018;24(Suppl 6):S19–22.
5. Sheu SM, Tsai CF, Yang HY, Pai HW, Chen SC. Comparison of age-specific hospitalization during pandemic and seasonal influenza periods from 2009 to 2012 in Taiwan: a nationwide population-based study. BMC Infect Dis. 2016;16:88. https://doi.org/10.1186/s12879-016-1438-x.
6. Perez-Padilla R, de la Rosa-Zamboni D, Ponce de Leon S, Hernandez M, Quiñones-Falconi F, Bautista E, et al. Pneumonia and respiratory failure from swine-origin influenza A (H1N1) in Mexico. N Engl J Med. 2009;361:680–9.
7. Reed C, Chaves SS, Perez A, D'Mello T, Kirley PD, Aragon D, et al. Complications among adults hospitalized with influenza: a comparison of seasonal influenza and the 2009 H1N1 pandemic. Clin Infect Dis. 2014;59:166–74.
8. Ho YC, Wang JL, Wang JT, Wu UI, Cahng CW, Wu HS, et al. Prognostic factors for fatal adult influenza pneumonia. J Infect. 2009;58:439–45.
9. Luzuriaga K, Sullivan JL. Infectious mononucleosis. N Engl J Med. 2010;362:1993–2000.
10. Beck CR, Sokal R, Arunachalam N, Puleston R, Cichowska A, Kessel A, et al. (UK antiviral effectiveness review group). Neuraminidase inhibitors for influenza: a review and public health perspective in the aftermath of the 2009 pandemic. Influenza Other Respir Viruses. 2013;7(Suppl 1):14–24.
11. Burch J, Paulden M, Conti S, Stock C, Corbett M, Welton NJ, et al. Antiviral drugs for the treatment of influenza: a systematic review and economic evaluation. Health Technol Assess. 2009;13(58):1–265. https://doi.org/10.3310/hta13580.
12. Jain S, Kamimoto L, Bramley AM, Schmitz AM, Benoit SR, Louie J, et al. Hospitalized patients with 2009 H1N1 influenza in the United States, April–June 2009. N Engl J Med. 2009;361:1935–44.
13. Siston AM, Rasmussen SA, Honein MA, Fry AM, Seib K, Callaghan WM, et al. Pandemic 2009 influenza A(H1N1) virus illness among pregnant women in the United States. JAMA. 2010;303:1517–25.
14. von Itzstein M, Wu WY, Kok GB, Pegg MS, Dyason JC, et al. Rational design of potent sialidase-based inhibitors of influenza virus replication. Nature. 1993;363:418–23.
15. Woods JM, Bethell RC, Coates JA, Healy N, Hiscox SA, Pearson BA, et al. 4-Guanidino-2,4-dideoxy-2,3-dehydro-N-acetylneuraminic acid is a highly effective inhibitor both of the sialidase (neuraminidase) and of growth of a wide range of influenza A and B viruses in vitro. Antimicrob Agents Chemother. 1993;37:1473–9.
16. Hayden FG. Developing new antiviral agents for influenza treatment: what does the future hold? Clin Infect Dis. 2009;48(Suppl 1):S3–13. https://doi.org/10.1086/591851.
17. Li W, Escarpe PA, Eisenberg EJ, Cundy KC, Sweet C, Jakeman K, et al. Identification of GS 4104 as an orally bioavailable prodrug of the influenza virus neuraminidase inhibitor GS 4071. Antimicrob Agents Chemother. 1998;42:647–53.
18. Nakamura Y, Sugawara T, Ohkusa Y, Taniguchi K, Miyazaki C, Momoi M, et al. Life-threatening abnormal behavior incidence in 10–19 year old patients administered neur-

aminidase inhibitors. PLoS One. 2015;10(7):e0129712. Published: July 1, 2015. https://doi.org/10.1371/journal.pone.0129712.
19. Toovey S, Rayner C, Prinssen E, Chu T, Donner B, Thakrar B, et al. Assessment of neuropsychiatric adverse events in influenza patients treated with oseltamivir: a comprehensive review. Drug Saf. 2008;31:1097–114.
20. Bantia S, Arnold CS, Parker CD, Upshaw R, Chand P. Anti-influenza virus activity of peramivir in mice with single intramuscular injection. Antivir Res. 2006;69:39–45.
21. Yamashita M. Laninamivir and its prodrug, CS-8958: long-acting neuraminidase inhibitors for the treatment of influenza (Review). Antivir Chem Chemother. 2010;21:71–84. https://doi.org/10.3851/IMP1688.
22. Furuta Y, Takahashi K, Kuno-Maekawa M, Sangawa H, Uehara S, Kozaki K, et al. Mechanism of action of T-705 against influenza virus. Antimicrob Agents Chemother. 2005;49:981–6.
23. PMDA: report on the deliberation results. https://www.pmda.go.jp/files/000210319.pdf.
24. Decroly E, Canard B. Biochemical principles and inhibitors to interfere with viral capping pathways. Curr Opin Virol. 2017;24:87–96.
25. Hayden FG, Sugaya N, Hirotsu N, Lee N, De Jong MD, Hurt AC, et al. Baloxavir marboxyl for uncomplicated influenza in adults and adolescents. N Engl J Med. 2018;379:913–23.
26. Ison MG, Portsmouth S, Yoshida Y, Shishido T, Hayden F, Uehara T. LB16. Phase 3 trial of baloxavir marboxil in high-risk influenza patients (CAPSTONE-2 study). Open Forum Infect Dis. 2018;5(Suppl 1):S764–5. Published 2018 Nov 26. https://doi.org/10.1093/ofid/ofy229.2190.
27. Hirotsu N, Sakaguchi H, Sato C, Ishibashi T, Baba K, Omoto S, et al. Baloxavir marboxyl in Japanese pediatric patients with influenza: safety and clinical and virological outcome. Clin Infect Dis. 2019;71(4):971–81. https://doi.org/10.1093/cid/ciz908.
28. Uehara T, Hayden FG, Kawaguchi K, Omoto S, Hurt AC, De Jong MD, et al. Treatment-emergent influenza variant viruses with reduced baloxavir susceptibility: impact on clinical and virologic outcomes in uncomplicated influenza. J Infect Dis. 2020;221:346–55. https://doi.org/10.1093/infdis/jiz244.
29. Morens DM, Taubenberger JK, Fauci AS. Predominant role of bacterial pneumonia as a cause death in pandemic influenza: implications for pandemic influenza preparedness. J Infect Dis. 2008;198:962–70.

Chapter 15
How to Use Anti-influenza Drugs: Zanamivir and Oseltamivir

Naoki Kawai

Abstract Zanamivir and oseltamivir have been used worldwide for the treatment of influenza for about 20 years, zanamivir as an inhaled and oseltamivir as an oral drug, with both administered twice daily for 5 days. For prophylaxis, both are administered once daily for 7–10 days. They are almost equally effective for influenza A. Oseltamivir is less effective against influenza B than against influenza A; however, it is sufficiently effective that it is much better than using no drug at all. The oseltamivir-resistant (H274Y mutated) seasonal H1N1 virus was prevalent in the 2008–2009 season, and the effectiveness of oseltamivir was less than that of zanamivir in that season; however, the oseltamivir-resistant seasonal H1N1 virus disappeared after the emergence of the novel N1N1 pandemic influenza virus (H1N1pdm09) in 2009. Of note, oseltamivir has shown continued effectiveness against H1N1pdm09 since the 2009–2010 season, as effective as against seasonal H1N1 in the 2007–2008 season and before. Zanamivir has been effective for 20 years, and no resistant virus has been found to date.

Zanamivir and oseltamivir continue to be effective and safe, and they are relatively cheaper than the newer NA inhibitors, laninamivir and peramivir. In today's Japan, the share of zanamivir has eroded, being replaced by the single administration drug laninamivir, which is structurally like zanamivir, but oseltamivir has continued to be widely used for patients of all ages, including infants. Zanamivir is recommended for patients without complications and oseltamivir for patients with or without complications, such as pneumonia and other diseases.

Keywords Oseltamivir · Zanamivir · Efficacy · H274Y mutated virus · Influenza type and subtypes

N. Kawai (✉)
Influenza Study Group of the Japan Physicians Association, Tokyo, Japan
e-mail: nkawai@city.gifu.med.or.jp

J. Fujita (ed.), *Influenza*, Respiratory Disease Series: Diagnostic Tools and Disease Managements, https://doi.org/10.1007/978-981-15-9109-9_15

1 Introduction

Von Itzstein et al. reported in 1993 that they had designed potent inhibitors based on the crystal structure of influenza virus sialidase [1]. Zanamivir (Relenza in powder form for oral inhalation) was the first neuraminidase inhibitor to be marketed (Dec, 2000 in Japan), followed a few months later by oseltamivir (Tamiflu) (Feb, 2001 in Japan) [2], a capsulated oral medication used for the treatment and prevention of influenza that has a similar mechanism to zanamivir. Both suppress and decrease the spread of influenza A and B viruses by blocking the action of neuraminidase, an enzyme produced by the virus that enables it to spread from infected cells to healthy cells.

2 Medical Use

Zanamivir and oseltamivir are approved for the treatment of the acute, uncomplicated illness of influenza A and B virus patients who have been symptomatic for no more than 2 days. Because of the risk of neuropsychiatric symptoms, it is recommended that teenage patients be carefully observed by family for 2 days. The safety of zanamivir and oseltamivir have been confirmed for pregnant woman and newborn babies, and it has been recommended for use by the Japan Society of Obstetrics and Gynecology.

2.1 *Zanamivir*

Zanamivir (10 mg) is inhaled twice per day for 5 days, both for adults and children who are capable of inhaling (usually 5 years or older). For prophylaxis, both for adults and children, 10 mg is used once daily for 10 days.

In 2006, the Food and Drug Administration (FDA) reported breathing problems (bronchospasm), including deaths, for some patients after inhalation. Most of these patients had asthma or chronic obstructive pulmonary disease, so zanamivir is not recommended for treatment or prophylaxis of patients with these diseases. For patients with asthma, it is recommended that the asthma drug be taken before zanamivir. Zanamivir is not recommended for hospitalized patients in serious condition with pneumonia or other complications.

2.2 *Oseltamivir*

Oseltamivir phosphate (Tamiflu) is an oral anti-viral drug approved for patients 2 weeks of age and older. It is administered orally twice daily for 5 days at 75 mg (1 capsule) for adults or children weighing 37.5 kg or over; 2 mg/kg (66.7 mg/kg as dry syrup, maximally 75 mg) for children aged over 1 year; and 3 mg/kg (100 mg/kg as dry syrup) for infants aged 2 weeks to 1 year. Dosage modification is recommended for adults with an estimated creatinine clearance less than or equal to 30 mL per minute.

For prophylaxis, 75 mg (1 capsule) for adults or 2 mg/kg for children is administrated once daily for 7–10 days. Common adverse drug reactions include nausea and vomiting and are experienced by over 1% of patients treated with oseltamivir. It is recommended for patients with or without serious disease complications, such as pneumonia.

3 Efficacy

3.1 Efficacy of Zanamivir and Oseltamivir Before the 2008–2009 Season

Hayden et al. did a clinical study in 1997 and reported a median time to the alleviation of major symptoms of 4 days for two zanamivir groups and 7 days for a placebo group ($p \leq 0.01$). The viral titers of nasal washings of the groups given inhaled or intranasal zanamivir were significantly lower than those of the placebo group. Topically administered zanamivir was well tolerated [3].

Nicholson et al. reported in a randomized trial that the duration of illness was significantly shorter, by 29 h ($p = 0.02$) with oseltamivir 75 mg and by 35 h ($p = 0.01$) with oseltamivir 150 mg, than with placebo. Oseltamivir was associated with less viral shedding and improved health and activity, and it was well tolerated [4].

Kashiwagi et al. in a Japanese Phase III trial of oseltamivir phosphate [5] found that the duration of illness was significantly reduced, by 1 day (23.3 h) ($p = 0.0216$), and that the main side effects associated with oseltamivir were gastrointestinal disorders such as stomachache, nausea, and vomiting.

Another investigation by Kashiwagi et al. of the efficacy of oseltamivir for prophylaxis showed that the incidence of laboratory-confirmed influenza with both fever of 37.5 °C or higher and at least two influenza symptoms was 1.3% in an oseltamivir group and 8.5% in a placebo group and that oseltamivir prophylaxis inhibited 85% of infection ($p = 0.00323$) [6].

3.2 Efficacy for Influenza B

Much data are available on the effectiveness of oseltamivir for influenza A, but its efficacy for influenza B and by subtype of influenza A has not been fully investigated because of a lack of patients with influenza B or because the subtype of influenza A was not routinely determined.

Table 15.1 Duration of fever by time to the first administration of oseltamivir after the onset of fever [8]

	Influenza A		Influenza B		
Time from onset to first dose (h)	No. of patients	Duration of fever (h)	No. of patients	Duration of fever (h)	*P*
Duration of fever after administration of the first dose of oseltamivir					
0–12	696	32.3 ± 25.8	518	47.9 ± 31.3	<0.001
13–24	709	31.0 ± 23.2	577	48.4 ± 30.3	<0.001
25–36	256	28.4 ± 20.6	200	43.5 ± 26.7	<0.001
37–48	157	31.5 ± 20.3	190	44.7 ± 34.7	<0.001
Duration of fever from the onset					
0–12	696	37.6 ± 25.9	518	53.1 ± 31.2	<0.001
13–24	709	49.1 ± 23.3	577	66.5 ± 30.3	<0.001
25–36	256	57.1 ± 21.0	200	72.9 ± 27.2	<0.001
37–48	157	73.3 ± 20.0	190	87.5 ± 34.9	<0.001

Duration of fever: mean h ± SD

Kawai et al. reported for 2002–2003 influenza season that the duration of fever (body temperature < 37.5 °C) of patients who had been administered oseltamivir after confirmed diagnosis by antigen detection test kit was significantly longer for 684 influenza B patients than for 803 influenza A patients [7]. A prospective, multicenter study of the 2003–2004 and 2004–2005 influenza seasons [8] found that the time, in hours, until the patient became afebrile after the initial administration of oseltamivir was significantly longer for patients with B than with A at 0–12, 13–24, 25–36, and 37–48 h from the onset of symptoms to the start of administration ($p < 0.001$) (Table 15.1).

Interestingly, the time from the initial administration of oseltamivir to the resolution of fever was comparable to the time from onset to the start of treatment at all four time points. Because a similar clinical course was seen for most patients after the initial administration of oseltamivir, these results indicate that inhibiting the increase of infected cells is important for quickly reducing symptoms and accelerating recovery from illness. The benefit of the early administration of oseltamivir was also demonstrated, shown by longer duration of fever from the onset according to the time lapsed from the start of therapy.

3.3 *Efficacy and Susceptibility for Each Type and Subtype of Influenza*

In further study of the 2003–2004 and 2004–2005 influenza seasons, the persistence, susceptibility, and resistance of the influenza A and influenza B viruses to oseltamivir was determined for outpatients of various ages [9]. Virus isolation was done before and 5 days after the initiation of oseltamivir therapy for 148 patients with influenza A/H3N2 and for 66 with influenza B, and the 50% inhibitory concentration (IC_{50}) of oseltamivir carboxylate was calculated. The virus isolation rate after oseltamivir therapy was significantly higher for influenza B (33.3%) than for influenza A/H3N2 (12.8%, $p < 0.001$). The mean IC_{50} values before oseltamivir therapy were significantly higher for patients with influenza B (10.82 nM) than for patients with influenza A/H3N2 (0.94 nM, $p < 0.001$). Sequence analysis revealed no known genotype with resistance to oseltamivir. We concluded that virus persistence after oseltamivir therapy was longer and IC_{50} values were higher for influenza B than for influenza A. This may explain our finding that oseltamivir is less effective against influenza B than against influenza A in a clinical setting.

The duration of fever after the first dose of oseltamivir was significantly longer for influenza B than for influenza A/H1N1 or A/H3N2 from 2003–2004 to 2007–2008 (Fig. 15.1) [10]. No statistically significant differences were found in the effectiveness of zanamivir during this period among patients with influenza A/H1N1, A/H3N2, or B (Fig. 15.1). The respective mean IC_{50}s of zanamivir and oseltamivir reported by Boivin et al. were 1.14 and 0.90 nM for influenza A/H1N1, 2.09 and 0.73 nM for influenza A/H3N2, and 4.15 and 11.53 nM for influenza B [11]. These findings may explain our results that show oseltamivir to be slightly more effective than zanamivir against influenza A/H3N2, but less effective against influenza B [12].

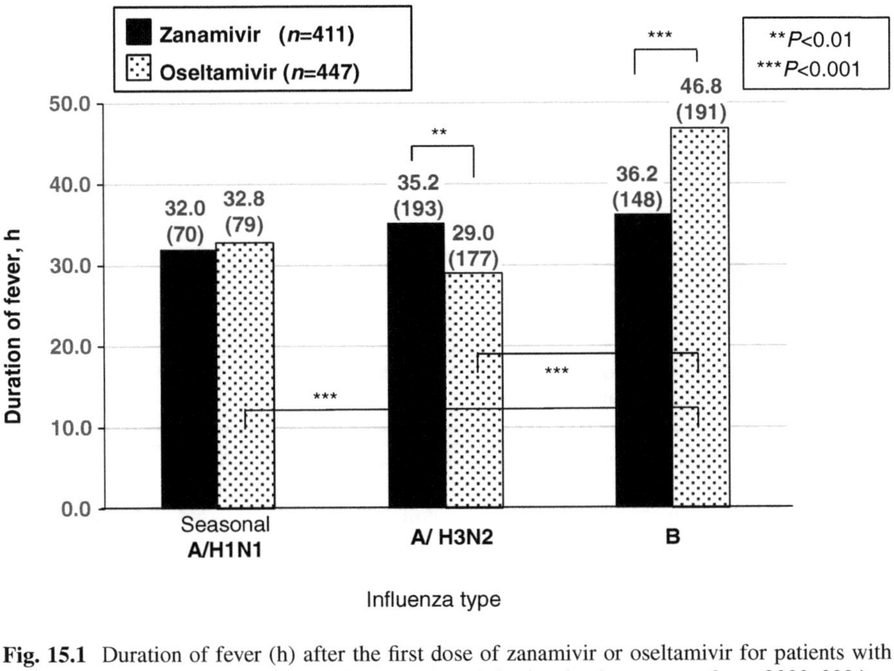

Fig. 15.1 Duration of fever (h) after the first dose of zanamivir or oseltamivir for patients with seasonal influenza A/H1N1, A/H3N2, or B virus infection in the seasons from 2003–2004 to 2007–2008 [10]

4 Efficacy for H274Y Mutated Virus

4.1 Efficacy of Oseltamivir for H274Y Mutated Virus in the 2008–2009 Season

The World Health Organization (WHO) announced a marked increase of the oseltamivir-resistant A(H1N1) virus with the N1 NA mutation H274Y (N2 numbering; H275Y in N1 numbering) in Japan from 3% in the 2007–2008 season to 97% in the 2008–2009 season [13]. In our study, NA sequence analysis found no H274Y mutation in the 2007–2008 season (44 patients), but all 29 patients in the 2008–2009 season had the mutation [14]. The mean IC_{50} before oseltamivir treatment was significantly higher (200-fold) in 2008–2009 (319.3 ± 185.4 nM) than in 2007–2008 (1.5 ± 0.8 nM; $p < 0.001$) (Fig. 15.2). After oseltamivir treatment, patients ≤15 years with oseltamivir-resistant virus infection in the 2008–2009 season had a higher rate of viral persistence than patients >15 years (50% and 11.8%, respectively, $p = 0.038$). The patients with oseltamivir resistance also showed a significantly higher body temperature during oseltamivir treatment than did patients ≤15 years without resistance (Fig. 15.2). From this, we concluded that the clinical effectiveness of

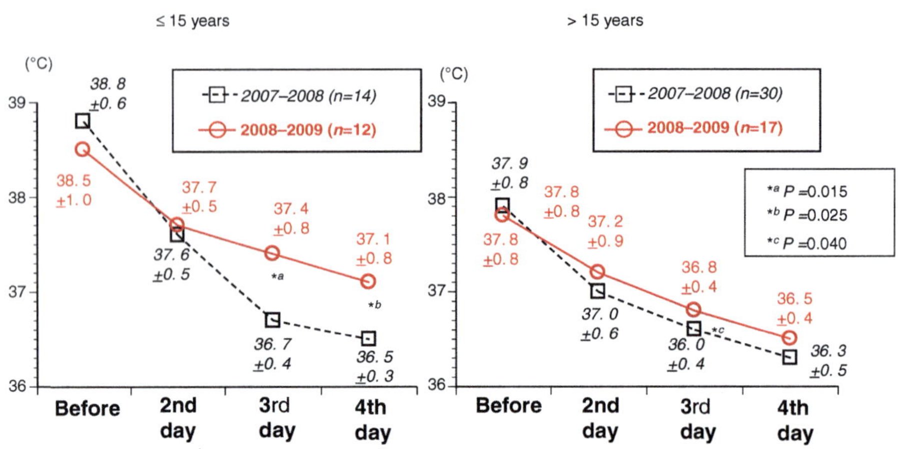

IC50 and H274Y mutation before oseltamivir treatment for A(H1N1) virus			
	2007-2008 season	2008-2009 season	p
IC_{50} (nM)	1.5 ± 0.8 (n=44)	319.3 ±185.4 (n=29)	<0.001
H274Y mutation	(−)	(+)	

Fig. 15.2 Body temperature before oseltamivir treatment and on the second, third, and fourth days after treatment in the 2007–2008 and 2008–2009 influenza seasons [14]. Body temperature before treatment and at either 8:00 AM or 8:00 PM, whichever was highest, on the second, third, and fourth days after starting oseltamivir treatment were analyzed. The mean IC_{50} before oseltamivir treatment was significantly (almost 200-fold) higher in the 2008–2009 than in 2007–2008 season, and H274Y mutation was detected in all cases in the 2008–2009 season

oseltamivir for the A(H1N1) virus was reduced in the 2008–2009 season compared with the previous season, especially for children, probably due to the H274Y mutation.

4.2 *Comparison of Oseltamivir and Zanamivir for H274Y Mutated Virus*

In another study, during the 2007–2008 season 68 patients had H1N1 virus infection (41 treated with oseltamivir and 27 with zanamivir) [15], and in the 2008–2009 season 164 had H1N1 (77 oseltamivir and 87 zanamivir) and 59 had H3N2 (31 oseltamivir and 28 zanamivir). All 49 analyzed H1N1 virus isolates obtained during the 2008–2009 season contained the H274Y mutation, but none was found in the isolates of the 2007–2008 season. The mean duration of fever (h) after the start of oseltamivir therapy was significantly longer for patients with H1N1 than for patients with H3N2 (49.1 ± 30.2 h vs. 33.7 ± 20 h, $p < 0.01$) during the 2008–2009 season and for patients with H1N1 during the 2007–2008 season (32.0 ± 18.9 h, $p < 0.001$) (Table 15.2). The duration of fever for H1N1 was longer for children ≤15 years of

Table 15.2 Duration of fever after oseltamivir or zanamivir administration for patients with influenza virus A subtypes H1N1 and H3N2

A. Seasonal comparisons [15, 17]

	Seasonal A(H1N1)		Pandemic A(H1N1)[a]	A(H3N2)
Virus type	2007–2008 (a)	2008–2009 (b)	2009–2010 (c)	2008–2009 (d)
Oseltamivir (Os)	32.0 ± 18.9 (*n* = 41)	49.1 ± 30.2 (*n* = 77)	23.0 ± 11.6 (*n* = 149)	33.7 ± 20.1 (*n* = 31)
Zanamivir (Zn)	31.5 ± 14.9 (*n* = 27)	27.5 ± 18.5 (*n* = 87)	26.9 ± 15.4 (*n* = 212)	30.1 ± 18.0 (*n* = 28)
P between Os & Zn	NS	<0.001	<0.001	NS

B. A(H1N1) by age [15]

	Oseltamivir		Zanamivir	*P*	
Patient's age	2007–2008 (e)	2008–2009 season (f)	2008–2009 season (g)	(e) and (f)	(f) and (g)
≤ 15 years	32.0 ± 19.0 (*n* = 20)	54.5 ± 34.0 (*n* = 38)	26.5 ± 18.6 (*n* = 46)	<0.01	< 0.001
>15 years	32.0 ± 18.7 (*n* = 21)	43.9 ± 24.9 (*n* = 39)	28.5 ± 18.3 (*n* = 41)	<0.05	< 0.01
P between ≤15 years and >15 years	NS	NS	NS		

Oseltamivir: for A(H1N1) in consecutive 3 seasons; (a) vs. (b), (b) vs. (c) $p < 0.001$; (a) vs. (c) $p < 0.01$

Oseltamivir: between A(H1N1) and A(H3N2) in the 2008–2009 season; (b) vs. (d) $p < 0.01$

[a]Citation from [17], other data cited from [15]

Duration of fever: mean h ± SD

age during 2008–2009 (54.5 ± 34.0 h) than for children during 2007–2008 (32.0 ± 19.0 h). For high-risk patients, H274Y mutated H1N1 infection was sometimes fatal [16]. Notably, the efficacy of zanamivir did not differ for patients with or without the H1N1 H274Y mutation (Table 15.2) [15]. This indicates that zanamivir would be a better recommendation than oseltamivir for children and adults with high-risk, underlying diseases who are infected with H274Y mutated A(H1N1) virus.

5 Efficacy After Emergence of H1N1pdm in the 2009–2010 Season and After

5.1 Restored Efficacy of Oseltamivir After Emergence of H1N1pdm09

Following the emergence of H1N1pdm09 in 2009, the seasonal H1N1 virus disappeared in the 2009–2010 season. None of the 34 analyzed pandemic H1N1 virus isolated in the 2009–2010 season contained the H274Y mutation, which had been commonly detected in the 2008–2009 season. The duration of fever after the start of oseltamivir therapy was significantly shorter for patients with pandemic (23.0 ± 11.6 h) than with seasonal H1N1 in both the 2008–2009 and 2007–2008 seasons (Table 15.2) [15, 17]. The mean duration of fever after the first dose of zanamivir was not different among the three seasons. The effectiveness of oseltamivir for the H1N1pdm09 that replaced seasonal H1N1 was similar to that of zanamivir after the 2009–2010 season [17, 18].

5.2 Recent Efficacy of Both Drugs Compared with Newly Developed Anti-influenza Drugs

In 2010, new neuraminidase inhibitors (NAIs), peramivir and laninamivir, came onto the market [19, 20], but oseltamivir has continued to be the most widely used anti-influenza drug in Japan because it is sold in both capsule and dry syrup forms and can be used easily for patients of all ages, including infants. In Japan, oseltamivir was prohibited for use by teens between 2006 and 2018 because of the risk of neuropsychiatric symptoms. However, when it became clear that these neuropsychiatric symptoms were found in patients who took other NAIs and others who had not taken any anti-influenza drug, oseltamivir use was again allowed for teens beginning in the 2018–2019 season. In addition, inexpensive generics of oseltamivir came onto the market in the 2018–2019 season. In contrast, the share of zanamivir has decreased since the appearance of laninamivir. This is because although the basic structural formula of laninamivir is similar to zanamivir, laninamivir has the advantage of being a single inhalation therapy.

During the 2018–2019 season, the durations of fever after the first administration of the four NAIs for influenza A were not significantly different: 27.7 h for oseltamivir ($n = 425$), 32.8 h for zanamivir ($n = 50$), 27.4 h for laninamivir ($n = 154$), and 30.5 h for peramivir ($n = 24$), (unpublished data). It is notable that the efficacy of oseltamivir and zanamivir are almost equal to the newer NA inhibitors, laninamivir and peramivir.

5.3 *Recent Safety Profiles of Both Drugs*

We measured the IC_{50}s of influenza virus isolates taken during the 2010–2011 to 2017–2018 seasons (Fig. 15.3). Viral isolation was done with specimen obtained prior to treatment, and the type and subtype were determined by RT-PCR using

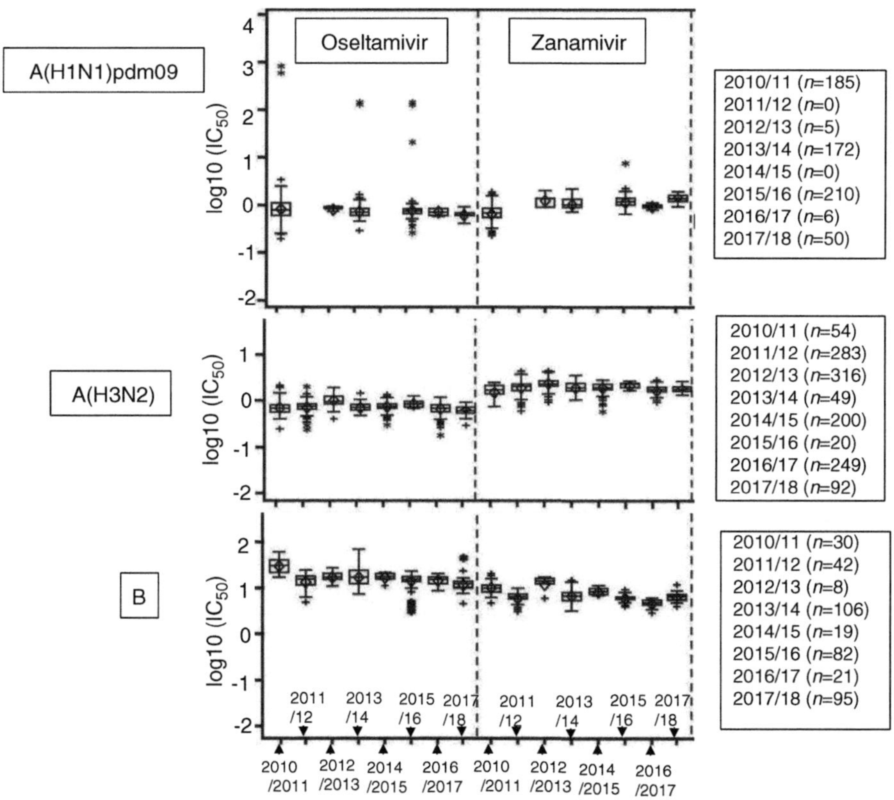

Fig. 15.3 Box and whisker plot analysis of the IC_{50}s of oseltamivir and zanamivir by virus type/subtype from 2010–2011 to 2017–2018 [21]. The bottom and top of the box are Q1 and Q3, and the band near the middle of the box is the median. The ends of the whiskers are the lowest datum still within a 1.5 interquartile range (IQR) of the lower quartile and the highest datum still within 1.5 IQR of the upper quartile. Open diamond: arithmetic mean. +: 1.5–3 interquartile range from the box. Asterisk: a more than 3 interquartile range from the box

type- and subtype-specific primers. In the latest reported 2017–2018 season, 237 virus isolates were measured, with 50 A(H1N1)pdm09, 92 A(H3N2), and 95 B. No A(H1N1)pdm09 found to have highly reduced sensitivity to oseltamivir. No isolates with highly reduced sensitivity to the four NAIs were found for A(H3N2) or B between 2010 and 2018. The geometric mean IC_{50}s of the four NAIs were consistent over the eight studied seasons. These results indicate that the sensitivity to the four commonly used NAIs has been maintained [21].

6 Conclusion

Zanamivir and oseltamivir are recommended for use within 48 h of the onset of influenza. Zanamivir is recommended for adults without serious disease complications and for children who can inhale (usually 5 years or older). Oseltamivir is recommended for adults and children, including infants less than 1 year (over 2 months) both with and without serious disease complications, such as pneumonia.

References

1. von Itzstein M, Wu WY, Kok GB, et al. Rational design of potent sialidase-based inhibitors of influenza virus replication. Nature. 1993;363:418–23.
2. Eisenberg EJ, Bidgood A, Cundy KC. Penetration of GS4071, a novel influenza neuraminidase inhibitor, into rat bronchoalveolar lining fluid following oral administration of the prodrug GS4104. Antimicrob Agents Chemother. 1997;41:1949–52.
3. Hayden FG, Osterhaus AD, Treanor JJ, et al. Efficacy and safety of the neuraminidase inhibitor zanamivir in the treatment of influenzavirus infections. GG167 Influenza Study Group. N Engl J Med. 1997;337:874–80.
4. Nicholson KG, Aoki FY, Osterhaus AD, et al. Efficacy and safety of oseltamivir in treatment of acute influenza: a randomised controlled trial. Lancet. 2000;355:1845–50.
5. Kashiwagi S, Kudoh S, Watanabe A, Yoshimura I. Clinical efficacy and safety of the selective oral neuraminidase inhibitor oseltamivir in treating acute influenza--placebo-controlled double-blind multicenter phase III trial. Kansenshogaku Zasshi. 2000;74:1044–61. (in Japanese)
6. Kashiwagi S, Kudoh S, Watanabe A, Yoshimura I. Efficacy and safety of the selective oral neuraminidase inhibitor oseltamivir for prophylaxis against influenza--placebo-controlled double-blind multicenter phase III trial. Kansenshogaku Zasshi. 2000;74:1062–76. (in Japanese)
7. Kawai N, Ikematsu H, Iwaki N, et al. Factors influencing the effectiveness of oseltamivir and amantadine for the treatment of influenza: a multicenter study from Japan of the 2002-2003 influenza season. Clin Infect Dis. 2005;40:1309–16.
8. Kawai N, Ikematsu H, Iwaki N, et al. A comparison of the effectiveness of oseltamivir for the treatment of influenza A and influenza B: a Japanese multicenter study of the 2003-2004 and 2004-2005 influenza seasons. Clin Infect Dis. 2006;43:439–44.
9. Kawai N, Ikematsu H, Iwaki N, et al. Longer virus shedding in influenza B than in influenza A among outpatients treated with oseltamivir. J Infect. 2007;55:267–72.
10. Kawai N, Ikematsu H, Iwaki N, et al. Comparison of the effectiveness of zanamivir and oseltamivir against influenza A/H1N1, A/H3N2, and B. Clin Infect Dis. 2009;48:996–7.

11. Boivin G, Goyette N. Susceptibility of recent Canadian influenza A and B virus isolates to different neuraminidase inhibitors. Antivir Res. 2002;54:143–7.
12. Kawai N, Ikematsu H, Iwaki N, et al. A comparison of the effectiveness of zanamivir and oseltamivir for the treatment of influenza A and B. J Infect. 2008;56:51–7.
13. World Health Organization. Influenza A(H1N1) virus resistance to oseltamivir 2008-2009 influenza season. http://www.who.int/csr/disease/influenzA(H1N1)20090122_final.pdf; 22 January 2009.
14. Kawai N, Ikematsu H, Iwaki N, et al. Clinical effectiveness of oseltamivir for influenza A(H1N1) virus with H274Y neuraminidase mutation. J Infect. 2009;59:207–12.
15. Kawai N, Ikematsu H, Hirotsu N, et al. Clinical effectiveness of oseltamivir and zanamivir for treatment of influenza A virus subtype H1N1 with the H274Y mutation: a Japanese, multicenter study of the 2007-2008 and 2008-2009 influenza seasons. Clin Infect Dis. 2009;49:1828–35.
16. Gooskens J, Jonges M, Claas EC, et al. Morbidity and mortality associated with nosocomial transmission of oseltamivir-resistant influenza A(H1N1) virus. JAMA. 2009;301:1066–9.
17. Kawai N, Ikematsu H, Tanaka O, et al. Comparison of the clinical symptoms and the effectiveness of neuraminidase inhibitors for patients with pandemic influenza H1N1 2009 or seasonal H1N1 influenza in the 2007-2008 and 2008-2009 seasons. J Infect Chemother. 2011;17:375–81.
18. Kawai N, Ikematsu H, Iwaki N, et al. Persistence of pandemic influenza H1N1 virus in young patients after oseltamivir therapy in the 2009-2010 season: a comparison with seasonal H1N1 with or without H275Y mutation. J Infect Chemother. 2012;18:180–6.
19. Kohno S, Kida H, Mizuguchi M, et al. Efficacy and safety of intravenous peramivir for treatment of seasonal influenza virus infection. Antimicrob Agents Chemother. 2010;54:4568–74.
20. Watanabe A, Chang SC, Kim MJ, et al. Long-acting neuraminidase inhibitor laninamivir octanoate versus oseltamivir for treatment of influenza: a double-blind, randomized, noninferiority clinical trial. Clin Infect Dis. 2010;51:1167–75.
21. Ikematsu H, Kawai N, Chong Y, et al. In vitro neuraminidase inhibitory concentration (IC_{50}) of four neuraminidase inhibitors in the Japanese 2017-18 season: comparison with the 2010-11 to 2016-17 seasons. J Infect Chemother. 2019;25:649–52.

Chapter 16
How to Use Anti-influenza Drugs: Laninamivir Octanoate

Hideyuki Ikematsu

Abstract A neuraminidase inhibitor, laninamivir octanoate (Inavir®; Daiichi Sankyo, Tokyo, Japan) is an inhaled drug with unique characteristics. The inhaled laninamivir octanoate is converted into its active form, laninamivir, in the lungs where a high concentration continues for a long period of time. The concentration of laninamivir exceeds the level necessary for virus replication inhibition for at least 5 days, thus treatment for influenza can be completed with only a single administration through inhalation.

Clinical trials have shown comparable efficacy for laninamivir octanoate and oseltamivir, but an advantage of laninamivir octanoate is that it has sufficient antiviral effect against A(H1N1) with NA/H275Y mutated oseltamivir resistant virus. Clinical observation showing a consistent duration of fever after inhalation and continued susceptibility of epidemic viruses to laninamivir over several Japanese influenza season supports the continued clinical effectiveness of laninamivir octanoate. No resistant virus has been clinically observed for laninamivir octanoate even though it has been widely used. The prophylactic efficacy of laninamivir octanoate has been shown both in animal models and post-exposure prophylaxis in household contacts.

A major clinical benefit of this drug is that the single administration provides great convenience for both the patient and doctor, which leads to improved compliance. No emergence or transmission of resistant virus had been observed, resulting in freedom from anxiety about resistant virus. Further, this drug shows great promise for the treatment of influenza in future pandemics because of its effectiveness against all types of influenza viruses investigated in preclinical studies.

Keywords Neuraminidase inhibitor · Inhale · Long acting · Resistance

---

H. Ikematsu (✉)
Ricerca Clinica Co., Influenza Study Group, Japan Physicians Association, Fukuoka, Japan
e-mail: ikematsu@gray.plala.or.jp

J. Fujita (ed.), *Influenza*, Respiratory Disease Series: Diagnostic Tools and Disease Managements, https://doi.org/10.1007/978-981-15-9109-9_16

1 Introduction

The treatment of influenza with neuraminidase inhibitors (NAIs) has become the most popular treatment among primary care doctors in Japan. In the pandemic of A(H1N1)pdm09 in 2009, the number of reported influenza associated deaths was only about 200 in Japan, far fewer than in other countries [1]. The early start of treatment with antiviral is considered for documented or suspected influenza patients presently [2]. Laninamivir octanoate (Inavir®; Daiichi Sankyo, Tokyo, Japan) was approved and available for the treatment of influenza from 2010 in Japan, but not yet in other countries including the EU and USA. The clinical outcomes of early start of treatment with NAIs including laninamivir octanoate, within 48 h of onset, have been well demonstrated in Japan [3–5].

2 Mechanism

Laninamivir inhibits the neuraminidase (NA) of influenza viruses. The chemical structures of laninamivir octanoate (CS-8958) and its active form (R-125489) are shown in Fig. 16.1 [6]. Laninamivir octanoate is a prodrug of laninamivir with octanoic acid ester at the C-3 position of its side chain ((2*R*, 3*R*, 4*S*)-3-Acetamido-4-guanidino-2-[(1*R*, 2*R*)-2-hydroxy-1-methoxy-3-(octanoyloxy) propyl]-3,4-dihydro-2*H*-pyran-6-carboxylic acid) (Fig. 16.1, left). The laninamivir octanoate is inhaled, then converted to laninamivir in the lung (Fig. 16.1, right). The binding stability of laninamivir to various virus NAs was experimentally assessed. Although considerable differences in the dissociation rates of the NAIs were observed among the virus strains, the binding of laninamivir to virus NA was relatively more stable than was observed for oseltamivir and zanamivir [7].

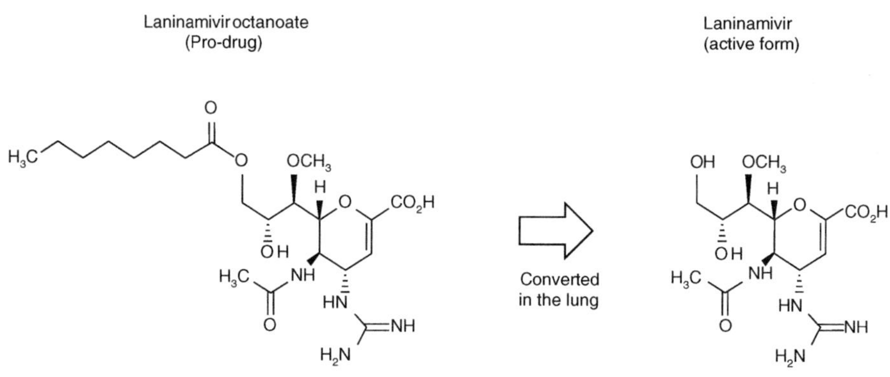

Fig. 16.1 Chemical structures of the prodrug, laninamivir octanoate (left) and the active form, laninamivir (right)

The good inhibitory activity of laninamivir to the NAs of various types of influenza virus including highly pathogenic avian influenza, H5N1 viruses and A(H1N1) pdm09, has been reported [7–10]. Thus, laninamivir is thought to be effective for all current human influenza viruses and should be effective against future strains, including those with NA subtypes other than N1 and N2.

3 **Pharmacokinetics** (Fig. 16.2)

In the pharmacokinetic study of healthy male volunteers [11], laninamivir octamic acid (prodrug) appeared in plasma immediately after inhalation, peaked at 0.5 h, and disappeared from plasma with a half-life of about 2 h. In contrast, laninamivir in its active form, detected in plasma, peaked at 4 h after inhalation, lasting for up to 144 h with a half-life of about 3 days. The cumulative urinary excretion of inhaled prodrug and laninamivir were 2.3–3.6% and 10.7–14.6% of the dose, respectively.

The lung concentration-time profiles of laninamivir and its efficacy have been investigated in mice [6, 12]. After a single intranasal administration, the lung prodrug concentration increased rapidly and then declined, with a *t*1/2 of 0.833 h (Fig. 16.2, prodrug). In contrast, the lung concentration of laninamivir increased

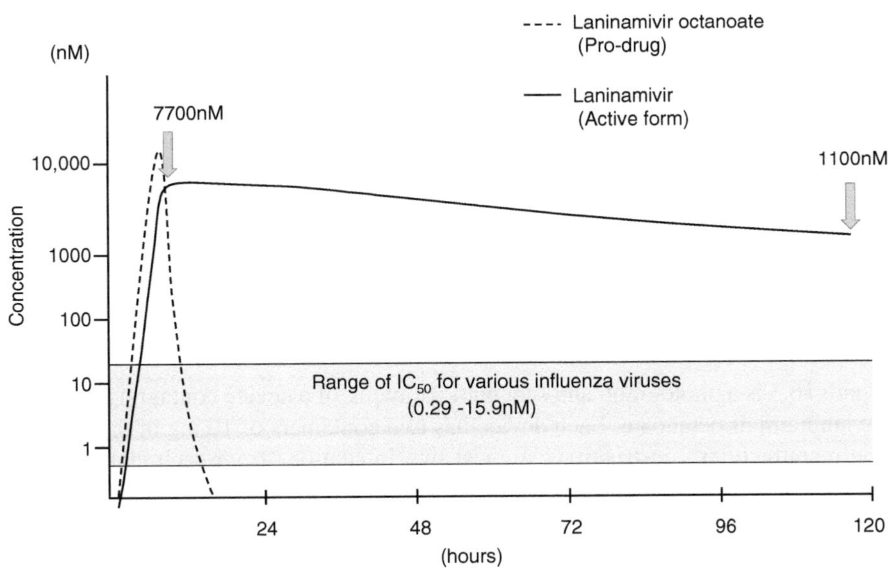

Fig. 16.2 Time course of the concentration of laninamivir in the lung after inhalation. After a single intranasal administration of prodrug, laninamivir octanoate, at a dose of 0.5 μmol/kg (0.236 mg/kg), the lung prodrug concentration increased rapidly and then declined, with a *t*1/2 of 0.833 h. In contrast, the lung concentration of laninamivir increased soon after, and it had a *t*1/2 of as long as 41.4 h. Even at 120 h post-dose, laninamivir remained in the mouse lung at a concentration of 0.915 nmol/g, equivalent to 1100 nM

soon after. At 120 h post-dose, laninamivir remained in the mouse lung at a high concentration and the expected concentration of laninamivir is much higher than its 50% inhibitory concentration (IC_{50}) for various influenza viruses (Fig. 16.2, active form). The mechanism of the long-lasting action of laninamivir has not been well elucidated. A hypothetical mechanism has been proposed that laninamivir octanoate may associate with the epithelial cells via hydrophobic moiety and move to the endoplasmic reticulum/Golgi where localized esterase hydrolyzes to generate laninamivir and retains as the active form [13]. These pharmacokinetic features, observed in mice, suggest a high concentration of laninamivir in the human lungs that lasts for at least 5 days that may work suppressively to generate low-susceptibility mutants.

4 In Vivo Efficacy

The virus titer in the lung of mice infected with influenza virus A/PR/8/34 was measured after a single intranasal administration of laninamivir octanoate, a twice daily oral administration of oseltamivir, or a twice daily intranasal administration of zanamivir [14]. The laninamivir group showed a more rapid, statistically significant reduction in virus titer compared to the oseltamivir group at a dose of 10 mg/kg. Laninamivir octanoate at a dose of 0.24 mg/kg (equivalent to 0.5 μmol/kg) showed a similar reduction in virus titer compared to zanamivir at a dose of 0.17 mg/kg (equivalent to 0.5 μmol/kg).

The prophylactic efficacy of laninamivir has also been shown in animal models [14]. Half of the mice administered laninamivir octanoate once 7 days before infection survived. The efficacy of laninamivir by a single administration was shown in a mouse infection model, including against H5N1 and H7N9 [7, 15].

5 Clinical Efficacy

Figure 16.3 is a photograph and schematic drawing of a device containing 20 mg of the laninamivir octanoate. Each device has two containers of 10 mg of dry powder. The manufacturer's instructions suggest two inhalations from each chamber. For children, four inhalations from one device are necessary, and eight inhalations from two devices are required for adults.

The results of a multicenter, double-blind, randomized control trial for adults have been reported [16]. Laninamivir octanoate was inhaled on Day 1 or oseltamivir (75 mg) was administered twice daily for 5 days. The median times to illness alleviation in the 20-mg, 40-mg laninamivir octanoate, and oseltamivir groups were 85.8, 73.0, and 73.6 h, respectively. The percentage of patients in the total and H1N1-infected subpopulations who had shed virus on day 3 was significantly lower for the 40-mg laninamivir octanoate group.

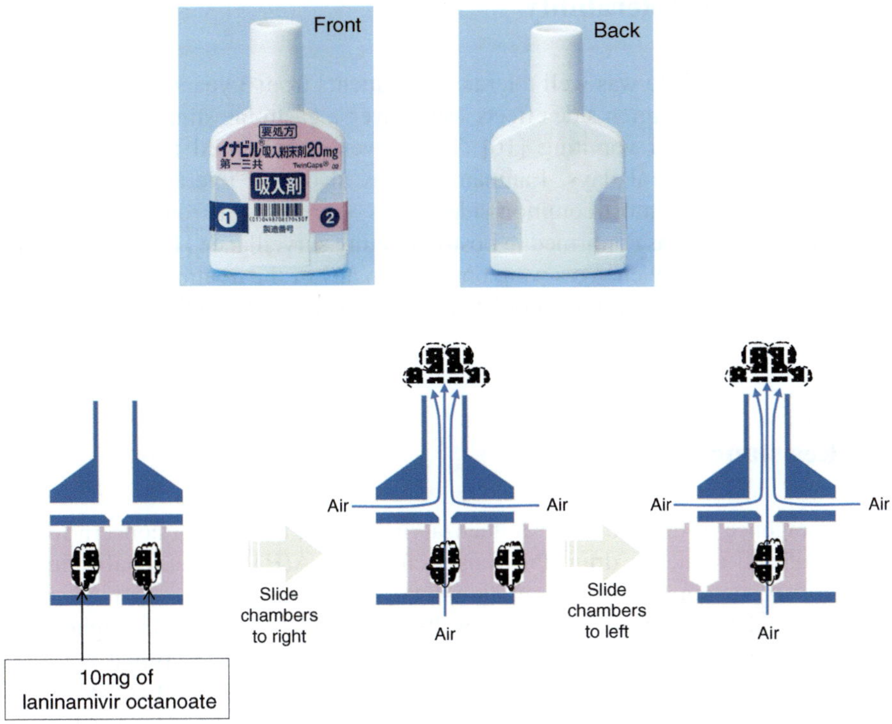

Fig. 16.3 Photograph and schematic drawing of a laninamivir octanoate inhaler. Each device has two chambers of 10 mg dry powder. The manufacturer's instructions suggest two inhalations from each chamber to insure a sufficient dose is inhaled. For children, four inhalations from one device are necessary, and eight inhalations from two devices are required of adults

Study results for pediatric patients in Japan have also been reported [17]. The median time to alleviation of influenza was shorter in the 20 and 40 mg of laninamivir octanoate groups than in the oseltamivir group (56.4, 55.4, and 87.3 h, respectively). When the cases were restricted to patients infected with H1N1 that was presumably H275Y mutated, the median times to alleviation of influenza were 44.3, 49.6, and 110.5 h, in the 20 and 40 mg of laninamivir octanoate groups and the oseltamivir group, respectively. The percentage of patients who had shed the virus on day 6 was significantly lower in the 20-mg laninamivir octanoate group than in the oseltamivir group in the H1N1-infected subpopulation.

According to a report by the Japan Physicians Association Influenza Study Group, laninamivir was used for approximately 50% of the prescriptions made by primary care physicians in the recent influenza seasons, mainly for adults. The rate of prescription to children under 3 years old was relatively low compared to oseltamivir. Duration of fever and symptoms after laninamivir octanoate inhalation was observed from the 2011–2012 to the 2016–2017 influenza seasons and constant results had been obtained, suggesting the continuing clinical effectiveness for all circulating influenza viruses, A(H1N1)pdm09, A(H3N2), and B of the Yamagata and Victoria lineages [18].

6 Safety and Tolerability

Laninamivir octanoate was well tolerated by patients from 3 years to over 70 years of age. The most common side effects were adverse gastrointestinal events such as diarrhea, nausea, and vomiting [16]. These events were mild to moderate and resolved within several days. Laninamivir was also well tolerated by pediatric patients [17], whose most common side effects were also gastrointestinal events. This safety profile was confirmed in post-marketing surveillance [19]. No clinically meaningful laboratory changes were observed in any of the treatment groups. Thus far, there have been no serious problems in the safety or tolerability of laninamivir for healthy adults or children.

7 Resistance

The emergence of drug resistant influenza viruses will be of great concern for the choice of anti-influenza drug. Previously circulated A(H1N1) seasonal influenza viruses that contain an H275Y mutation in the NA, the so-called oseltamivir resistant seasonal H1N1 strain, emerged in 2008 and quickly spread throughout the world [20]. The clinical efficacy of oseltamivir to this mutated seasonal A(H1N1) influenza virus was reduced, especially for children [21, 22]. In the 2009–2010 influenza seasons, this H275Y mutated seasonal A(H1N1) was replaced as the predominant strain by the pandemic H1N1 2009 virus, A(H1N1)pdm09. The substantial number of A(H1N1)pdm09 carried the H275Y NA mutation.

The virus with reduced susceptibility to oseltamivir and peramivir has been consistently observed in Japan [23]. The IC_{50} of the drug for a virus is a marker of virus susceptibility to NAIs. The IC_{50} of virus isolated from patients prior to anti-influenza drug administration was surveyed from the 2010–2011 season to the 2017–2018 influenza season [24]. A(H1N1)pdm09 virus with increased IC_{50} to oseltamivir was observed in around 1% of the viruses measured. However, no virus with elevated IC_{50} to laninamivir was observed (Fig. 16.4). The distribution of the IC_{50} to laninamivir was constant from the 2010–2011 season to the 2017–2018 season and no trend was found for elevation of the IC_{50}s of laninamivir. The high level of laninamivir use in Japan is not a driving force in the emergence of resistant influenza viruses or the elevation of the IC_{50}s.

8 Efficacy for Prophylaxis

Close contact with an influenza patient increases the risk of subsequent infection. In such cases, antiviral chemoprophylaxis should be considered for persons at high risk from serious illness or death related to influenza (the elderly or those with

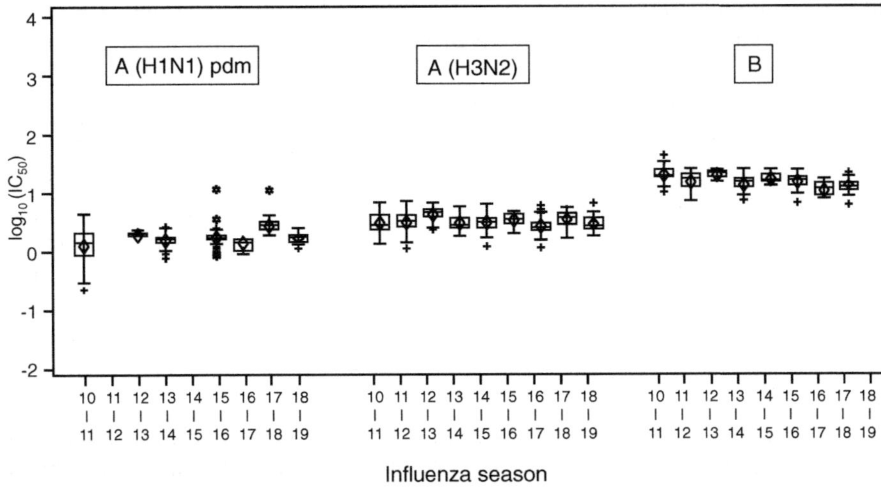

Fig. 16.4 Box and whisker plot analysis of the IC_{50}s of the four tested NAIs by virus type/subtype. The bottom and top of the box are Q1 and Q3, and the band near the middle of the box is the median. The ends of the whiskers are the lowest datum still within 1.5 IQR of the lower quartile and the highest datum still within 1.5 IQR of the upper quartile. Open diamond: arithmetic mean, +: 1.5–3 interquartile ranges from the box

chronic respiratory illness or metabolic disorders, including diabetes mellitus, chronic heart disease, or immunodeficiency) [25, 26]. A pharmacokinetics finding that a relatively high laninamivir concentration persisted in the lungs for 10 days after a single inhalation suggested the effectiveness of laninamivir octanoate inhalation for post-exposure prophylaxis. In a double-blind, multicenter, randomized, placebo-controlled study of post-exposure prophylaxis in household setting, a single administration of laninamivir octanoate, equivalent to the dose used for treatment, showed significantly reduced development of influenza compared with placebo [27]. No safety concerns have been found in the use of laninamivir octanoate for prophylaxis.

9 Conclusions

Laninamivir octanoate (a prodrug) is inhaled and hydrolyzed in the lung where it is retained in its active form for a long period of time at a high concentration, sufficient to inhibit the proliferation of influenza virus. Thus, only a single inhalation is required for the treatment of influenza. Completing treatment for influenza with an inhalation process that can be done at a single sitting would be of great benefit and convenience.

The continued clinical efficacy of laninamivir for both adults and children has been confirmed in the clinical setting including A(H1N1)pdm virus carrying the

H275Y mutation. Laninamivir octanoate has been widely used by primary care physicians in Japan and the clinical effectiveness has been shown to be quite comparable to that of oseltamivir and zanamivir. No serious problems in the safety or tolerability have been observed. Laninamivir octanoate is the first-line option for the treatment of influenza. Its effectiveness to the NAs of various influenza viruses including HPAI H5N1 viruses suggest that laninamivir is a promising candidate for use against future pandemics.

References

1. WHO. Transmission dynamics and impact of pandemic influenza A(H1N1) 2009 virus. Wkly Epidemiol Rec. 2009;46:481–4. http://www.who.int/wer/2009/wer8446.pdf.
2. Uyeki TM, Bernstein HH, Bradley JS, Englund JA, File TM, Fry AM, et al. Clinical practice guidelines by the Infectious Diseases Society of America: 2018 update on diagnosis, treatment, chemoprophylaxis, and institutional outbreak management of seasonal influenza. Clin Infect Dis. 2019;68:895–902.
3. Kawai N, Ikematsu H, Iwaki N, Maeda T, Satoh I, Hirotsu N, et al. A comparison of the effectiveness of oseltamivir for the treatment of influenza A and influenza B: a Japanese multicenter study of the 2003-2004 and 2004-2005 influenza seasons. Clin Infect Dis. 2006;43:439–44.
4. Kawai N, Ikematsu H, Iwaki N, Maeda T, Kawashima T, Hirotsu N, et al. Comparison of the effectiveness of zanamivir and oseltamivir against influenza A/H1N1, A/H3N2, and B. Clin Infect Dis. 2009;48:996–7.
5. Ikematsu H, Kawai N, Iwaki N, Kashiwagi S, Ishikawa Y, Yamaguchi H, et al. Duration of fever and other symptoms after the inhalation of laninamivir octanoate hydrate in the 2016/17 Japanese influenza season; comparison with the 2011/12 to 2015/16 seasons. J Infect Chemother. 2018;24:718–24.
6. Koyama K, Takahashi M, Oitate M, Nakai N, Takakusa H, Miura S, et al. CS-8958, a prodrug of the novel neuraminidase inhibitor R-125489, demonstrates a favorable long retention profile in the mouse respiratory tract. Antimicrob Agents Chemother. 2009;53:4845–51.
7. Kiso M, Kubo S, Ozawa M, Le QM, Nidom CA, Yamashita M, et al. Efficacy of the new neuraminidase inhibitor CS-8958 against H5N1 influenza viruses. PLoS Pathog. 2010;6:e1000786.
8. Yamashita M, Tomozawa T, Kakuta M, Tokumitsu A, Nasu H, Kubo S. CS-8958, a prodrug of the new neuraminidase inhibitor R-125489, shows long-acting anti-influenza virus activity. Antimicrob Agents Chemother. 2009;53:186–92.
9. Itoh Y, Shinya K, Kiso M, Sakoda Y, Hatta M, Muramoto Y, et al. In vitro and in vivo characterization of new swine-origin H1N1 influenza viruses. Nature. 2009;460:1021–5.
10. Kubo S, Kakuta M, Yamashita M. In vitro and in vivo effects of a long-acting anti-influenza agent CS-8958 (laninamivir octanoate, Inavir) against pandemic (H1N1) 2009 influenza viruses. Jpn J Antibiot. 2010;63:337–46.
11. Ishizuka H, Yoshiba S, Okabe H, Yoshihara K. Clinical pharmacokinetics of laninamivir, a novel long-acting neuraminidase inhibitor, after single and multiple inhaled doses of its prodrug, CS-8958, in healthy male volunteers. J Clin Pharmacol. 2010;50:1319–20.
12. Kubo S, Tokumitsu A, Tomozawa T, Kakuta M, Yamashita M. High and continuous exposure of laninamivir, an anti-influenza drug, may work suppressively to generate low-susceptibility mutants in animals. J Infect Chemother. 2012;18:69–74.
13. Yamashita M, Hirai T, Kubota K, Kubo S. Unique characteristics of long acting neuraminidase inhibitor laninamivir octanoate (CS-8958) that explains its long-lasting activity. Influenza Other Respir Viruses. 2010;5(Suppl 1):93–5.

14. Kubo S, Tomozawa T, Kakuta M, Tokumitsu A, Yamashita M. Laninamivir prodrug CS-8958, a long-acting neuraminidase inhibitor, shows superior anti-influenza virus activity after a single administration. Antimicrob Agents Chemother. 2010;54:1256–64.
15. Watanabe T, Kiso M, Fukuyama S, Nakajima N, Imai M, Yamada S, et al. Characterization of H7N9 influenza A viruses isolated from humans. Nature. 2013;501:551–5.
16. Watanabe A, Chang SC, Kim MJ, Chu DW, Ohashi Y. Long-acting neuraminidase inhibitor laninamivir octanoate versus oseltamivir for treatment of influenza: a double-blind, randomized, noninferiority clinical trial. Clin Infect Dis. 2010;51:1167–75.
17. Sugaya N, Ohashi Y. Long-acting neuraminidase inhibitor laninamivir octanoate (CS-8958) versus oseltamivir as treatment for children with influenza virus infection. Antimicrob Agents Chemother. 2010;54:2575–82.
18. Ikematsu H, Kawai N, Iwaki N, Kashiwagi S, Ishikawa Y, Yamaguchi H, Shiosakai K. Duration of fever and other symptoms after the inhalation of laninamivir octanoate hydrate in the 2016/17 Japanese influenza season; comparison with the 2011/12 to 2015/16 seasons. J Infect Chemother. 2018;24:718–24.
19. Kashiwagi S, Yoshida S, Yamaguchi H, Niwa S, Mitsui N, Tanigawa M, et al. Safety of the long-acting neuraminidase inhibitor laninamivir octanoate hydrate in post-marketing surveillance. Int J Antimicrob Agents. 2012;40:381–8.
20. Lackenby A, Hungnes O, Dudman SG, et al. Emergence of resistance to oseltamivir among influenza A(H1N1) viruses in Europe. Eur Secur. 2008;13:1–2.
21. Kawai N, Ikematsu H, Hirotsu N, Maeda T, Kawashima T, Tanaka O, et al. Clinical effectiveness of oseltamivir and zanamivir for treatment of influenza A virus subtype H1N1 with the H274Y mutation: a Japanese multicenter study of the 2007-2008 and 2008-2009 influenza seasons. Clin Infect Dis. 2009;49:1828–35.
22. Kawai N, Ikematsu H, Iwaki N, Kondou K, Hirotsu N, Kawashima T, et al. Clinical effectiveness of oseltamivir for influenza A(H1N1) virus with H274Y neuraminidase mutation. J Infect. 2009;59:207–12.
23. https://www.niid.go.jp/niid/en/influ-resist-e.html.
24. Ikematsu H, Kawai N, Chong Y, Bando T, Iwaki N, Kashiwagi S. In vitro neuraminidase inhibitory concentration (IC_{50}) of four neuraminidase inhibitors in the Japanese 2017–18 season: comparison with the 2010–11 to 2016–17 seasons. J Infect Chemother. 2019;25:649–52.
25. Harper SA, Bradley JS, Englund JA, File TM, Gravenstein S, Hayden FG, et al. Seasonal influenza in adults and children--diagnosis, treatment, chemoprophylaxis, and institutional outbreak management: clinical practice guidelines of the Infectious Diseases Society of America. Clin Infect Dis. 2009;48:1003–32.
26. Fiore AE, Fry A, Shay D, Gubareva L, Bresee JS, Uyeki TM. Antiviral agents for the treatment and chemoprophylaxis of influenza --- recommendations of the Advisory Committee on Immunization Practices (ACIP). MMWR. 2011;60:1–24.
27. Kashiwagi S, Watanabe A, Ikematsu H, Uemori M, Awamura S. Long-acting neuraminidase inhibitor laninamivir octanoate as post-exposure prophylaxis for influenza. Clin Infect Dis. 2016;63:330–7.

Chapter 17
How to Use Anti-influenza Drugs: Baloxavir Marboxil

Takeki Uehara

Abstract Baloxavir marboxil (hereafter referred to as baloxavir), the prodrug of baloxavir acid, is a novel inhibitor of the cap-dependent endonuclease in the polymerase PA subunit of the influenza virus. Taken orally as a single dose, baloxavir was first approved in Japan for the treatment of influenza in 2018. Baloxavir has activity against influenza A and B viruses including neuraminidase inhibitors (NAIs) resistant viruses. Baloxavir showed efficacy in alleviating influenza symptoms compared to placebo both in otherwise healthy adolescents and adults, and in those at higher risk of influenza complications in randomized, double-blind, placebo- and oseltamivir-controlled phase III trials without evident safety concerns. The baloxavir effectiveness in otherwise healthy pediatric patients was also shown in a single arm, non-controlled phase III trial, compared with outcomes of previous placebo-controlled pediatric studies for NAIs. Furthermore, baloxavir showed efficacy in ameliorating influenza symptoms against influenza B, more rapid reduction in influenza viral load, less frequent influenza-related complications compared to placebo or oseltamivir. The emergence of reduced susceptibility viruses to baloxavir following exposure to the drug warrants further investigation. However, currently available evidence suggests that baloxavir, with the benefits of a single dose oral regimen, provides a new and convenient therapeutic option for the treatment of influenza patients.

Keywords Baloxavir marboxil · Cap-dependent endonuclease

T. Uehara (✉)
Project Management Department, Shionogi & Co., Ltd., Osaka, Japan
e-mail: takeki.uehara@shionogi.co.jp

J. Fujita (ed.), *Influenza*, Respiratory Disease Series: Diagnostic Tools and Disease Managements, https://doi.org/10.1007/978-981-15-9109-9_17

1 Introduction

Baloxavir is an anti-influenza virus drug with a novel mechanism of action that was discovered by Shionogi & Co., Ltd. The first marketing approval of baloxavir was in Japan for the treatment of influenza A or B virus infection for treatment in children weighing 10 kg or more and in adults on 23 February 2018.

Baloxavir represents an important advance in the antiviral treatment of influenza. As demonstrated in non-clinical *in vitro* and *in vivo* studies, it is a very potent antiviral with broad activity against all types and subtypes of influenza, including influenza resistant to existing antivirals, and those with highly pathogenic and pandemic potential. Baloxavir with a simple dosing regimen (single oral dose) could also improve patient adherence.

1.1 Mechanism of Action

Baloxavir marboxil is a prodrug and is converted pre-systemically to the active form, baloxavir acid through metabolism (hydrolysis) [1]. Baloxavir selectively inhibits the cap-dependent endonuclease (CEN), an influenza virus-specific enzyme coded in the polymerase acidic (PA) protein, a subunit of the viral RNA polymerase complex, which thereby inhibits influenza virus replication (Fig. 17.1). The PA protein, a subunit of the viral RNA polymerase, is essential for virus RNA transcription, and its inhibition by baloxavir blocks virus replication. Baloxavir showed a high inhibitory potency against the influenza CEN activity in an enzymatic assay, with mean 50% inhibitory concentration (IC_{50}) values of 1.4–3.1 nM for PA protein from influenza A viruses and 4.5–8.9 nM for that from influenza B viruses [2].

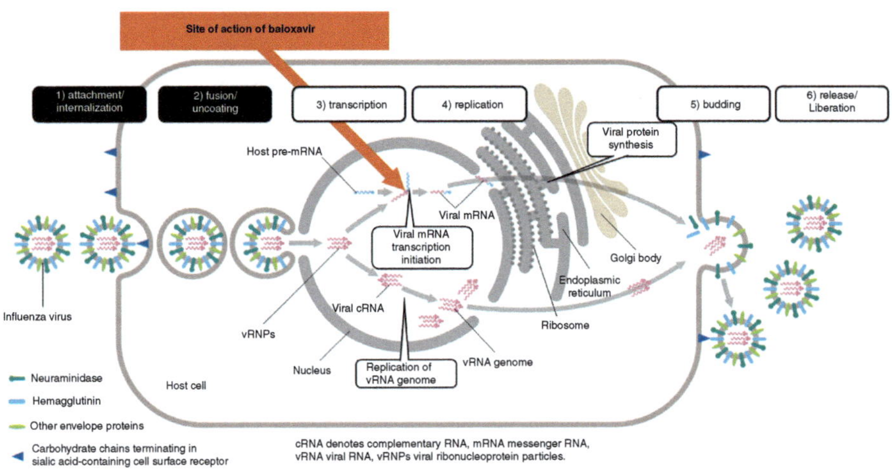

Fig. 17.1 Mechanism of action

1.2 US Indication

In the US, baloxavir is currently approved by the FDA for treatment of acute uncomplicated influenza within 2 days of illness onset in patients 12 years and older who are otherwise healthy, or at high risk of developing influenza-related complications. Baloxavir is the first drug that is FDA-approved in the United States for treatment of patients at risk for influenza complications. In 2018/2019 and 2019/2020 season, CDC recommended use of baloxavir as one of four influenza antiviral medications approved in the US [3].

Baloxavir works differently than the other currently recommended influenza antiviral drugs, which are neuraminidase inhibitors (oseltamivir, zanamivir, and peramivir). Given how frequently flu viruses change and the potential for influenza viruses to develop resistance or reduced susceptibility to one or more influenza antiviral drugs, it is good to have more options for treating flu. For example, flu viruses that are resistant to oseltamivir should still be susceptible to baloxavir. Note, however that CDC does not recommend use of baloxavir in pregnant women, breastfeeding mothers, outpatients with complicated or progressive illness, severely immunosuppressed people, or hospitalized patients because of the lack of information on use of baloxavir for these groups to date.

2 Non-clinical

A broad spectrum of baloxavir activity against influenza including A, B, C, and D was shown *in vitro* study [2, 4]. In an *in vitro* cellular assay, baloxavir inhibited replication of representative seasonal influenza A and B viruses. The 90% effective concentration (EC_{90}) was 0.63–0.95 nM against influenza A (n = 5) and 6.1 and 6.5 nM against influenza B. Similar activity was also observed against zoonotic influenza A viruses of subtypes H1N2, H5N1, H5N2, H5N6, H7N9, and H9N2, with EC_{90} values of baloxavir between 0.73 and 1.6 nM [2]. Additionally, baloxavir also showed similar activity against NAI resistant viruses in influenza A with the neuraminidase H274Y substitution [2]. These findings were confirmed in another study, using neuraminidase inhibitor-resistant variants and their parental wild-type [5].

In lethal mouse models infected with influenza A(H1N1) or B, baloxavir protected against mortality with greater antiviral reduction compared with oseltamivir [6]. In a mouse model infected with A(H7N9), baloxavir demonstrated protection against mortality to greater extent than oseltamivir [7]. Synergistic efficacy of baloxavir in combination with oseltamivir was observed on mortality compared with monotherapy in the A(H1N1) infection model [8].

3 Clinical

The efficacy of baloxavir in the treatment of acute uncomplicated influenza in adults and adolescents was demonstrated in two randomized, double-blind placebo- and oseltamivir-controlled phase III trials.

CAPSTONE-1 involved otherwise healthy outpatients aged 12–64 years within ≤48 h from influenza onset [9]. Baloxavir demonstrated significantly shorter time of symptom alleviation compared with placebo. The difference in the median time was −26.5 h between baloxavir (53.7 h) and placebo (80.2 h). Median times of symptom alleviation were similar for baloxavir (53.5 h) and oseltamivir (53.8 h) groups containing patients aged ≥20 years. Baloxavir was associated with significantly greater reductions in virus titer (1 day after dosing: over 4 log $log_{10}TCID_{50}$/mL) than placebo or oseltamivir at early time points (Fig. 17.2).

CAPSTONE-2 involved outpatients aged ≥12 years within ≤48 h from onset of influenza who were at higher risk for influenza complications (e.g., asthma or other chronic lung disease; an endocrine disorder, including diabetes mellitus; an age of ≥65 years) [10]. Baloxavir demonstrated significantly shorter time to improvement of symptom with placebo, resulted in shorter median time (73.2 h), fewer complications (2.8%), and significantly greater reductions in viral titer (3.45 $log_{10}TCID_{50}$/mL) 1 day after dosing compared to placebo (102.3 h, 10.4% and 1.20 $log_{10}TCID_{50}$/mL, respectively). CAPSTONE-2 was conducted in 2017/2018 influenza season which had an influenza B epidemic, and baloxavir also showed shorter time to improvement of symptom compared with placebo and oseltamivir in patients with influenza B virus infections associated with rapid virus titer reduction (Fig. 17.3).

The effectiveness of baloxavir in otherwise healthy children aged <12 years was also shown in an open-label trial in Japan [11] compared with outcomes of previous

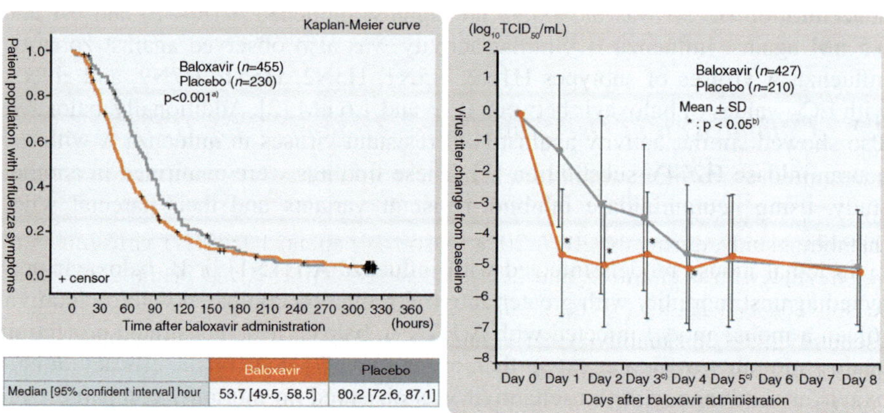

	Baloxavir	Placebo
Median [95% confident interval] hour	53.7 [49.5, 58.5]	80.2 [72.6, 87.1]

Fig. 17.2 Kaplan–Meier curves of the time to alleviation symptoms and virus titer change in CAPSTONE-1. [a] vs. placebo, generalized Wilcoxon test with stratification according to a composite symptom score (<12, ≥12) at baseline and country (Japan, USA). [b]vs. placebo, van Elteren test with stratification according to a composite symptom score (<12, ≥12) at baseline and country (Japan, USA). No multiplicity adjustments were conducted. [c]Optional visit

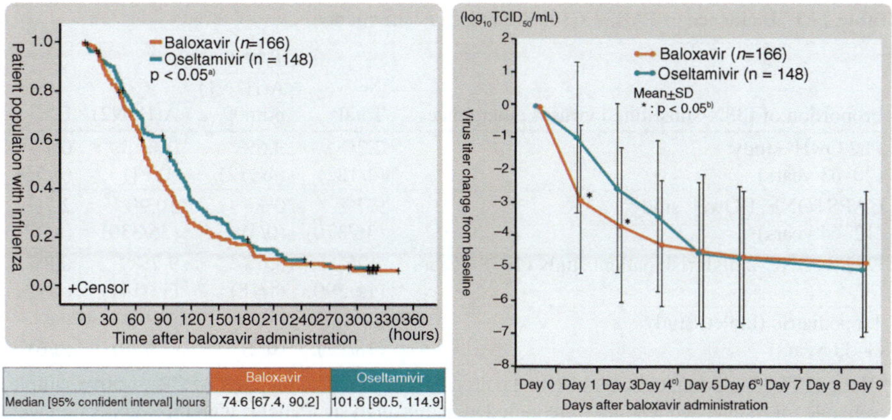

Fig. 17.3 Kaplan–Meier curves of the time to symptom improvement and virus titer change in influenza B infected patients in CAPSTONE-2. [a] vs. oseltamivir, generalized Wilcoxon test with stratification according to a composite symptom score at baseline (<15, ≥15), country (Asia, Northern hemisphere except Asia, Southern hemisphere), and pre-existing and worsened symptom. [b] vs. oseltamivir, van Elteren test with stratification according to a composite symptom score at baseline (<15, ≥15), country (Asia, Northern hemisphere except Asia, Southern hemisphere), and pre-existing and worsened symptom. No multiplicity adjustments were conducted. [c] Optional visit

pediatric studies for NAI in Japan [12, 13] and placebo-controlled studies in countries other than Japan [14–16]. The median time to illness alleviation was 44.6 h associated with similar reduction in viral titer in early time points (1 day after dosing: over 4 $\log_{10}TCID_{50}$/mL) compared to adult and adolescent trials.

4 Resistance

All antiviral treatments exert a selective pressure on a virus, which can lead to the emergence of resistant virus to the antiviral. Baloxavir treatment resulted in emergence of PA-substituted viruses with substitutions at position I38 (PA/I38X) conferring reduced susceptibility in clinical trials. Incidences of PA/I38X-substituted virus in baloxavir recipients were 2.2–23.4% in clinical trials (Table 17.1). Emergence of PA/I38X-substituted virus is thought to be affected by factors such as influenza type/subtype, patients age, or seasons (more likely in patients with A(H3N2) and in children). These factors have been shown to play a role in emergence of variants resistant to neuraminidase inhibitors, such as oseltamivir [17]. The higher incidence of resistant variants in children may reflect the immaturity of their immune systems [11]. The influenza susceptibility surveillance conducted by the National Institute of Infectious Disease in Japan also reported similar incidence in 2018/2019 season, 8.0% in patients with A(H3N2) and 2.3% in those with A(H1N1)pdm09 [18]. As eight cases of PA/I38X-substituted virus were detected in patients who had not received baloxavir, limited cases of variant virus transmission were

Table 17.1 Incidence of PA/I38X-substituted virus emergence

Proportion of I38X-substituted viruses emergence	Total[a]	Type (subtype)[b] A(H1N1) pdm09	A(H3N2)	B
Ph2 OwH[c] study (20–63 years)	2.2% (4/182)	3.6% (4/112)	0% (0/14)	0% (0/56)
CAPSTONE-1 OwH[c] study (12–64 years)	9.7% (36/370)	0% (0/4)	10.9% (36/330)	2.7% (1/37)
CAPSTONE-2 high risk patient study (12–84 years)	5.2% (15/290)	5.6% (1/18)	9.2% (13/141)	0.8% (1/131)
1st pediatric (tablet) study (1–11 years)	23.4% (18/77)	0% (0/2)	25.7% (18/70)	0% (0/6)

[a]Of the ITTI population, patients who had paired baseline and follow-up RT-PCR-positive samples evaluable for Sanger sequencing were included in this analysis. Patients with mixed infection were counted once in the total number of patients

[b]Patients with mixed infection with paired sequencing data were counted once by each virus type/subtype category

[c]OwH: otherwise-healthy

suspected. In 2019/2020 season, the risk of transmission of PA/I38X-substituted virus was limited, because surveillance reported only one case of PA/I38X-substituted A(H1N1)pdm09 virus in non-treated patient [19].

To assess the clinical impact of PA/I38X-substituted virus emergence, we had a post hoc analysis of CAPSTONE-1. The median time to symptom alleviation in baloxavir recipients with PA/I38X-substituted viruses (63.1 h) was 12 h longer than in those without PA/I38X-substituted viruses (51.0 h), but 17.2 h shorter than in the placebo recipients (80.2 h) [20]. Differences in the proportions with symptom alleviation between the baloxavir-treated subgroups observed from 24 h post-dose, but after approximately 60 h the proportions were similar between subgroups with or without PA/I38X-substituted viruses. As the virus titer in patients with PA/I38X-substituted virus began to increase around 72 h, the proportion difference of symptom alleviation arose prior to the virus increase. When the PA/I38X-substituted virus increase observed (96–120 h), the immune system is already activated and can effectively suppress viral replication. Actually, after 120 h the virus was decreasing and cleared around 192 h. It indicates that the PA/I38X-substituted virus emergence prolonged time of virus detection but does not prevent clearance. No differences in symptom scores over time were found between the baloxavir subgroups, and no late increases in score were noted in those with PA/I38X-substituted viruses (Fig. 17.4). Additionally, the same post hoc analysis of CAPSTONE-2 showed that the median time to improvement of symptom was not longer in baloxavir recipient with PA/I38X-substituted viruses (65.2 h) than those without PA/I38X-substituted viruses (76.8 h) [10]. These post hoc analyses indicate that clinical benefit of baloxavir was still observed in adults and adolescents despite the transient emergence of resistant virus.

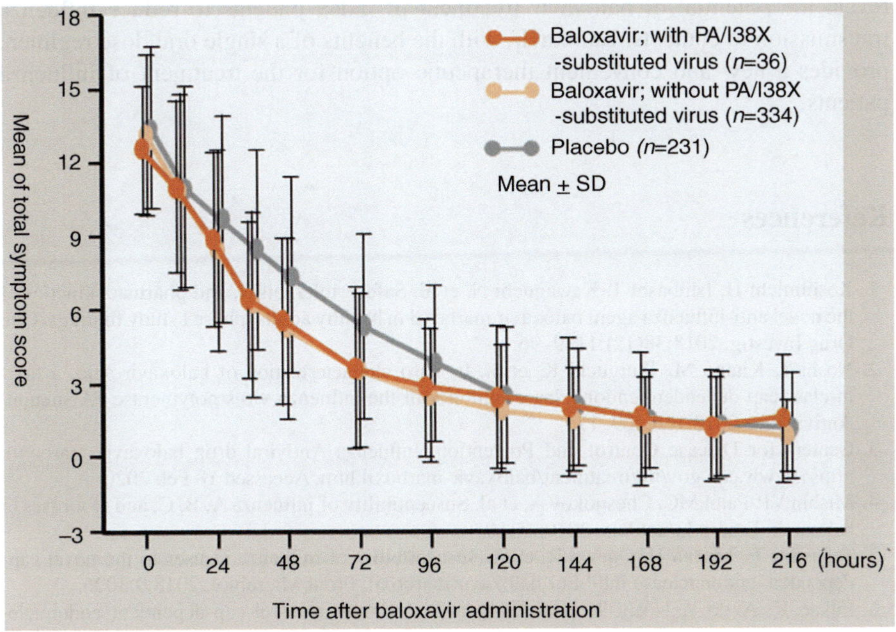

Fig. 17.4 Change of composite symptom score in baloxavir-treated patients in CAPSTONE-1

5 Conclusion

Oral baloxavir is a well-tolerated, easily administered influenza cap-dependent endonuclease inhibitor that is active against influenza A and B viruses, including variants resistant to NAIs. Baloxavir showed efficacy in alleviating influenza symptoms with rapid reduction of virus load compared to placebo both in otherwise healthy adolescents and adults, and in those at higher risk of influenza complications in randomized, double-blind, placebo- and oseltamivir-controlled phase III trials, and was without evident safety concerns. Baloxavir effectiveness was also shown in otherwise healthy pediatric patients in a single arm, non-controlled phase III trial. Furthermore, baloxavir demonstrated efficacy in ameliorating influenza symptoms against influenza B, more rapid reduction in influenza viral load, less frequent influenza-related complications compared to both placebo and oseltamivir.

Virus with PA substitution conferring reduced susceptibility was observed after baloxavir treatment; the pathogenicity and transmission fitness of these variants remain to be determined. Baloxavir's efficacy will be confirmed in ongoing trials for children (NCT03629184, NCT03653364), and hospitalized and severely ill influenza patients (NCT03684044). Also, an ongoing trial (NCT03969212) will reveal the potential of baloxavir treatment of index patients to reduce influenza transmission to contacts. Baloxavir, with the benefits of a single oral dose regimen, provides a new and convenient therapeutic option for the treatment of influenza patients.

References

1. Koshimichi H, Ishibashi T, Kawaguchi N, et al. Safety, tolerability, and pharmacokinetics of the novel anti-influenza agent baloxavir marboxil in healthy adults: phase I study findings. Clin Drug Investig. 2018;38(12):1189–96.
2. Noshi T, Kitano M, Taniguchi K, et al. In vitro characterization of baloxavir acid, a first-in-class cap-dependent endonuclease inhibitor of the influenza virus polymerase PA subunit. Antivir Res. 2018;160:109–17.
3. Centers for Disease Control and Prevention. Influenza Antiviral drug baloxavir marboxil. https://www.cdc.gov/flu/treatment/baloxavir-marboxil.htm. Accessed 18 Feb 2020.
4. Mishin VP, Patel MC, Chesnokov A, et al. Susceptibility of influenza A, B, C, and D viruses to baloxavir. Emerg Infect Dis. 2019;25:10.
5. Takashita E, Morita H, Ogawa R, et al. Susceptibility of influenza viruses to the novel cap-dependent endonuclease inhibitor baloxavir marboxil. Front Microbiol. 2018;9:3026.
6. Fukao K, Ando Y, Noshi T, et al. Baloxavir marboxil, a novel cap-dependent endonuclease inhibitor potently suppresses influenza virus replication and represents therapeutic effects in both immunocompetent and immunocompromised mouse models. PLoS One. 2019;14(5):e0217307.
7. Taniguchi K, Ando Y, Nobori H, et al. Inhibition of avian-origin influenza A(H7N9) virus by the novel cap-dependent endonuclease inhibitor baloxavir marboxil. Sci Rep. 2019;9(1):3466.
8. Fukao K, Noshi T, Yamamoto A, et al. Combination treatment with the cap-dependent endonuclease inhibitor baloxavir marboxil and a neuraminidase inhibitor in a mouse model of influenza A virus infection. J Antimicrob Chemother. 2019;74(3):654–62.
9. Hayden FG, Sugaya N, Hirotsu N, et al. Baloxavir marboxil for uncomplicated influenza in adults and adolescents. N Engl J Med. 2018;379(10):913–23.
10. Ison MG, Portsmouth S, Yoshida Y, et al. A randomized placebo-controlled phase 3 study of early treatment with baloxavir marboxil in high-risk adolescent and adult outpatients with uncomplicated influenza. Lancet Infect Dis. 2020;20(10):1204–14, accepted for publication.
11. Hirotsu N, Sakaguchi H, Sato C, et al. Baloxavir marboxil in Japanese pediatric patients with influenza: safety, pharmacokinetics and clinical and virologic outcomes. Clin Infect Dis. 2020;71(4):971–81.
12. Sugaya N, Kohno S, Ishibashi T, et al. Efficacy, safety, and pharmacokinetics of intravenous peramivir in children with 2009 pandemic H1N1 influenza A virus infection. Antimicrob Agents Chemother. 2012;56:369–77.
13. Sugaya N, Ohashi Y. Long-acting neuraminidase inhibitor laninamivir octanoate (CS-8958) versus oseltamivir as treatment for children with influenza virus infection. Antimicrob Agents Chemother. 2010;54:2575–82.
14. Whitley RJ, Hayden FG, Reisinger KS, et al. Oral oseltamivir treatment of influenza in children. Pediatr Infect Dis J. 2001;20:127–33.
15. Heinonen S, Silvennoinen H, Lehtinen P, et al. Early oseltamivir treatment of influenza in children 1-3 years of age: a randomized controlled trial. Clin Infect Dis. 2010;51:887–94.
16. Fry AM, Goswami D, Nahar K, et al. Efficacy of oseltamivir treatment started within 5 days of symptom onset to reduce influenza illness duration and virus shedding in an urban setting in Bangladesh: a randomised placebo-controlled trial. Lancet Infect Dis. 2014;14:109–18.

17. Lina B, Boucher C, Osterhaus A, et al. Five years of monitoring for the emergence of oseltamivir resistance in patients with influenza A infections in the influenza resistance information study. Influenza Other Respir Viruses. 2018;12(2):267–78.
18. National Institute Infectious Disease. Antiviral resistance surveillance in Japan. 2018/2019 influenza season. https://www.niid.go.jp/niid/en/influ-resist-e/9439-flu-r-e20200228.html. Accessed 10 Mar 2020.
19. National Institute Infectious Disease. Antiviral resistance surveillance in Japan. 2019/2020 influenza season. https://www.niid.go.jp/niid/en/influ-resist-e/9439-flu-r-e20200228.html. Accessed 10 Mar 2020.
20. Uehara T, Hayden FG, Kawaguchi K, et al. Treatment emergent influenza variant viruses with reduced baloxavir susceptibility: impact on clinical and virologic outcomes in uncomplicated influenza. J Infect Dis. 2020;221(3):346–55.

Chapter 18
How to Use Anti-influenza Drugs: Peramivir

Yutaka Saisho

Abstract Peramivir (Rapiacta®) is an intravenous neuraminidase (NA) inhibitor prescribed for the treatment of the influenza virus. A basic profile of the drug and the significance of peramivir in the treatment of influenza has been obtained in clinical studies. Of these studies, recent studies have focused on evaluating peramivir's antiviral effects early in an infection. In this chapter, noteworthy characteristics of the drug in terms of immune response to viral infection are summarized. The clinical studies showed the basic profile, pharmacokinetics, the safety of peramivir, and early antipyretic effects in parallel with the early antiviral effect. The more recent study also demonstrated a strong antiviral effect, which was a primary goal in showing possible clinical benefits, such as a virus reduction in the infection independent of the host's memory immunity due to previous infections with same type/subtype virus. It is expected that further clinical benefits, based on the rapid reduction of viral load will be demonstrated in future clinical studies.

Keywords Rapiacta · Peramivir · Influenza · Neuraminidase

1 Introduction

Up to the present, four inhibitors of the influenza virus neuraminidase (NA) have been clinically used in Japan, including oseltamivir (Tamiflu®, oral agent), zanamivir (Relenza®, inhalant), peramivir (Rapiacta®, intravenous agent), and laninamivir (Inavir®, inhalant). Since NA inhibitors have a mechanism of action that shows virustatic but not viruscidal effects, they need to be administered at the earliest possible stage of the infection, to prevent further multiplication of the virus so that the host immune response, enhanced (antigen-specific) later, can work successfully.

The original version of this chapter was revised. The correction to this chapter can be found at https://doi.org/10.1007/978-981-15-9109-9_23

Y. Saisho (✉)
Shionogi & Co., Ltd., Osaka, Japan
e-mail: yutaka.saisho@shionogi.co.jp

J. Fujita (ed.), *Influenza*, Respiratory Disease Series: Diagnostic Tools and Disease Managements, https://doi.org/10.1007/978-981-15-9109-9_18

Such effects of NA inhibitors are expected to prevent the disease from becoming severe especially in high-risk patients with immunity problems and pediatric patients with poor immunological memory due to lower exposure to previous infections (including subclinical infection).

Peramivir has facilitated the treatment of patients who had difficulty in receiving oral and inhaled agents. Moreover, evidence has been established for the early antiviral effect of peramivir in a recent study in which the virus titer, not conventionally used symptoms, was used as the primary endpoint [1]. We here present an outline of the drug profile of peramivir and description of the evidence of the early antiviral effect from recent clinical studies in the context of immunity against viral infection.

2 Indications and Dosage and Administration of Peramivir

The following are the indications for dosage and administration of peramivir on the package insert in Japan [2]. Descriptions of the mechanism of action include prevention of budding of progeny viruses from infected host cells and, in addition, a recently-proposed mechanism of action, entry inhibition [3].

- Mechanism of Action: NA inhibition[1]
- Indications: Influenza A or B virus infection
- Dosage and Administration (Japan):

Adults: The typical dose is 300 mg of peramivir administered as a single intravenous infusion over 15 min. For patients who may have complications suspecting severe (or suspected severe infections), peramivir 600 mg should be administered once daily over 15 min as a single intravenous infusion but may be repeated daily if the patient's symptoms persist. The dose may be reduced depending on the age and symptoms of the individual patient.

Children: Peramivir should be intravenously infused at a dose of 10 mg/kg (600 mg in patients whose body weight is 60 kg or more) over more than 15 min once and a repeated dose (treated for >1 day) administered in accordance with persisting symptoms in pediatric patients.

[1] NA inhibitors prevent the budding of progeny viruses from host cells by binding the active site of NA, a spiked protein on the surface of the influenza virus. Additionally, entry inhibition is a recently reported mechanism of action, in which binding of the drug to the NA active site leads to the functional imbalance of hemagglutinin and NA, interfering with viral activities on the cell surface, thereby blocking entry into the cells during the endocytosis process [3].

3 Positional Relationship of Contribution to Healing Between NA Inhibitor and Immune Response

Influenza is a self-limited disease that does not require further treatment when the host has a healthy immune response. In normal (uncomplicated) patients, the clinical effect of the drug depends on not only the drug itself but also host immunity. After the middle stage of the infection, the host immune response is primarily responsible for the healing of an influenza infection. While acquired immunity, produced against the causative virus during the end stage of the infection (IgG antibody generated by long-lived plasmablasts), is highly specific to the virus antigen, immunity already acquired during past infections (including subclinical infections), against viruses with similar antigenicity to the causative virus (i.e., memory immunity) plays an active role until start of antigen-specific IgG generation. In the acute to middle stage, antibodies produced by short-lived plasmablasts derived from memory B cells contribute to the body's defense against the virus and keep symptoms mild if the hosts are infected. Since influenza epidemics occur every year, memory immunity based on common epitope among the previous viruses seems to play a critical role in influenza treatment.

In this light, NA inhibitors should be used in the early stage of infection, during which immunity against the causative virus is immature (Fig. 18.1) [4]. It is known that the use of NA inhibitors in the early stage of infection (within 48 h of onset)

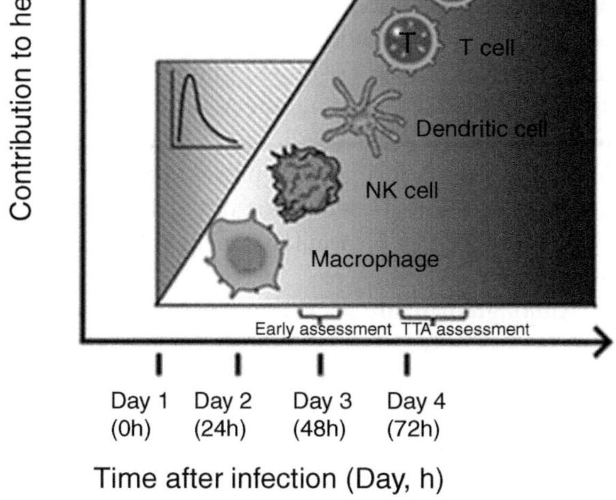

Fig. 18.1 Positional relationship showing the contribution to healing between NA inhibitor and the immune response. Diagrams express a rough magnitude of efficacious activity. *NA* neuraminidase, *NK* natural killer. TTA* time to alleviation symptom

reduces the duration of an influenza illness by approximately 1 day, as compared with an untreated case [5].

The early effect in the initial stage of infection is also important from an antiviral viewpoint as well. Specifically, as severe conditions such as encephalopathy triggered by influenza are known to be caused by an overreaction of the innate immune system to rapidly growing viruses (or tissue-derived substances damaged by viruses) [6], it is considered necessary to control viral load in the initial stage of infection to prevent critical illness especially in at-risk patients.

In addition, from a public health perspective, the early antiviral effect also is a noteworthy profile of the drug in that influenza transmission can be suppressed by reducing viral load, during which patients are most likely to transmit the virus to others.

4 End Points for Anti-influenza Treatments

The duration of influenza illness based on self-assessed seven influenza symptoms used as an endpoint, when evaluating NA inhibitors, is approximately 60–80 h (median) in normal adult patients. This includes the period between antigen presentation and when antigen-specific immune systems start acting. Innate immune responses start acting immediately upon the entry of a virus into the host body. Once the antigen is presented, acquired immune systems start getting ready and become enhanced (antigen-specific). As a rough indication, B cells aggregate to form a germinal center on Day 4 [7], and IgG antibody titers begin increasing on Days 5–6 [8], during which antigen-specific acquired immune responses begin establishing. Therefore, the above end point based on symptom alleviation seems to be an add-on evaluation indicator mainly affected by immune activity, and not appropriate for evaluating the effect of the drug [4]. The contribution of immune responses to healing is therefore important, considering that significant involvement of host immunity improves symptoms from the middle to the end stages of infection, resulting in healing. Memory immunity [9] also plays a full role from the initial stage through to the establishment of acquired immunity. In addition to that, onset prevention by split vaccines (i.e., vaccine effect) was not activated in patients without previous influenza infection history but activated with previous infection [10], so memory immunity also contributes to prevention of disease onset, severe disease, and to healing. Therefore, a calculation of the duration of an influenza illness based on the symptoms may not be a suitable method to evaluate the effect of the drug appropriately [4].

Although there are some arguments that NA inhibitors reduce the duration of an infection by only 1 day, as compared with no treatment, a decrease in the virus load still makes sense, considering that it takes time for immune cells to differentiate regardless of volume and types of antigens. On the assumption that the duration of influenza illness is used as the end point, between-group comparison of drug efficacy seems to be difficult, especially in high-risk patients because the effect of immunity differs by individual [4]. On the other hand, pediatric patients seem to be a suitable population for drug evaluation, in whom the effect of the drug on healing will be more significant, because they have fewer experiences of influenza virus and thus less effect from memory immune responses.

5 Pharmacokinetics and Safety of Peramivir

The pharmacokinetics of peramivir are characterized by rapid, systemic exposure, in the sense that all the active sites of NA are thoroughly covered. When intravenous peramivir is administered at the typical dose of 300 mg, it is distributed to the whole body, rapidly reaching an approximately 100-fold blood concentration and 15-fold AUC greater than the active metabolite of oseltamivir [4]. Therefore, peramivir can treat influenza infection with a single dose because the early, high exposure completely covers the active site of NA before viral proliferation and remains in place for a long time without being dissociated [11]. Concentrations of distributed peramivir at infected sites (nasal cavity, pharynx) and IC_{50} of epidemic viruses during the clinical trial period (2007–2010) are summarized in Fig. 18.2 [4]. Even in 2008–2009, when an oseltamivir-resistant strain with NA/H275Y mutation spread, the concentration of distributed peramivir at the upper airway was a hundredfold greater than the IC_{50} of the epidemic virus, which shows possibility that peramivir can be effective on even oseltamivir-resistant viruses [4]. The high exposure may be a safety concern, but it is known that peramivir remains in the body for as short a time as 3 h or less, and that excess peramivir which has not bound to the NA of the affected cells is rapidly excreted in urine [4]. In fact, peramivir of the usual dose of

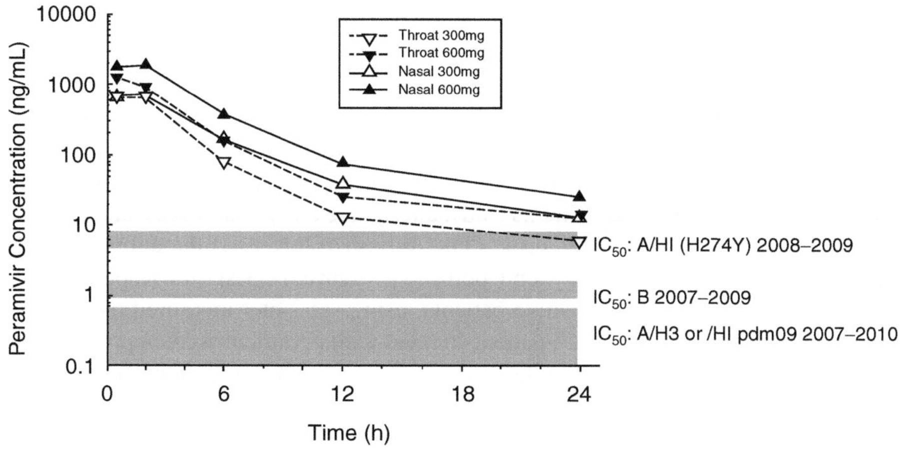

Fig. 18.2 Relationship between peramivir concentration at infected sites in humans (estimated (The value for 300 mg was the average of the 200 and 400 mg treatment groups, and for 600 mg was the average of the 400 and 800 mg treatment groups)) and IC50 of the epidemic strain

300 mg was shown to be significantly safer compared with oseltamivir, when considering adverse reactions in the phase 3 study. (Incidence of adverse reactions: 14% [peramivir 300 mg group] vs. 20% [oseltamivir group] [12])

6 Clinical Study Results of Peramivir

The following are results of two phase 3 studies of peramivir (randomized, double-blind, comparative study with oseltamivir [12] and a randomized, double-blind study in high-risk patients [13]). Although peramivir was found to be comparable to oseltamivir with regard to symptom alleviation, it significantly improved viral titers 24 h after administration (600 mg) and antipyretic effect (both 300 and 600 mg) compared with oseltamivir, demonstrating the earlier effectiveness of peramivir [12]. Moreover, there was no difference in the duration of the illness between the 300 mg group and 600 mg group in both studies [5] (peramivir groups in both studies showed significant improvement over placebo). Meanwhile, in a study with high-risk patients [13], the duration of the influenza illness was significantly reduced in the 600 mg group compared with the 300 mg group (repeat doses were allowed in both groups) in high-risk patients, even though, as described above, demonstrating the between-group difference is normally difficult to obtain. The results suggest that multiple administrations of the 600 mg dose (73% of the accumulated patients received peramivir over 2 days) acted to supplement the effect of the patients' otherwise-reduced immune responses, leading to earlier healing.

7 Recent Clinical Studies of Peramivir

We recently reported the result of a collaborative clinical study with Hirotsu Medical Clinic (Kawasaki, Japan), in which we randomized 123 children aged 4–12 years with influenza infection into groups receiving 1 of 4 NA inhibitors, to evaluate the relationship between viral dynamics and clinical effects. While the duration of the influenza illness is generally employed as the primary end point in clinical trials to indicate efficacy of treatment, in this study, alternative end points were established to verify the characteristics of the drug. Our study therefore used the antiviral effect (i.e., virus titer) as the primary end point [1]. Figure 18.3 shows Kaplan–Meier curves for the rate of virus-positive patients, using viral titer measured dairy as an indicator. As shown in Fig. 18.3, patients treated with peramivir were approximately 80% viral negative in 2 days after the start of treatment, whereas patients treated with other drugs remained approximately 40–60% viral positive, and peramivir exhibited an antiviral effect significantly earlier compared to oseltamivir (adjusted $p = 0.035$) [1]. Although no correlation was found between the antiviral effect and the secondary end points of the duration of influenza illness and duration of fever, the rate of relapse was lower with peramivir than with other drugs numerically (Table 18.1).

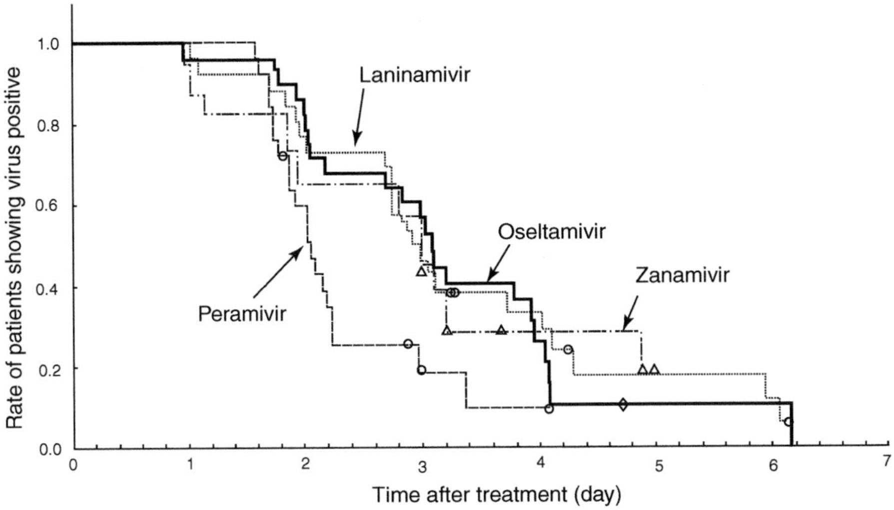

Fig. 18.3 Rate of pediatric patients testing positive for the virus after treatment with four different NA inhibitors

Table 18.1 Rate of patients with relapse

		Treatment group			
		Peramivir	Oseltamivir	Zanamivir	Laninamivir
Virus recurrence	*n*	19	15	11	17
	No. of cases of recurrence	2	5	3	4
	Rate of recurrence	10.5%	33.3%	27.3%	23.5%
	95% CI for recurrence	(1.3, 33.1)	(11.8, 61.6)	(6.0, 61.0)	(6.8, 49.9)
Fever recurrence	*n*	27	29	25	30
	No. of cases of recurrence	0	0	2	5
	Rate of recurrence	0.0%	0.0%	8.0%	16.7%
	95% CI for recurrence	(0.0, 12.8)	(0.0, 11.9)	(1.0, 26.0)	(5.6, 34.7)

Next, this study found a correlation between virologic effects and memory immune responses (antibody titer at baseline) [10]. Presumably, the higher the baseline antibody titer, the lower the likelihood of influenza onset. Although the correlation between the baseline antibody titer and prevention of illness is unknown, we usually have no opportunity to investigate healthy conditions including subclinical infections which do not become symptomatic. And at a hospital, a high correlation was detected between viral dynamics and baseline antibody titer in influenza-infected patients [10]. In particular, when viral dynamics are examined for a history of previous infection with the same type or subtype of the influenza virus, patients with a history, and thus assumed to have memory immunity are shown to have greater virus reduction (Fig. 18.4) [10]. Evaluating the antiviral effect of four anti-influenza drugs by the presence of a history of previous infection with A/H3N2

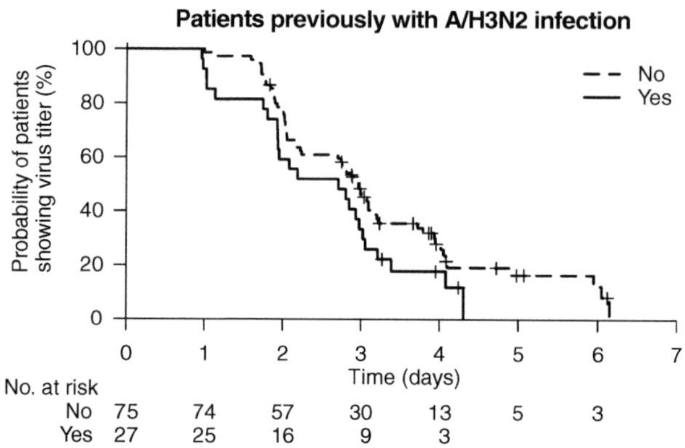

Fig. 18.4 Kaplan–Meier curves of the time from the start of treatment with neuraminidase inhibitor to the influenza virus titer showing clear, according to the presence (bold line) or absence (dotted line) of previous influenza A/H3N2 infection in the patient, adjusted hazard ratio:1.72, $P = 0.03$

virus revealed that while two types of NA inhibitors (oseltamivir and zanamivir) had a memory immunity-dependent antiviral effect [10], peramivir had equivalent virus reduction [1, 10] regardless of the presence of memory immunity (Fig. 18.5) [10]. It may be considered that peramivir maximizes the antiviral effect at the early stage of infection, which is a requirement for effective antiviral agents.

8 Possible Clinical Benefit of Early Antiviral Effect

If an early antiviral effect is demonstrated, but does not improve the duration of influenza illness, the question arises about what the benefit is to patients. Although an early antiviral effect is assumed to prevent severe disease, it is difficult to show the relationship between the preventive effect and difference in antiviral effect among NA inhibitors, even in retrospective database research, where a considerable number of samples can be researched. This is because there are fewer patients with severe disease in Japan, where early treatment is usually available, unlike some other countries, and because patient characteristics can vary the drugs used (for example, peramivir is more commonly used for patients with severe disease).

On the other hand, the early antiviral effect is considered to play a role in the control of transmission within the population, and this leads to public health benefits. The evidence of this transmission control has been shown in a recent study [14]. We also conducted a prospective observational study jointly with Hirotsu Medical Clinic over six seasons (2010–2016) to evaluate household transmission depending on drugs and viral types/subtypes, in 3400 patients with adjustment for other influential factors such as age [14]. The results can be found in Part 1. Transmission of influenza virus in home, in this journal.

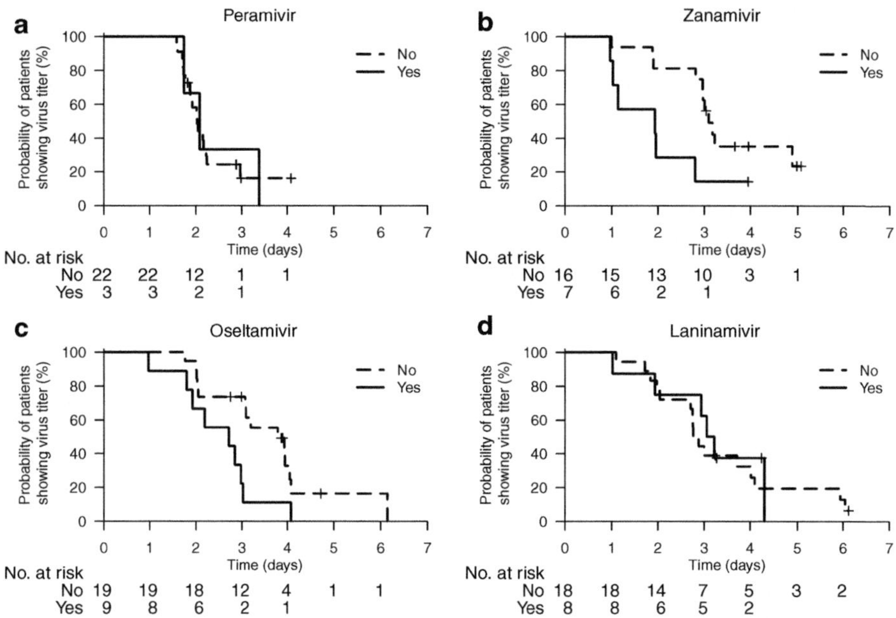

Fig. 18.5 Kaplan–Meier curves of the time from the start of treatment with a neuraminidase inhibitor to the influenza virus titer showing clear, according to the presence (bold line) or absence (dotted line) of previous influenza A/H3N2 infection: (**a**) peramivir, (**b**) zanamivir, (**c**) oseltamivir, or (**d**) laninamivir. (adjusted hazard ratio, *P*) = (**a**) (5.24, 0.09), (**b**) (3.22, 0.03), (**c**) (3.43, 0.01), (**d**) (0.80, 0.68)

In current clinical practice, NA inhibitors (other than peramivir) are used for post-exposure prophylaxis to prevent the onset of the disease in, for example, family members in close contact with the patient, and health care professionals. However, when it comes to prophylaxis, NA inhibitors are used in multiple patients prior to disease onset. Additionally, if treating affected already infected patients can reduce transmission to others, it is reasonable from both health, economic and infection control perspectives.

9 Conclusion

The noteworthy characteristic of peramivir in terms of aiding the immune response to viral infection is summarized. Hopefully, early administration of NA inhibitors brings both clinical benefits, with regard to obtaining the additional benefits as well as a rapid improvement in symptoms. It is desirable to select NA inhibitors so that the advantage of the early antiviral effect can be utilized.

References

1. Hirotsu N, Saisho Y, Hasegawa ST. Clinical and virologic effects of four neuraminidase inhibitors in influenza A virus-infected children (aged 4–12 years): an open-label, randomized study in Japan. Expert Rev Anti-Infect Ther. 2018;16:173–82. https://doi.org/10.1080/14787210.2018.1421945. Epub 2017.
2. Rapiacta® for intravenous drip infusion. Package insert 2019. The Pharmaceuticals and Medical Devices Agency(PMDA), Tokyo, Japan. https://www.info.pmda.go.jp/go/pack/6250405A1032_1_11/. (Updated Sep 2019. Accessed 6 Mar 2020).
3. Sakai T, Nishimura SI, Naito T, Saito M. Influenza A virus hemagglutinin and neuraminidase act as novel motile machinery. Sci Rep. 2017;7:45043. https://doi.org/10.1038/srep45043.
4. Saisho Y, Ishibashi T, Fukuyama H, Fukase H, Shimada J. Pharmacokinetics and safety of intravenous peramivir, neuraminidase inhibitor of influenza virus in healthy Japanese subjects. Antivir Ther. 2017;22:313–23.
5. Kohno S, Kida H, Mizuguchi M, Shimada J, S-021812 Clinical Study Group. Efficacy and safety of intravenous peramivir for treatment of seasonal influenza virus infection. Antimicrob Agents Chemother. 2010;54:4568.
6. Imai Y, Sakuma T, Imai H, Kuba K, Fujiwara S. Potential cellular targets for anti-influenza drug development. Cell Immunol Immunother. 2016;1:1–12.
7. Kitano M, Moriyama S, Ando Y, Hikida M, Mori Y, Kurosaki T, Okada T. Bcl6 protein expression shapes pre-germinal center Bcell dynamics and follicular helper T cell heterogeneity. Immunity. 2011;34:961–72.
8. Sato M, Hashimoto K, Kawasaki Y, Hosoya M. Immune response after a single intravenous peramivir administration in children with influenza. Antivir Ther. 2018;23:435–41. https://doi.org/10.3851/IMP3222.
9. Alt F W., Honjo T, Radbruch A, Reth Ml. Molecular Biology of B Cells. 2015.
10. Hirotsu N, Saisho Y, Hasegawa T, Kitano M, Shishido T. Antibody dynamics in Japanese paediatric patients with influenza A infection treated with neuraminidase inhibitors in a randomised trial. Sci Rep. 2019;9:11891. https://doi.org/10.1038/s41598-019-47884-0.
11. Bantia S, Upshaw R, Babu YS. Charaterization of the binding affinities of peramivir and oseltamivir carboxylate to the neuraminidase enzyme. Antivir Res. 2011;91:288–91.
12. Kohno S, Yen MY, Cheong HJ, Hirotsu N, Ishida T, Kadota J, Mizuguchi M, Kida H, Shimada J, S-021812 Clinical Study Group. Phase III randomized, double-blind study comparing single-dose intravenous peramivir with oral oseltamivir in patients with seasonal influenza virus infection. Antimicrob Agents Chemother. 2011;55:5267.
13. Kohno S, Kida H, Mizuguchi M, Hirotsu N, Ishida T, Kadota J, Shimada J, S-021812 Clinical Study Group. Intravenous peramivir for treatment of influenza A and B virus infection in high-risk patients. Antimicrob Agents Chemother. 2011;55:2803.
14. Hirotsu N, Saisho Y, Hasegawa T. The effect of neuraminidase inhibitors on household transmission in Japanese patients with influenza A and B infection: a prospective, observational study. Influenza Other Respir Viruses. 2019;13:123–32. . Published online 2018 Dec 28. https://doi.org/10.1111/irv.12590.

Chapter 19
Prophylaxis of Influenza Viral Transmission: What Is the Current Prophylaxis?

Nobuhiro Asai and Hiroshige Mikamo

Abstract Influenza is one of the most common infectious diseases that, in humans, is caused by influenza A or influenza B viruses. Typically characterized by annual seasonal epidemics, sporadic pandemic outbreaks involve influenza A virus strains of zoonotic origin. Flu could cause morbidity and mortality with high socioeconomic burden in Japan as well as worldwide. We focus on why the mortality rate of flu-related disease in Japan is the lowest in the world. Still, we worry that the Japanese government will go against a global trend of an influenza strategy. In practice, for influenza, antiviral agents newly developed such as peramivir and baloxavir are focused and are expected to achieve better results. We should be aware that the best strategy for flu is preventive methods such as vaccination or personal protective measures. Non-pharmaceutical interventions like school/work closure or adjusting room humidity are also effective methods for limiting a flu epidemic. This article describes the trends and topics regarding influenza preventive strategies.

Keywords Vaccine · Personal protective measurement · Hand hygiene · Medical mask · School/work closure · Respiratory etiquette · Post-exposure prophylaxis

1 Introduction

Flu (Influenza) is one of the most common infections caused by the influenza virus, and the WHO estimates that annual epidemics of influenza result in ~1 billion infections, three to five million cases of severe illness and 300,000–500,000 deaths

N. Asai · H. Mikamo (✉)
Department of Clinical Infectious Diseases, Aichi Medical University Hospital, Nagakute, Aichi, Japan

Department of Infection Control and Prevention, Aichi Medical University Hospital, Nagakute, Aichi, Japan
e-mail: mikamo@aichi-med-u.ac.jp

J. Fujita (ed.), *Influenza*, Respiratory Disease Series: Diagnostic Tools and Disease Managements, https://doi.org/10.1007/978-981-15-9109-9_19

worldwide [1] and could cause morbidity and mortality resulting in a high socioeconomic burden [1, 2]. Prevention is the best strategy for seasonal flu, and vaccination is the most important preventive method. Unfortunately, the Japanese government shifted to not focusing on the prevention in 1994, stopping a universal vaccination among school children [3]. This resulted in the increase in the number of influenza patients in Japan. Additionally, in recent years, tourists coming from foreign countries [4] and many Japanese visiting outside Japan brought about an epidemic flu in the summer season in Japan [5]. It is time to reconsider the preventive strategy for flu.

2 Epidemiology of Seasonal Influenza

The prevalence of influenza in Japan is the same as in the United States. However, the mortality rate of influenza-related diseases in the USA is 20 times higher than in Japan [6]. Although there must be advocates and detractors for neuraminidase inhibitors (NAIs) overuse for flu patients in Japan [7], the early intervention could contribute to favorable outcomes among the patients. During the 2009 pandemic season, the mortality rate of flu in Japan was the lowest in the world as shown in Table 19.1 [8]. This result may be attributable to the specific aspects in the Japanese healthcare system. Japanese medical service is based on a free-access policy just as in the USA. Medical cost could be covered by a universal public insurance system for every citizen as well as for inhabitants from abroad. On the other hand, an increase in costs and efforts among medical staffs should be a social problem to be improved.

3 Prophylaxis

3.1 Vaccine

One of the best ways for influenza prevention is flu vaccination. Flu vaccine prevents millions of illnesses and flu-related doctor's visits each year. In the USA, during 2017–2018, flu vaccination prevented an estimated 6.2 million influenza

Table 19.1 Comparison with the mortality rate caused by influenza A (H1N1 pdm2009) virus

Country	USA	Canada	Mexico	Australia	UK	Singapore
Number of deaths	12,000	428	1111	191	457	257
Death rate (%)	3.96	1.92	1.05	0.95	0.76	0.57
Country	Korea	France	NZ	Thai	Germany	Japan
Number of deaths	257	312	20	225	255	199
Death rate (%)	0.53	0.51	0.46	0.35	0.91	0.16

USA United States of America, *UK* United Kingdom, *NZ* New Zealand, *Thai* Thailand
Death rate was mortality rate per 100,000 population

illnesses, 3.2 million influenza-associated medical visits, 91,000 influenza-associated hospitalizations, and 5700 influenza-associated deaths [9]. During influenza season, flu vaccine has been shown to reduce the occurrence of influenza by 40–60% [9]. Because these rates are lower than those of other vaccines, some people do not get immunized. Japan started a universal vaccination program for schoolchildren in the 1960s. The Japanese Government abandoned this program in 1994 due to lack of evidence for flu prevention in schoolchildren [3]. Consequently, a significant inverse correlation between the vaccine coverage rates and both the number of class cancellation days and absentee rates were confirmed. In addition, some documented that the universal vaccination program associated with substantial indirect mortality benefits in seniors [10, 11]. After abandoning the vaccination program in 1994, the vaccination rates in Japan have been declining year by year and is about 50%, which is lower compared with other OECD member countries in 2003 [12]. Unfortunately, this trend completely goes against the global trend for flu prevention. The Japanese should be aware of the importance of flu prevention by vaccination.

Currently available influenza vaccines licensed for use are Trivalent Inactivated Influenza Vaccine (TIV, IIV3), Quadrivalent Inactivated Influenza Vaccine (QIV, IIV4), Trivalent Live Attenuated Influenza Vaccine (LAIV3), and Quadrivalent Live Attenuated Influenza Vaccine (LAIV4). LAIVs are administered intranasally, while IIVs are given by intramuscular or subcutaneous injection [13–15]. Despite that vaccination strategies vary in many countries, vaccination programs were more effective than no vaccination in all studies to prevent a substantial number of hospitalizations and death by influenza virus infections. A systematic review of influenza vaccination showed that it is cost-effective in a range of countries as well as in subgroups of patients such as the elderly or pregnant women, even though most of the studies were performed in high-income countries [15].

3.2 *Personal Protective Measures (PPMs)*

Personal protective measures (PPMs) such as the use of a medical mask, frequent hand hygiene, and respiratory etiquette are not costly and easy to implement for everyone, and should be recommended. Doing all of these is important and effective for flu prevention.

3.2.1 Hand Hygiene

Flu viruses can survive on hand surfaces for 24 h and are capable of being transmitted to hands resulting in infections. Additionally, it is well known that a hand sanitizer can kill flu virus on surfaces rapidly [16]. Because of this, hand hygiene against flu seems effective. In fact, some report that a recent meta-analysis showed that regular hand hygiene was significantly protective in preventing a pandemic influenza infection, while facemask use alone was not significantly protective [17–20].

On the other hand, Wong et al. documented that a combination of hand hygiene and facemask was found to have a significant protective effect, but hand hygiene alone did not have any significant effect in preventing influenza infection [19].

3.2.2 Medical Mask

Some studies and a meta-analysis found a non-significant protective effect of medical mask for flu prevention [17, 21, 22]. These results could be explained due to the heterogeneities of the studies of medical masks. In a sub-analysis, if the RCTs and cohorts were pooled with case-control study, the heterogeneity decreased and a significant protective effect was confirmed [20]. In the studies, participants were not instructed to wear protective devices. Lewis et al. reported that medical masks are not inferior to N95 respiratory mask in preventing influenza [23]. This suggests that wearing a face mask properly is more important than what kind of mask is worn. There might be errors of mask fitting in the study. We suggest that a medical mask is one of the most useful methods in preventing flu because it is easy to handle and is inexpensive. Both hand hygiene and medical mask are useful protective methods and should be used simultaneously.

3.2.3 Respiratory Etiquette

Respiratory etiquette is a manner and a method which is cost free and everyone can do it for prevention of infectious respiratory diseases such as influenza infections or tuberculosis. Although no studies were found which evaluated the effectiveness of respiratory etiquette, a recent study reported that the efficacy of cough-etiquette maneuvers in blocking aerosol particles revealed that it did not block the release or dispersion of aerosol droplets, particularly those smaller than 1 μm in size [24]. Particles of influenza virus are extremely small, measuring 0.08–0.12 μm in diameter [25] and could be carried in small droplets by cough or sneezing. Nevertheless, cough etiquette could reduce droplets, leading to prevention for influenza infection. While people in the United States and in European countries seldom wear a facemask, Japanese tend to wear one to protect from infectious droplets for any infectious disease [26]. This habitual difference may reflect the difference of the culture.

3.3 Others

School/Work closure, another non-pharmaceutical measurement, appeared effective for preventing an influenza epidemic, even though socioeconomic damage should be considered [27]. In addition, adjusting room humidification is an effective non-pharmaceutical intervention to reduce influenza virus infection, as compared to a control room [28].

3.4 Post-exposure Prophylaxis (PEP)

Four NAIs, oseltamivir (Tamiflu1, Chugai Pharmaceutical Co., Ltd., Tokyo, Japan), zanamivir (Relenza1, GlaxoSmithKline plc, London, United Kingdom), laninamivir (Inavir1, Daiichi Sankyo Co., Ltd., Tokyo, Japan), and peramivir (Rapiactal, Shionogi & Co., Ltd., Osaka, Japan) are available for clinical use in Japan [29]. These NAIs are prescribed to seven to eight million influenza-infected outpatients and inpatients annually [29]. Previous surveillance of influenza reported that Japan is the greatest oseltamivir consumer, which consumed 75% of prescriptions worldwide during 1999–2007, followed by 20% in the United States [7]. As above mentioned in **20.2**, this phenomenon in Japan could be influenced by the Japanese medical service which allows free access to every medical institute and coverage by a universal public insurance system. In addition, Japanese people tend to favor being prescribed medication when they visit a doctor.

There are three types of NAIs (oseltamivir, zanamivir, and laninamivir) which are available for post-exposure prophylaxis (PEP) for influenza. While appropriate PEP by oseltamivir is cost-effective in the healthcare setting [30, 31], some are overconfident as to its effectiveness for prevention of influenza. The primary prevention for flu is a standard protective strategy such as medical mask and hand hygiene. The second one is vaccination. The order of priority of PEP is low and healthy people basically do not need medication of PEP for influenza. However, it is generally believed that patients at high risk for severe flu complications (as shown in Table 19.2) who have been exposed to flu patients should receive antiviral agents as PEP. Likewise, people residing in group living facilities such as a nursing home or a long-term facility should be considered to receive PEP for influenza when they are exposed to flu patients, since an outbreak of influenza could easily occur in such facilities [32, 33].

Table 19.2 Patients at high risk of severe flu complications

• People older than 65 years
• Heart disease (chronic heart failure, coronary artery disease)
• Chronic pulmonary diseases (chronic obstructive pulmonary disease, asthma)
• Diabetes mellitus
• Malignancy
• Kidney disorder
• Immune system diseases
• Neurologic and neurodevelopment conditions
• Pregnant woman
• Obese (body mass index of 40 or higher)

4 Conclusion

The best strategy of influenza is prevention. PPMs are inexpensive and easy to implement for everyone. We do recommend that a combination of vaccine and all of PPMs such as hand hygiene, use of facemasks, and respiratory etiquette are the best strategies for flu prevention. On a case by case basis, work/school close should be performed even if the socioeconomic burden would be high. PEP should be considered for patients with high risk for severe influenza complications, or for those living in specific facilities such as nursing homes.

Acknowledgments We are grateful for the diligent and thorough critical reading of our manuscript by Dr. Yoshihiro Ohkuni, Chief Physician, Taiyo and Mr. John Wocher, Executive Vice President and Director, International Affairs/International Patient Services, Kameda Medical Center (Japan).

References

1. Krammer F, Smith GJD, Fouchier RAM, Peiris M, Kedzierska K, Doherty PC, et al. Influenza. Nat Rev Dis Primers. 2018;4:3.
2. Murakami Y, Hashimoto S, Kawado M, Ohta A, Taniguchi K, Sunagawa T, et al. Estimated number of patients with influenza A(H1)pdm09, or other viral types, from 2010 to 2014 in Japan. PLoS One. 2016;11:e0146520. Epub 2016/01/20.
3. Kawai S, Nanri S, Ban E, Inokuchi M, Tanaka T, Tokumura M, et al. Influenza vaccination of schoolchildren and influenza outbreaks in a school. Clin Infect Dis. 2011;53:130–6.
4. Japan National Tourism Organization website. <https://www.jnto.go.jp/jpn/statistics/data_info_listing/index.html>. Accessed 11 Feb 2020.
5. Sunagawa S, Iha Y, Taira K, Okano S, Kinjo T, Higa F, et al. An epidemiological analysis of summer influenza epidemics in Okinawa. Intern Med. 2016;55:3579–84.
6. Centers for Disease control and Prevention: Weekly U.S. Influenza Surveillance Report. <https://www.cdc.gov/flu/weekly/index.htm>. Accessed 16 Feb 2020.
7. Tashiro M, McKimm-Breschkin JL, Saito T, Klimov A, Macken C, Zambon M, et al. Surveillance for neuraminidase-inhibitor-resistant influenza viruses in Japan, 1996-2007. Antivir Ther. 2009;14:751–61.
8. The Japanese Association for Infectious Diseases. Homepage. <http://www.kansensho.or.jp/modules/en/index.php?content_id=1>. Accessed 16 Feb 2020.
9. Centers for Disease control and Prevention: estimated influenza illnesses, medical visits, and hospitalizations averted by vaccination. <https://www.cdc.gov/flu/vaccines-work/burden-averted.htm>. Accessed 25 Dec 2019.
10. Charu V, Viboud C, Simonsen L, Sturm-Ramirez K, Shinjoh M, Chowell G, et al. Influenza-related mortality trends in Japanese and American seniors: evidence for the indirect mortality benefits of vaccinating school children. PLoS One. 2011;6:e26282.
11. Sugaya N, Takeuchi Y. Mass vaccination of schoolchildren against influenza and its impact on the influenza-associated mortality rate among children in Japan. Clin Infect Dis. 2005;41:939–47.
12. Organization for Economic Co-operation and Development. Influenza vaccination rates. OECD website. <http://www.oecd.org/>. Accessed 11 Feb 2020.
13. Raviotta JM, Smith KJ, DePasse J, Brown ST, Shim E, Nowalk MP, et al. Cost-effectiveness and public health effect of influenza vaccine strategies for US elderly adults. J Am Geriatr Soc. 2016;64:2126–31.

14. Centers for Disease Control and Prevention NCfIaRDN. United States, 2016–2017 influenza season. 2017. www.cdc.gov/flu/protect/vaccine/vaccines.htm.
15. D'Angiolella LS, Lafranconi A, Cortesi PA, Rota S, Cesana G, Mantovani LG. Costs and effectiveness of influenza vaccination: a systematic review. Ann Ist Super Sanita. 2018;54:49–57.
16. Boyce JM, Pittet D, Healthcare Infection Control Practices Advisory Committee, HICPAC/SHEA/APIC/IDSA Hand Hygiene Task Force. Guideline for hand hygiene in health-care settings. Recommendations of the Healthcare Infection Control Practices Advisory Committee and the HICPAC/SHEA/APIC/IDSA Hand Hygiene Task Force. Society for Healthcare Epidemiology of America/Association for Professionals in Infection Control/Infectious Diseases Society of America. MMWR Recomm Rep. 2002;51:1–45.
17. Suess T, Remschmidt C, Schink S, Luchtenberg M, Haas W, Krause G, et al. Facemasks and intensified hand hygiene in a German household trial during the 2009/2010 influenza A(H1N1) pandemic: adherence and tolerability in children and adults. Epidemiol Infect. 2011;139:1895–901.
18. Azor-Martínez E, Gonzalez-Jimenez Y, Seijas-Vazquez ML, Cobos-Carrascosa E, Santisteban-Martínez J, Martínez-López JM, et al. The impact of common infections on school absenteeism during an academic year. Am J Infect Control. 2014;42:632–7.
19. Wong VW, Cowling BJ, Aiello AE. Hand hygiene and risk of influenza virus infections in the community: a systematic review and meta-analysis. Epidemiol Infect. 2014;142:922–32.
20. Saunders-Hastings P, Crispo JAG, Sikora L, Krewski D. Effectiveness of personal protective measures in reducing pandemic influenza transmission: a systematic review and meta-analysis. Epidemics. 2017;20:1–20.
21. Cheng VC, Tai JW, Wong LM, Chan JF, Li IW, To KK, et al. Prevention of nosocomial transmission of swine-origin pandemic influenza virus A/H1N1 by infection control bundle. J Hosp Infect. 2010;74:271–7.
22. Jaeger JL, Patel M, Dharan N, Hancock K, Meites E, Mattson C, et al. Transmission of 2009 pandemic influenza A (H1N1) virus among healthcare personnel-Southern California, 2009. Infect Control Hosp Epidemiol. 2011;32:1149–57.
23. Radonovich LJ Jr, Simberkoff MS, Bessesen MT, Brown AC, Cummings DAT, Gaydos CA, et al. N95 respirators vs medical masks for preventing influenza among health care personnel: a randomized clinical trial. JAMA. 2019;322:824–33.
24. Zayas G, Chiang MC, Wong E, MacDonald F, Lange CF, Senthilselvan A, et al. Effectiveness of cough etiquette maneuvers in disrupting the chain of transmission of infectious respiratory diseases. BMC Public Health. 2013;13:811.
25. Stanley WM. The size of influenza virus. J Exp Med. 1944;79:267–83.
26. Hayashi K, Sunayama M, Imai M. A survey of preventive and coping behavior for influenza among foreigners staying in the Kaga area of Ishikawa prefecture. Ishikawa J Nurs. 2014;11:83–92. In Japanese.
27. Bin Nafisah S, Alamery AH, Al Nafesa A, Aleid B, Brazanji NA. School closure during novel influenza: a systematic review. J Infect Public Health. 2018;11:657–61.
28. Reiman JM, Das B, Sindberg GM, Urban MD, Hammerlund MEM, Lee HB, et al. Humidity as a non-pharmaceutical intervention for influenza A. PLoS One. 2018;13:e0204337.
29. Zaraket H, Saito R. Japanese surveillance systems and treatment for influenza. Curr Treat Options Infect Dis. 2016;8:311–28.
30. Hagihara M, Kato Y, Kurumiya A, Takahashi T, Sakata M, Kato H, et al. The prophylactic effect of anti-influenza agents for an influenza outbreak in a university hospital. Intern Med. 2018;57:497–501.
31. Vecoso LVZ, Silva MT, Resende MR, da Silva EN, Galvao TF. Cost-effectiveness analysis of influenza A (H1N1) chemoprophylaxis in Brazil. Front Pharmacol. 2019;10:945.
32. Parker R, Loewen N, Skowronski D. Experience with oseltamivir in the control of a nursing home influenza B outbreak. Can Commun Dis Rep. 2001;27:37–40.
33. Booy R, Lindley RI, Dwyer DE, Yin JK, Heron LG, Moffatt CR, et al. Treating and preventing influenza in aged care facilities: a cluster randomised controlled trial. PLoS One. 2012;7:e46509.

Part VI
Topics

Chapter 20
Influenza Vaccine Efficacy/Effectiveness: With Special Reference to Current Epidemiological Methodology

Wakaba Fukushima

Abstract Influenza vaccination is the primary strategy for preventing influenza and its severe complications. Because influenza vaccine has been used internationally for a long time, the methodologies used to evaluate influenza vaccine efficacy/effectiveness have also changed over time. In this chapter, we provide an overview of the epidemiological approaches to assess influenza vaccine efficacy/effectiveness with reference to the fundamental principles of epidemiology. We also highlight the test-negative design, a modified case-control study, because it is currently the most desirable epidemiological approach for evaluating influenza vaccine effectiveness against laboratory-confirmed influenza. Evidence of vaccine effectiveness from test-negative design studies, global trends to monitor vaccine effectiveness using test-negative design across the seasons, inherent limitations of the current influenza vaccines in terms of effectiveness, available influenza vaccines worldwide, as well as future perspectives for vaccine development are also discussed.

Keywords Influenza vaccine · Efficacy · Effectiveness · Test-negative design Vaccine development

1 Introduction

Influenza is an acute febrile respiratory disease that causes annual epidemics, typically in the winter in Japan. Persons who are known to be at higher risk for severe complications from influenza include young children, the elderly, persons with

W. Fukushima (✉)
Department of Public Health, Osaka City University Graduate School of Medicine, Osaka, Japan

Research Center for Infectious Disease Sciences, Osaka City University Graduate School of Medicine, Osaka, Japan
e-mail: wakaba@med.osaka-cu.ac.jp

J. Fujita (ed.), *Influenza*, Respiratory Disease Series: Diagnostic Tools and Disease Managements, https://doi.org/10.1007/978-981-15-9109-9_20

certain chronic diseases, and pregnant women [1]. Vaccination is the primary strategy for preventing influenza and its severe complications. In the United States, annual influenza vaccination is recommended for all persons aged ≥6 months who do not have contraindications [1]. In Europe, those requiring vaccination vary between countries: the elderly and pregnant women are generally recommended to have the vaccination, whereas guidelines for children and adolescents are variable [2]. In Japan, influenza vaccination is designated as a national immunization program under the Immunization Law. The target population are those aged ≥65 years and those aged 60–64 years with a specific underlying disease. Otherwise vaccination is performed voluntarily.

Influenza vaccine has been used internationally for a long time. Methodologies to evaluate influenza vaccine efficacy/effectiveness have also changed over time. In this chapter, we provide an overview of influenza vaccine efficacy/effectiveness with special reference to current epidemiological methodology. Available vaccines overseas and future perspectives for vaccine development are also discussed.

2 Epidemiological Approaches to Evaluate Influenza Vaccine Efficacy/Effectiveness

The best evidence for vaccine efficacy (i.e., the extent of disease prevention under experimental settings) in a human population comes from randomized controlled trials (RCTs). The study subjects are randomly allocated (or assigned) by the investigator to either the vaccine group or the comparison group, and they are followed up over time to estimate the vaccine efficacy by comparing the incidence of influenza between the groups (Fig. 20.1a). However, RCTs cannot be performed ethically in populations for which vaccination is already recommended. Additionally, even an excellent RCT only provides time-, place-, and subject-specific observations and not conclusive findings because (1) the characteristics of circulating influenza viruses differ by time and place; (2) the proportion of patients with pre-existing immunity differ by time, place, and age group; and (3) vaccine strains differ by time (i.e., season) [3]. In this context, observational studies that assess vaccine effectiveness (i.e., the extent of disease prevention under non-experimental settings) also provide important evidence in a real-world setting. Hereafter, both "vaccine efficacy" and "vaccine effectiveness" are referred to as "VE."

Among observational epidemiological studies, cohort studies have the highest level of evidence for evaluating VE. The concept of calculating VE in cohort studies is the same as that for RCTs as shown in Fig. 20.1a. However, when the outcome measure is defined as laboratory-confirmed influenza, it is difficult for cohort studies to achieve an "equal intensity" of follow-up because of a disparity in healthcare-seeking attitudes between vaccinated and unvaccinated subjects. Furthermore, it is difficult for the investigators to provide active surveillance for outcome confirmation throughout the influenza season (e.g., all subjects are periodically surveyed for

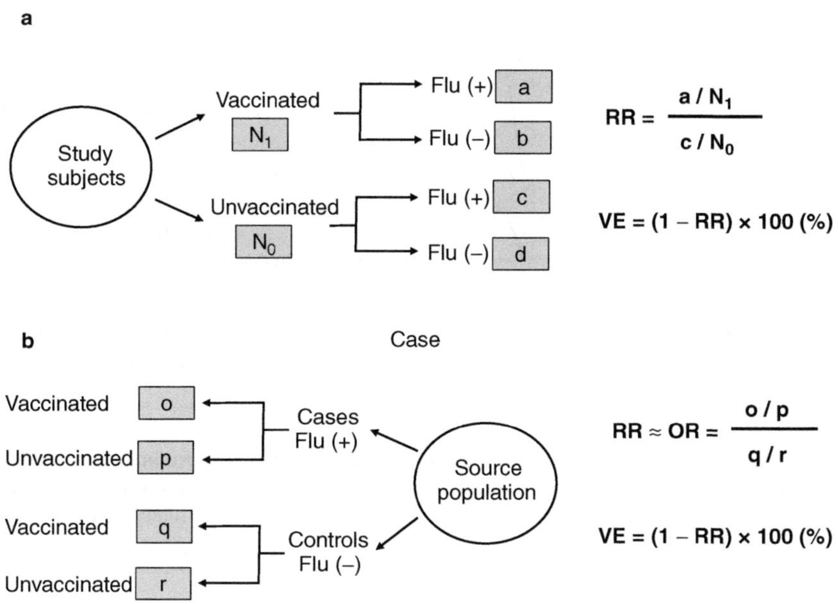

Fig. 20.1 Outline of intervention trials (including RCTs) or cohort studies (**a**), and case-control studies (**b**). General equations to calculate the vaccine effectiveness/efficacy are shown. *RCT* randomized controlled trial, *Flu* influenza, *RR* relative risk, *VE* vaccine effectiveness/efficacy, *OR* odds ratio. In epidemiological terms, the VE corresponds to the "prevented fraction" defined as "the extent to the relative reduction of attack rate among vaccinated in comparison to unvaccinated." In other words, it refers to "the proportion of those who would not become influenza positive among those who actually became influenza positive without vaccination, if they had been vaccinated"

the pre-defined influenza-like illness (ILI); once ILI onset is recognized, the researchers have to visit the subjects' homes to obtain a respiratory specimen for influenza diagnosis) [3].

The test-negative design, which was introduced in the mid-2000s, is currently the most desirable epidemiological approach for evaluating influenza VE against laboratory-confirmed influenza. Because the test-negative design is a modified case-control study, the starting point is not identifying vaccinated and unvaccinated individuals, but identifying subjects with the disease (cases) and without the disease (controls). Although VE cannot be directly calculated as shown in Fig. 20.1a, the odds ratio (i.e., ratio of the odds of vaccinations among cases to the odds among controls) can be calculated as an approximation of the relative risk (Fig. 20.1b). In the test-negative design, cases are defined as those with "positive test results for influenza" and controls are defined as those with "negative test results for influenza," both of which are selected from eligible subjects who visited a clinic or hospital due to pre-defined ILI during the influenza season (Fig. 20.2). A notable feature of the test-negative design is its ability to minimize the misclassification of diseases and confounding by healthcare-seeking attitudes when evaluating

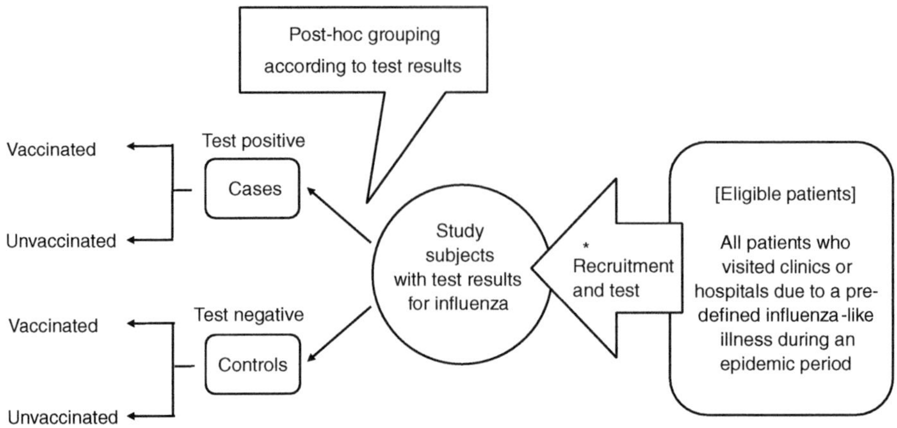

Fig. 20.2 Adapted from [3, 7]. Outline of the test-negative design to evaluate influenza vaccine effectiveness. To avoid selection bias occurring at "recruitment and test" (asterisk), all eligible patients (or a subset of eligible patients selected in a random or systematic manner) have to be recruited in the study and all study subjects (or a subset who are selected in a random or systematic manner) have to be tested

influenza VE. Because patients with ILI are expected to visit a clinic or hospital immediately after the onset of symptoms, healthcare-seeking attitude is likely to be similar between cases and controls, which can solve potential problems in cohort studies. The detailed principles of this method have been discussed elsewhere [3–7].

3 Influenza Vaccine Effectiveness Using the Test-Negative Design

After the introduction of the test-negative design, evidence has accumulated regarding influenza VE. A meta-analysis showed that inactivated influenza vaccines provide moderate protection against laboratory-confirmed influenza [8]. They summarized 56 studies that recruited patients (largely outpatients) on the basis of pre-defined ILI criteria and used real-time reverse-transcriptase polymerase chain reaction (PCR) to confirm the influenza diagnosis. Pooled VE according to type or subtype is shown in Table 20.1. A low VE for A(H3N2) was indicated (33%), which might be partly explained by the antigenic mismatch between vaccine strains and circulating strains due to egg-induced mutations in hemagglutinin, particularly for the A(H3N2) strain [9, 10]. However, additional analyses showed that the VE for A(H3N2) was still low (33%) in a season where the vaccine strains and circulating strains were antigenically similar. Furthermore, the VE for A(H3N2) was not uniform across age groups: the highest estimate was for pediatric age groups (43%, 95% confidence interval [CI]: 28–55%) and the lowest estimate was for older adults (24%, 95% CI: −6% to 45%). Recent reports have emphasized the importance of

Table 20.1 Pooled vaccine effectiveness against laboratory-confirmed influenza: results from a meta-analysis that summarized 56 test-negative design studies, published between January 2004 and March 2015 [8]

	Vaccine type	Pooled VE (%)	Pooled standard error	VE estimates (*n*)	*p* value for heterogeneity	I^2
Without age restriction						
Type B	Seasonal	54% (46–61)	0.083	36	<0.0001	61.3
H3N2	Seasonal	33% (26–39)	0.050	34	0.005	44.4
H1N1pdm09	Seasonal	61% (57–65)	0.048	29	0.783	0.0
H1N1pdm09	Monovalent	73% (61–81)	0.188	10	0.217	31.4
H1N1 (pre-2009)	Seasonal	67% (29–85)	0.397	5	0.093	57.6

VE vaccine effectiveness. Data in parentheses are the 95% confidence intervals

factors other than antigenic match in the interpretation of influenza VE [11, 12]. Another meta-analysis focused on preventing hospitalization with influenza-associated conditions and summarized 30 test-negative design studies [13]. Overall, the pooled VE showed moderate protection against laboratory-confirmed hospitalized influenza among adults (Table 20.2).

In several developed countries, test-negative designs are currently used to "monitor" influenza VE across the seasons, in which influenza is diagnosed by PCR to estimate VE against laboratory-confirmed influenza [14–18]. These studies have contributed to the Global Influenza Vaccine Effectiveness (GIVE) Collaboration, which is led by the World Health Organization (WHO) and provided VE data at a WHO meeting where seasonal influenza vaccine strains were recommended [19]. Factors considered at the meeting included worldwide seasonal influenza activity, antigenic and genetic characteristics of recent circulating influenza viruses, proliferation of candidate vaccine strains, and results from the antigenic analysis of candidate vaccine strains by hemagglutination inhibition assay using post-infection ferret antisera or post-vaccination human antisera. The data from the GIVE Collaboration, although confidential, will be an important indicator of VE in a human population during the latest season.

4 Inherent Limitations of the Current Influenza Vaccine in Terms of Effectiveness

Evidence shows that when inactivated influenza vaccines function at full ability, they reduce the risk of developing influenza by about two-thirds (i.e., VE of 60–70%) and the risk of hospitalization from influenza by about half (i.e., VE of 50%).

Table 20.2 Pooled vaccine effectiveness against laboratory-confirmed hospitalized influenza among adults: results from a meta-analysis that summarized 30 test-negative design studies, published between January 2009 and November 2016 [13]

	Pooled VE (%)	95%CI	Number of VE estimates	*p*-value for heterogeneity	I^2
Any influenza					
All adults	41	34;48	24	0.005	48
Under 65 years	51	44;58	14	0.762	0
65 years and above	37	30;44	21	0.137	26
A(H1N1)pdm09					
All adults	48	37;59	7	0.212	28
Under 65 years	55	34;76	3	0.948	0
65 years and above	54	26;82	5	0.026	64
A(H3N2)					
All adults	37	24;50	9	0.021	56
Under 65 years	50	38;62	7	0.775	0
65 years and above	33	21;45	11	0.137	33
B					
All adults	38	23;53	5	0.640	0
Under 65 years	45	8;81	2	0.907	0
65 years and above	31	11;51	4	0.812	0

VE vaccine effectiveness, *CI* confidence interval

Although this is "statistically significant," the public may consider this unsatisfactory. Reasons why the influenza vaccine is "not very effective" include the following: (1) despite yearly vaccine strain selections being based on the best scientific knowledge available, the extent of antigenic matching between the vaccine strains and the epidemic strains varies; (2) the inactivated influenza vaccine induces limited immunity due to its structure and administration route; and (3) from an epidemiological point of view, the most notable limitation is that even unvaccinated persons have a degree of immunity, because influenza epidemics occur every year. As shown in Fig. 20.1a, VE is theoretically the "contrast" of the disease incidence between unvaccinated and vaccinated individuals: the greater the difference, the higher the VE. For influenza, the presence of immunity among unvaccinated individuals results in a lower influenza incidence, which makes it difficult to obtain a clear VE. To achieve a high VE, an influenza vaccine should reduce disease incidence among those vaccinated to almost "zero," which is challenging.

5 Trends of Influenza Vaccination Worldwide and Future Perspectives

To date, all influenza vaccines currently approved in Japan are quadrivalent, standard-dose, egg-based, unadjuvanted, split-virus inactivated vaccines that contain 15 μg of hemagglutinin (HA) per vaccine virus in a 0.5-mL dose. However, a variety of influenza vaccines are available overseas. Table 20.3 shows the influenza vaccines available in the 2019–2020 season in the USA [1]. The use of a cell culture-based inactivated vaccine and recombinant vaccine can avoid antigenic changes of vaccine strain during egg adaptation. A high-dose trivalent influenza vaccine (containing 60 μg of hemagglutinin per vaccine virus) and adjuvanted influenza vaccine, both of which are approved for the elderly and currently available as a trivalent formulation, can improve immunogenicity. Live attenuated influenza vaccine (LAIV) is administered intranasally and induces mucosal immune responses (secretory IgA) in the upper respiratory tract, which theoretically prevent "infection" by influenza.

Global efforts are also ongoing to achieve a more effective influenza vaccine. Vaccines under development in Japan include an intranasal inactivated influenza vaccine that incorporates the advantages of classical inactivated vaccines and LAIV [20], and a whole virus inactivated influenza vaccine that can provide similar

Table 20.3 Influenza vaccines—United States, 2019–2020 influenza season [1]

Trade name (manufacturer)	Age indication	Route
IIV4–standard dose–egg based		
Afluria Quadrivalent (Seqirus)	≥6 months	IM
Fluarix Quadrivalent (GlaxoSmithKline)	≥6 months	IM
FluLaval Quadrivalent (GlaxoSmithKline)	≥6 months	IM
Fluzone Quadrivalent (Sanofi Pasteur)	≥6 months	IM
IIV4–standard dose–cell culture based		
Flucelvax Quadrivalent (Seqirus)	≥4 years	IM
IIV3–high dose–egg based		
Fluzone high-dose (Sanofi Pasteur)	≥65 years	IM
IIV3–standard dose–egg based with MF59 adjuvant		
Fluad (Seqirus)	≥65 years	IM
RIV4–recombinant HA		
Flublok Quadrivalent (Sanofi Pasteur)	≥18 years	IM
LAIV4–egg based		
FluMist Quadrivalent (AstraZeneca)	2–49 years	NAS

IIV3 inactivated influenza vaccine, trivalent; *IIV4* inactivated influenza vaccine, quadrivalent; *RIV4* recombinant influenza vaccine, quadrivalent; *LAIV4* live attenuated influenza vaccine, quadrivalent; *IM* intramuscular; *NAS* intranasal

immunity to the natural infection by retaining the original virus structure and components [21]. Overseas, a universal influenza vaccine that provides broad-spectrum cross-protection against influenza A and B by inducing humoral and cell-mediated immunity is under development [22].

6 Conclusions

Influenza vaccines are often criticized, probably because their VE is difficult to understand. However, it should be recognized that most infectious diseases do not have available vaccines. For influenza, it is important to make the best use of the current vaccines, while developing more effective vaccines. Given the current globalization, the benefit of influenza vaccine as a primary prevention tool should be better understood.

References

1. Grohskopf LA, Alyanak E, Broder KR, Walter EB, Fry AM, Jernigan DB. Prevention and control of seasonal influenza with vaccines: recommendations of the Advisory Committee on Immunization Practices—United States, 2019-20 influenza season. MMWR Recomm Rep. 2019;68(3):1–21.
2. Sheikh S, Biundo E, Courcier S, Damm O, Launay O, Maes E, et al. A report on the status of vaccination in Europe. Vaccine. 2018;36(33):4979–92.
3. Fukushima W, Hirota Y. Basic principles of test-negative design in evaluating influenza vaccine effectiveness. Vaccine. 2017;35(36):4796–800.
4. Jackson ML, Nelson JC. The test-negative design for estimating influenza vaccine effectiveness. Vaccine. 2013;31(17):2165–8.
5. Foppa IM, Haber M, Ferdinands JM, Shay DK. The case test-negative design for studies of the effectiveness of influenza vaccine. Vaccine. 2013;31(30):3104–9.
6. Sullivan SG, Tchetgen Tchetgen EJ, Cowling BJ. Theoretical basis of the test-negative study design for assessment of influenza vaccine effectiveness. Am J Epidemiol. 2016;184(5):345–53.
7. Ozasa K, Fukushima W. Commentary: test negative design reduces confounding by healthcare-seeking attitude in case-control studies. J Epidemiol. 2019;29(8):279–81.
8. Belongia EA, Simpson MD, King JP, Sundaram ME, Kelley NS, Osterholm MT, et al. Variable influenza vaccine effectiveness by subtype: a systematic review and meta-analysis of test-negative design studies. Lancet Infect Dis. 2016;16(8):942–51.
9. Skowronski DM, Janjua NZ, De Serres G, Sabaiduc S, Eshaghi A, Dickinson JA, et al. Low 2012-13 influenza vaccine effectiveness associated with mutation in the egg-adapted H3N2 vaccine strain not antigenic drift in circulating viruses. PLoS One. 2014;9(3):e92153.
10. Zost SJ, Parkhouse K, Gumina ME, Kim K, Diaz Perez S, Wilson PC, et al. Contemporary H3N2 influenza viruses have a glycosylation site that alters binding of antibodies elicited by egg-adapted vaccine strains. Proc Natl Acad Sci U S A. 2017;114(47):12578–83.
11. Skowronski DM, Chambers C, Sabaiduc S, De Serres G, Winter AL, Dickinson JA, et al. Beyond antigenic match: possible agent-host and immuno-epidemiological influences on influenza vaccine effectiveness during the 2015-2016 season in Canada. J Infect Dis. 2017;216(12):1487–500.

12. Cobey S, Gouma S, Parkhouse K, Chambers BS, Ertl HC, Schmader KE, et al. Poor immunogenicity, not vaccine strain egg adaptation, may explain the low H3N2 influenza vaccine effectiveness in 2012-2013. Clin Infect Dis. 2018;67(3):327–33.
13. Rondy M, El Omeiri N, Thompson MG, Levêque A, Moren A, Sullivan SG. Effectiveness of influenza vaccines in preventing severe influenza illness among adults: a systematic review and meta-analysis of test-negative design case-control studies. J Infect. 2017;75(5):381–94.
14. Ferdinands JM, Fry AM, Reynolds S, Petrie J, Flannery B, Jackson ML, et al. Intraseason waning of influenza vaccine protection: evidence from the US Influenza Vaccine Effectiveness Network, 2011-12 through 2014-15. Clin Infect Dis. 2017;64(5):544–50.
15. Kissling E, Rondy M, I-MOVE/I-MOVE+ study team. Early 2016/17 vaccine effectiveness estimates against influenza A(H3N2): I-MOVE multicentre case control studies at primary care and hospital levels in Europe. Euro Surveill. 2017;22(7):30464.
16. Skowronski DM, Zou M, Sabaiduc S, Murti M, Olsha R, Dickinson JA, et al. Interim estimates of 2019/20 vaccine effectiveness during early-season co-circulation of influenza A and B viruses, Canada, February 2020. Euro Surveill. 2020;25(7):2000103.
17. Cheng AC, Holmes M, Dwyer DE, Senanayake S, Cooley L, Irving LB, et al. Influenza epidemiology in patients admitted to sentinel Australian hospitals in 2018: the Influenza Complications Alert Network (FluCAN). Commun Dis Intell (2018). 2019:43. https://pubmed.ncbi.nlm.nih.gov/31738866/
18. Fukushima W, Morikawa S, Matsumoto K, Fujioka M, Matsushita T, Kubota M, et al. for the study group funded by Ministry of Health, Labour and Welfare Japan. Influenza vaccine effectiveness in Japanese children under 6 years: summary findings from 2013-14 season to 2017-18 season. IASR. 2019;40:194–5. [in Japanese]
19. World Health Organization. Recommended composition of influenza virus vaccines for use in the 2020-2021 northern hemisphere influenza season. https://www.who.int/influenza/vaccines/virus/recommendations/202002_recommendation.pdf?ua=1. Accessed 28 Mar 2020.
20. Sano K, Ainai A, Suzuki T, Hasegawa H. Intranasal inactivated influenza vaccines for the prevention of seasonal influenza epidemics. Expert Rev Vaccines. 2018;17(8):687–96.
21. Sekiya T, Mifsud EJ, Ohno M, Nomura N, Sasada M, Fujikura D, et al. Inactivated whole virus particle vaccine with potent immunogenicity and limited IL-6 induction is ideal for influenza. Vaccine. 2019;37(15):2158–66.
22. Pleguezuelos O, Dille J, de Groen S, Oftung F, Niesters HGM, Islam MA, et al. Immunogenicity, safety, and efficacy of a standalone universal influenza vaccine, FLU-v, in healthy adults: a randomized clinical trial. Ann Intern Med. 2020;172(7):453–62.

Chapter 21
The New Anti-influenza Drug Baloxavir Marboxil: Can Influenza Viruses with Reduced Susceptibility to Baloxavir Maintain Viral Fitness?

Masaki Imai and Yoshihiro Kawaoka

Abstract In 2018, baloxavir marboxil, which targets the polymerase acidic (PA) protein of influenza A and B viruses, was licensed in Japan and the United States. This anti-influenza drug is highly effective against these virus infections. During the 2018–2019 influenza season in Japan, however, influenza A viruses carrying an I38T mutation in PA that confers reduced susceptibility to baloxavir acid (the active form of baloxavir marboxil) were detected at a relatively high frequency in pediatric patients after treatment with this drug. In addition, influenza A virus PA-I38T variants were detected in patients before drug treatment. In animal models, the replicative abilities, pathogenicity, and transmissibility of influenza A virus PA-I38T variants isolated from patients have been shown to be comparable to those of wild-type isolates. In this chapter, we summarize recent findings regarding the fitness of influenza A viruses with reduced susceptibility to baloxavir acid isolated from patients.

Keywords Baloxavir marboxil · Baloxavir acid · Influenza virus variant · Reduced susceptibility

M. Imai
Division of Virology, Department of Microbiology and Immunology, Institute of Medical Science, University of Tokyo, Tokyo, Japan

Y. Kawaoka (✉)
Division of Virology, Department of Microbiology and Immunology, Institute of Medical Science, University of Tokyo, Tokyo, Japan

Influenza Research Institute, Department of Pathobiological Sciences, School of Veterinary Medicine, University of Wisconsin-Madison, Madison, WI, USA

Department of Special Pathogens, International Research Center for Infectious Diseases, Institute of Medical Science, University of Tokyo, Tokyo, Japan
e-mail: yoshihiro.kawaoka@wisc.edu

J. Fujita (ed.), *Influenza*, Respiratory Disease Series: Diagnostic Tools and Disease Managements, https://doi.org/10.1007/978-981-15-9109-9_21

1 Introduction

Influenza-specific antiviral drugs are important for managing influenza. By 2017, two classes of antiviral drugs were commercially available for the prophylaxis and treatment of seasonal influenza virus infections: inhibitors of the influenza A virus M2 protein (amantadine and rimantadine) and inhibitors of influenza A and B virus neuraminidases (NAs) (oseltamivir, zanamivir, peramivir, and laninamivir). In 2018, a new class of anti-influenza drug, baloxavir marboxil, was licensed in Japan and the United States. Oseltamivir, which is the most widely used treatment for influenza, is usually taken orally twice daily for 5 days. In contrast, baloxavir marboxil is a single-dose oral medication, which is easier and more convenient for influenza patients. Accordingly, during the 2018–2019 influenza season, baloxavir marboxil gained the largest share of the anti-influenza drug market in Japan.

However, influenza virus surveillance studies in Japan during the influenza season revealed that influenza A viruses with reduced susceptibility to baloxavir acid, the active form of baloxavir marboxil, were detected at a relatively high frequency (https://www.niid.go.jp/niid/images/flu/resistance/20191227/dr18-19j20191227-1.pdf). Here, we summarize recent characterization studies of influenza A viruses with reduced susceptibility to baloxavir acid isolated from patients.

2 Antiviral Mechanism of Baloxavir Marboxil and Effectiveness of Baloxavir Marboxil in Patients

The M2 channel blockers inhibit influenza A virus replication by blocking the ion-channel activity of that M2 protein that is required for the release of viral RNA into the cytoplasm of infected cells [1] (Fig. 21.1). In contrast, the ion-channel activity of influenza B virus BM2 protein is not affected by these drugs [1]. Unfortunately, the M2 channel blockers are not often used due to high levels of resistance [2–4]. In contrast, the NA inhibitors are effective against both influenza A and B viruses. During the budding process, the NA protein of influenza A and B viruses cleaves sialic acids from cellular receptors to facilitate the release of virus particles from the infected cell surface [5, 6]. NA inhibitors function by competitively binding (with sialic acids) to the NA enzyme active site, thereby resulting in a reduction in the amount of virus that is released from the infected cells [7, 8].

Influenza A and B viruses possess eight single-stranded negative-sense RNA segments; each segment associates with a heterotrimeric RNA polymerase complex and nucleoprotein (NP). The RNA polymerase complex consists of the polymerase basic 2 (PB2), polymerase basic 1 (PB1), and polymerase acidic (PA) subunits, which are responsible for the transcription and replication of the viral RNA genome. In 2014, favipiravir (also known as T-705) was licensed in Japan. It suppresses the RNA polymerase activity of influenza A and B viruses, thus inhibiting viral gene replication [9]. However, due to teratogenicity concerns, favipiravir is approved

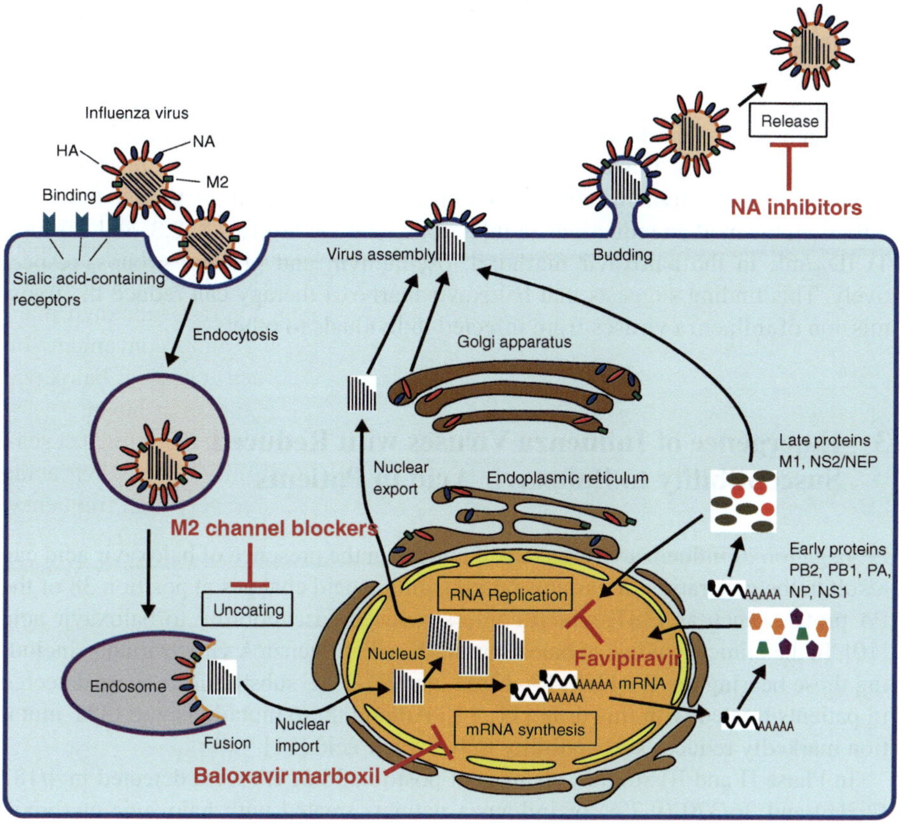

Fig. 21.1 Influenza A virus life cycle and targets for antiviral therapy. Influenza A virus binds to cells via an interaction between its HA and sialic acid-containing receptors on the host cell. The virus is subsequently endocytosed, and the low pH of the endosome initiates the fusion of the virus envelope with the endosomal membrane. After membrane fusion, viral ribonucleoprotein (vRNP) complexes are released into the cytoplasm and subsequently transported to the nucleus, where replication and transcription occur. Viral messenger RNAs (mRNAs) are exported to the cytoplasm for the translation of viral protein components. Newly synthesized viral proteins and vRNPs are transported to the plasma membrane, where progeny virions are assembled, formed, and released by budding. *PB2* polymerase basic protein 2, *PB1* polymerase basic protein 1, *PA* polymerase acidic protein, *HA* hemagglutinin, *NP* nucleoprotein, *NA* neuraminidase, *M1* matrix protein, *NS1* nonstructural protein 1, and *NS2/ NEP* nonstructural protein 2/nuclear export protein

only for the treatment of patients infected with a drug-resistant pandemic influenza virus.

The mechanism of action of baloxavir marboxil differs from that of other approved anti-influenza drugs. Baloxavir marboxil efficiently prevents the replication of influenza A and B viruses by inhibiting the cap-dependent endonuclease activity of their PA subunits, which is required for the generation of capped RNA primers for viral transcription [10, 11]. Therefore, this drug may be effective against NA inhibitor-resistant influenza virus infections.

In an international Phase III clinical trial for uncomplicated influenza patients (age range, 12–64 years), the median time to alleviation of influenza symptoms was shorter among individuals treated with baloxavir marboxil than those who received placebo (53.7 versus 80.2 h) [12]. However, it was not significantly different between baloxavir marboxil-treated patients and oseltamivir recipients (53.7 versus 53.8 h). Importantly, this clinical study demonstrated that baloxavir marboxil was superior to oseltamivir in terms of antiviral activity [12]; at 24 h after treatment initiation, the median reductions in infectious viral load were 4.8, 2.8, and 1.3 $\log_{10}$ $TCID_{50}$/mL in the baloxavir marboxil, oseltamivir, and placebo groups, respectively. This finding suggests that baloxavir marboxil therapy can reduce the transmission of influenza viruses from infected individuals to others.

3 Emergence of Influenza Viruses with Reduced Susceptibility to Baloxavir Acid in Patients

Propagation of influenza viruses in cell culture in the presence of baloxavir acid can result in the generation of variants bearing amino acid changes at position 38 of the PA protein, such as I38T, which confers reduced susceptibility to baloxavir acid [10]. In the clinical studies of baloxavir marboxil, influenza A virus variants, including those bearing the PA-I38T, PA-I38M, and PA-I38F substitutions, were detected in patients treated with this drug [11, 12]. Among these mutations, the I38T mutation markedly reduces susceptibility to baloxavir acid [11].

In Phase II and III studies, changes at position 38 of PA were detected in 4/182 (2.2%) and 36/370 (9.7%) of influenza patients treated with baloxavir marboxil, respectively [12]. Notably, in a pediatric study, PA-I38 variants were presented in 18 (23.4%) of 77 baloxavir marboxil-treated children with influenza [11]. In a Phase III trial, baloxavir marboxil-treated patients infected with PA-I38T/M mutant variants exhibited prolonged infectious viral shedding compared with baloxavir marboxil-treated patients infected with viruses that lacked these mutations and the placebo-treated group [12]. In addition, in the baloxavir marboxil-treated patients infected with PA-I38T/M mutant variants, the time to alleviation of influenza symptoms was longer than that for the baloxavir marboxil-treated group infected with viruses that lacked these mutations. In the clinical trial, a rapid decline in viral load was observed in patients treated with baloxavir marboxil within 24 h of treatment [12]. These findings suggest that limited viral replication in baloxavir marboxil-treated patients does not stimulate effective innate and adaptive immune responses, which are essential for viral clearance, and thus allows the emergence of PA-I38T variants, thereby causing prolonged virus shedding. Further investigations are required to determine whether the host immune response to viral infections is effectively induced in these specific patients.

Influenza virus surveillance studies in Japan during the 2018–2019 influenza season revealed that influenza A viruses carrying amino acid substitutions at position 38 of PA were detected in 9/395 (2.3%) and 34/424 (8.0%) of the A/H1N1 2009 pandemic (A/H1N1pdm)- and A/H3N2-positive patients, respectively (https://www.niid.go.jp/niid/images/flu/resistance/20191227/dr18-19j20191227-1.pdf). Most of the patients infected with A/H1N1pdm or A/H3N2 virus possessing a mutation at position 38 in PA were children under the age of 12 [13, 14]. Among the 43 influenza A virus variants, eight were collected from untreated patients: three A/H1N1pdm- and five A/H3N2-positive patients, indicating the possibility of person-to-person transmission of the variant [13]. Imai et al. [15] also analyzed respiratory specimens collected from patients during the 2018–2019 season in Japan (96 A/H1pdm-positive patients and 157 A/H3-positive patients). All of the clinical specimens from untreated patients with A/H1pdm encoded isoleucine at position 38 of PA. However, among untreated patients with A/H3, samples from two patients contained variants carrying the PA-I38T mutation. One of these two patients was found to have had contact with an influenza patient who was treated with baloxavir marboxil in their household, suggesting that person-to-person transmission of influenza A/H3N2 viruses carrying an I38T mutation in PA occurred within this family. In addition, when the post-treatment samples were analyzed, variants, including those bearing the PA-I38T, PA-I38T/N/S, PA-I38T/S, and/or PA-I38M substitutions, were detected in 5/22 (22.7%) and 4/16 (25.0%) of the A/H1pdm- and A/H3-positive patients, respectively. Consistent with the surveillance studies during the 2018–2019 season in Japan, most of the patients in whom variants were detected were children younger than 12 years of age. Taken together, these findings suggest that seasonal influenza A viruses possessing a mutation at position 38 in PA, which confers reduced susceptibility to baloxavir acid, may easily emerge in pediatric patients during treatment with baloxavir marboxil and that such variants appear to be transmissible from person to person.

4 Characterization of Influenza A Viruses with Reduced Susceptibility to Baloxavir Acid

Recombinant influenza A/H1N1 and A/H3N2 viruses expressing the I38T substitution in their PA protein in the background of old laboratory strains [A/WSN/33 (H1N1) or A/Victoria/2/75 (H3N2)] have been shown to be greatly attenuated in their replication in cell culture relative to their baloxavir acid-sensitive counterparts [10, 11], suggesting that the reduction in replicative fitness of influenza A viruses is caused by the I38T mutation. In contrast, recombinant influenza B viruses carrying this mutation in the background of the B/Maryland/1/59 strain replicate as efficiently as the wild-type virus in cell culture, suggesting that the PA-I38T mutation does not have a detrimental effect on the fitness of influenza B viruses in vitro. Recently, Checkmahomed et al. [16] generated recombinant viruses possessing the PA-I38T mutation in the background of A/H1N1pdm or A/H3N2 viruses that were isolated in 2009 or 2013, respectively. These mutant viruses replicated comparably to their wild-type counterparts in the lungs of mice and retained their pathogenicity in this animal model. Moreover, in competitive growth assays using mice, both the A/H1N1pdm and A/H3N2 mutant viruses showed a replicative advantage over each wild-type virus. Chesnokov et al. [17] isolated an A/H3N2 virus encoding PA-38T that emerged naturally, and performed competition experiments in a ferret model, which is exquisitely susceptible to infection with human influenza viruses. In ferrets, a control virus with PA-38I was shown to outcompete virus encoding PA-38T; however, the advantage was limited.

More recently, Imai et al. [15] showed that seasonal A/H1N1pdm and A/H3N2 viruses possessing the PA-I38T mutation isolated from patients grew as efficiently as their baloxavir acid-sensitive counterparts in cell culture. In addition, they found that these mutant isolates replicated comparably to baloxavir acid-sensitive isolates in the respiratory tracts of hamsters and mice and retained their pathogenicity in these animals (Fig. 21.2). They also demonstrated that the A/H1N1pdm and H3N2 mutant isolates carrying the PA-I38T substitution were efficiently transmitted via respiratory droplets among ferrets. Another recent study has reported that influenza A and B viruses with reduced susceptibility to baloxavir acid retained transmissibility. Jones et al. [18] generated nine recombinant viruses possessing the PA-I38T, PA-I38M, or PA-I38F mutations in the background of A/H1N1pdm, A/H3N2, or B viruses that were isolated in 2009, 2017, or 2008, respectively, and analyzed their

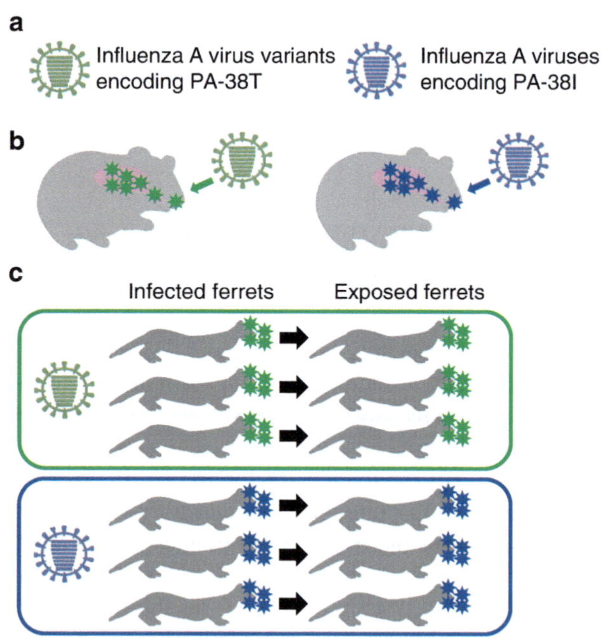

Fig. 21.2 Fitness of influenza A viruses with reduced susceptibility to baloxavir acid isolated from patients. (**a**) Influenza A viruses harboring a PA-I38T mutation (blue) or encoding PA-38I (green) recovered from patients. (**b**) Influenza A viruses with a PA-I38T mutation replicate efficiently in the respiratory organs of infected animals, similar to their wild-type counterparts. (**c**) Influenza A viruses with a PA-I38T mutation transmit efficiently from infected ferrets to naïve ferrets (exposed ferrets) via respiratory droplets

transmissibility in the ferret model. All recombinant viruses bearing a PA protein with the PA-I38T or PA-I38M mutation transmitted via respiratory droplets in ferrets; however, A/H3N2 and B viruses with the PA-I38F mutation failed to transmit via respiratory droplets. Collectively, these observations suggest that the currently circulating seasonal influenza A viruses could maintain their viral fitness even though they have evolved to a status with less susceptibility to baloxavir acid.

5 Conclusions and Perspectives

In animal models, the replicative abilities, pathogenicity, and transmissibility of PA-I38T variants isolated from patients were found to be comparable to those of wild-type isolates. The data suggest that influenza A viruses circulating in humans can rapidly acquire an I38T mutation in their PA, which confers reduced susceptibility to baloxavir acid, without a loss of viral fitness. It is therefore possible that widespread use of baloxavir marboxil will result in the circulation of influenza A viruses with this mutation. The appropriate use of this drug and continued close monitoring for the emergence or prevalence of seasonal influenza A virus PA-I38T variants are extremely important.

The clinical studies of baloxavir marboxil and surveillance for baloxavir acid-resistant influenza viruses in Japan indicate that the frequency of PA-I38 variants is higher in children than in adults. Importantly, baloxavir marboxil-treated pediatric patients with PA-I38 variants have been shown to shed the virus longer and take longer to recover from their clinical symptoms than those without the PA-I38 variants [19, 20]. Limited immunity to circulating influenza viruses in children may allow prolonged viral replication, promoting the emergence of PA-I38 variants. Given that the emergence of these variants is associated with increased duration of illness, the use of baloxavir marboxil in pediatric patients should be carefully considered. By contrast, in adults, influenza A viruses with reduced susceptibility to baloxavir acid have been detected at relatively a low level. Baloxavir marboxil, which can dramatically reduce the amount of virus in the body after a single dose, is a very useful antiviral drug for adults.

Acknowledgments We thank Susan Watson for scientific editing. This research was supported by Leading Advanced Projects for medical innovation (LEAP) from the Japan Agency for Medical Research and Development (AMED) (JP18am001007), by Grants-in-Aid for Scientific Research on Innovative Areas from the Ministry of Education, Culture, Science, Sports, and Technology (MEXT) of Japan (Nos. 16H06429, 16K21723, and 16H06434), by the Japan Initiative for Global Research Network on Infectious Diseases (J-GRID) from AMED (JP19fm0108006), by a Research Program on Emerging and Re-emerging Infectious Diseases from AMED (JP19fk0108031, JP19fk0108056, JP19fk0108058, and JP19fk0108066), and by the NIAID-funded Center for Research on Influenza Pathogenesis (CRIP, HHSN272201400008C).

References

1. Pinto LH, Lamb RA. The M2 proton channels of influenza A and B viruses. J Biol Chem. 2006;281(14):8997–9000. https://doi.org/10.1074/jbc.R500020200.
2. Bright RA, Medina MJ, Xu X, Perez-Oronoz G, Wallis TR, Davis XM, et al. Incidence of adamantane resistance among influenza A (H3N2) viruses isolated worldwide from 1994 to 2005: a cause for concern. Lancet. 2005;366(9492):1175–81. https://doi.org/10.1016/S0140-6736(05)67338-2.
3. Centers for Disease Control and Prevention (CDC). Update: drug susceptibility of swine-origin influenza A (H1N1) viruses, April 2009. MMWR Morb Mortal Wkly Rep. 2009;58(16):433–5.
4. Deyde VM, Xu X, Bright RA, Shaw M, Smith CB, Zhang Y, et al. Surveillance of resistance to adamantanes among influenza A(H3N2) and A(H1N1) viruses isolated worldwide. J Infect Dis. 2007;196(2):249–57. https://doi.org/10.1086/518936.
5. Liu C, Eichelberger MC, Compans RW, Air GM. Influenza type A virus neuraminidase does not play a role in viral entry, replication, assembly, or budding. J Virol. 1995;69(2):1099–106.
6. Palese P, Tobita K, Ueda M, Compans RW. Characterization of temperature sensitive influenza virus mutants defective in neuraminidase. Virology. 1974;61(2):397–410. https://doi.org/10.1016/0042-6822(74)90276-1.
7. Bossart-Whitaker P, Carson M, Babu YS, Smith CD, Laver WG, Air GM. Three-dimensional structure of influenza A N9 neuraminidase and its complex with the inhibitor 2-deoxy 2,3-dehydro-N-acetyl neuraminic acid. J Mol Biol. 1993;232(4):1069–83. https://doi.org/10.1006/jmbi.1993.1461.
8. Varghese JN, Epa VC, Colman PM. Three-dimensional structure of the complex of 4-guanidino-Neu5Ac2en and influenza virus neuraminidase. Protein Sci. 1995;4(6):1081–7. https://doi.org/10.1002/pro.5560040606.
9. Furuta Y, Gowen BB, Takahashi K, Shiraki K, Smee DF, Barnard DL. Favipiravir (T-705), a novel viral RNA polymerase inhibitor. Antivir Res. 2013;100(2):446–54. https://doi.org/10.1016/j.antiviral.2013.09.015.
10. Noshi T, Kitano M, Taniguchi K, Yamamoto A, Omoto S, Baba K, et al. In vitro characterization of baloxavir acid, a first-in-class cap-dependent endonuclease inhibitor of the influenza virus polymerase PA subunit. Antivir Res. 2018;160:109–17. https://doi.org/10.1016/j.antiviral.2018.10.008.
11. Omoto S, Speranzini V, Hashimoto T, Noshi T, Yamaguchi H, Kawai M, et al. Characterization of influenza virus variants induced by treatment with the endonuclease inhibitor baloxavir marboxil. Sci Rep. 2018;8(1):9633. https://doi.org/10.1038/s41598-018-27890-4.
12. Hayden FG, Sugaya N, Hirotsu N, Lee N, de Jong MD, Hurt AC, et al. Baloxavir marboxil for uncomplicated influenza in adults and adolescents. N Engl J Med. 2018;379(10):913–23. https://doi.org/10.1056/NEJMoa1716197.
13. Takashita E, Ichikawa M, Morita H, Ogawa R, Fujisaki S, Shirakura M, et al. Human-to-human transmission of influenza A(H3N2) virus with reduced susceptibility to baloxavir, Japan, February 2019. Emerg Infect Dis. 2019;25(11):2108–11. https://doi.org/10.3201/eid2511.190757.
14. Takashita E, Kawakami C, Ogawa R, Morita H, Fujisaki S, Shirakura M, et al. Influenza A(H3N2) virus exhibiting reduced susceptibility to baloxavir due to a polymerase acidic subunit I38T substitution detected from a hospitalised child without prior baloxavir treatment, Japan, January 2019. Euro Surveill. 2019;24(12):1900170. https://doi.org/10.2807/1560-7917.ES.2019.24.12.1900170.
15. Imai M, Yamashita M, Sakai-Tagawa Y, Iwatsuki-Horimoto K, Kiso M, Murakami J, et al. Influenza A variants with reduced susceptibility to baloxavir isolated from Japanese patients are fit and transmit through respiratory droplets. Nat Microbiol. 2020;5(1):27–33. https://doi.org/10.1038/s41564-019-0609-0.
16. Checkmahomed L, M'Hamdi Z, Carbonneau J, Venable MC, Baz M, Abed Y, et al. Impact of the baloxavir-resistant polymerase acid I38T substitution on the fitness of contemporary

influenza A(H1N1)pdm09 and A(H3N2) strains. J Infect Dis. 2020;221(1):63–70. https://doi.org/10.1093/infdis/jiz418.
17. Chesnokov A, Patel MC, Mishin VP, De La Cruz JA, Lollis L, Nguyen HT, et al. Replicative fitness of seasonal influenza A viruses with decreased susceptibility to baloxavir. J Infect Dis. 2020;221(3):367–71. https://doi.org/10.1093/infdis/jiz472.
18. Jones JC, Pascua PNQ, Fabrizio TP, Marathe BM, Seiler P, Barman S, et al. Influenza A and B viruses with reduced baloxavir susceptibility display attenuated in vitro fitness but retain ferret transmissibility. Proc Natl Acad Sci U S A. 2020;117:8593. https://doi.org/10.1073/pnas.1916825117.
19. Hirotsu N, Sakaguchi H, Sato C, Ishibashi T, Baba K, Omoto S, et al. Baloxavir marboxil in Japanese pediatric patients with influenza: safety and clinical and virologic outcomes. Clin Infect Dis. 2019;71:971. https://doi.org/10.1093/cid/ciz908.
20. Sato M, Takashita E, Katayose M, Nemoto K, Sakai N, Hashimoto K, et al. Detection of variants with reduced baloxavir marboxil susceptibility after treatment of children with influenza A during the 2018/2019 influenza season. J Infect Dis. 2020;222:121. https://doi.org/10.1093/infdis/jiaa061.

Chapter 22
Viruses Resistant to Oseltamivir or Baloxavir: What Do the Data Reveal About Resistance?

Emi Takashita

Abstract Three classes of antiviral drugs are approved for the treatment or prophylaxis of influenza: the M2 inhibitors (amantadine and rimantadine), the neuraminidase inhibitors (oseltamivir, peramivir, zanamivir, and laninamivir), and the polymerase inhibitors (favipiravir and baloxavir). These antiviral drugs are fully effective against drug-susceptible viruses but work less well or not at all against drug-resistant viruses. The clinical significance of antiviral drug-resistant viruses is influenced by many factors including their frequency of emergence, genetic stability, pathogenicity, transmissibility, and replication fitness. The emergence and global spread of M2 inhibitor-resistant viruses and oseltamivir-resistant viruses occurred in the early 2000s. Recently, human-to-human transmission of baloxavir-resistant viruses has been observed. These resistant viruses are genetically stable, show similar or higher pathogenicity, transmissibility, and replication fitness compared with their susceptible counterparts, and exhibit highly reduced antiviral susceptibility. The clinical efficacy of oseltamivir and baloxavir is limited in patients infected with these resistant viruses compared with those infected with wild-type viruses, indicating that antiviral-resistant viruses can lead to clinical resistance to antiviral drugs.

Keywords Influenza · Oseltamivir · Baloxavir · Amantadine · Resistance

1 Introduction

Three classes of antiviral drugs are approved for the treatment or prophylaxis of influenza: the M2 inhibitors (amantadine and rimantadine), the neuraminidase (NA) inhibitors (oseltamivir, peramivir, zanamivir, and laninamivir), and the polymerase inhibitors (favipiravir and baloxavir). The M2 inhibitors are active against influenza

E. Takashita (✉)
Influenza Virus Research Center, National Institute of Infectious Diseases, Tokyo, Japan
e-mail: emitaka@nih.go.jp

J. Fujita (ed.), *Influenza*, Respiratory Disease Series: Diagnostic Tools and Disease Managements, https://doi.org/10.1007/978-981-15-9109-9_22

A viruses, but not influenza B viruses. The NA inhibitors act against influenza A and B viruses, whereas the polymerase inhibitors are effective against influenza A, B, C, and D viruses. The emergence and spread of antiviral-resistant viruses are of great concern. Because global surveillance of antiviral resistance is essential, the World Health Organization (WHO) Global Influenza Surveillance and Response System (GISRS) Expert Working Group for Surveillance of Antiviral Susceptibility (WHO-AVWG) has been conducted a global analysis of circulating influenza viruses [1]. Antiviral-resistant viruses are monitored through a combination of phenotypic methods analyzing antiviral susceptibility and genotypic methods detecting amino acid substitutions associated with antiviral resistance. The antiviral drugs are fully effective against drug-susceptible viruses but not against drug-resistant viruses. The clinical significance of these antiviral-resistant viruses likely depends on factors such as their frequency of emergence, genetic stability, pathogenicity, transmissibility, and replication fitness. [2]. This review provides an overview of the viruses that are resistant to antiviral drugs, in particular two drugs that are widely used in Japan: the NA inhibitor oseltamivir and the polymerase inhibitor baloxavir.

2 M2 Inhibitors

The influenza virus M2 is a membrane protein that forms an ion channel. The M2 inhibitors—amantadine and its derivative rimantadine—block the M2 ion channel of influenza A viruses and inhibit virus replication within the infected cell [3]. Since the structures of the M2 ion channels are different in influenza A and B viruses, the M2 inhibitors are not effective against influenza B viruses.

Amantadine susceptibility of influenza viruses was evaluated on the basis of a therapeutic index, the ratio of the maximal concentration of drug not toxic to the tissue to the minimal concentration of drug inhibiting the virus [4]. Amantadine-resistant viruses were found to emerge rapidly in the presence of amantadine, and the therapeutic index of the resistant viruses was calculated as 1. Furthermore, more than a 100-fold higher drug concentration was required to inhibit the growth of the resistant viruses by 50% (IC_{50}) relative to that required to similarly inhibit the growth of amantadine-susceptible wild-type viruses in cell culture-based assays [5, 6] (Table 22.1). These results demonstrate that higher concentrations of amantadine are required to inhibit the replication of amantadine-resistant viruses.

M2 inhibitor resistance is associated with single amino acid substitutions at position 26, 27, 30, 31, or 34 in the M2 protein, which line the interior of the M2 ion channel [3]. In 2003–2004, the prevalence of M2 inhibitor-resistant A(H3N2) viruses significantly increased in China as a result of increased use of the M2 inhibitors, and the viruses spread globally during 2005–2006 [7]. Almost all of these resistant viruses possessed an S31N substitution in the M2 protein. Antigenic changes in the circulating A(H3N2) viruses, which contribute to evasion of the host immune system, were accompanied by the M2 S31N substitution and may have allowed the spread of the M2 inhibitor-resistant A(H3N2) viruses [7]. In 2009, a

Table 22.1 Amantadine susceptibility of influenza A(H3N2) viruses carrying the S31N amino acid substitution in the M2 protein

Isolate name	M2 substitution	GISAID isolate ID	IC_{50}, nM (fold-change)[a]
A/MIE/16/2017	S31N	EPI ISL 267066	75.32 (260)
A/MIE/23/2019	S31N	EPI ISL 392482	53.18 (180)
A/YOKOHAMA/187/2019	S31N	EPI ISL 395536	62.77 (220)
A/SAPPORO/58/2019	S31N	EPI ISL 400577	38.47 (130)
A/NAGANO/2599/2019	S31N	EPI ISL 400583	47.84 (160)
A/MIE/18/2017	None (wild type)	EPI ISL 273503	0.29

GISAID Global Initiative on Sharing All Influenza Data, *IC_{50}* 50% inhibitory concentration
[a]IC_{50} values were determined by use of a focus reduction assay. Fold-change in IC_{50} values compared with the wild-type virus

novel A(H1N1)pdm09 virus emerged and has been circulating as a seasonal influenza virus. The A(H1N1)pdm09 virus M2 protein was derived from the Eurasian lineage of swine viruses, which contained the M2 S31N substitution [8]. Therefore, the currently circulating influenza A viruses are resistant to the M2 inhibitors. Consequently, the WHO does not currently recommend the use of the M2 inhibitors for the treatment or prophylaxis of influenza A virus infections.

The M2 inhibitor-resistant viruses were genetically stable and showed similar pathogenicity, transmissibility, and replication fitness to M2 inhibitor-susceptible wild-type viruses [3]. Prolonged virus shedding was observed in patients infected with these resistant viruses [9]. Children infected with these resistant viruses showed a significant recurrence of fever [10], and their illness was prolonged compared with that of those infected with the wild-type viruses [9, 10]. These findings demonstrated that the M2 inhibitor-resistant viruses can lead to clinical resistance to M2 inhibitors.

3 NA Inhibitors

The influenza virus NA is a membrane glycoprotein that mainly functions to release progeny viruses from infected cells via its enzyme activity. The NA inhibitors—oseltamivir, peramivir, zanamivir, and laninamivir—bind to the NA enzyme active site and inhibit virus release from infected cells [3]. Since the NA enzyme active site is conserved between influenza A and B viruses, the NA inhibitors are active against both influenza A and B viruses.

The WHO-AVWG has been conducting global surveillance of NA inhibitor resistance since the 2012–2013 period [1]. Cell culture-based assays are not currently recommended for evaluation of NA inhibitor susceptibility of influenza viruses because the receptor-binding properties of the viruses can affect NA inhibitor susceptibility in these assays [3]. Therefore, NA inhibitor susceptibility is evaluated based on the drug concentration required to inhibit the NA enzyme activity by 50% (IC_{50}) in an NA inhibition assay. To standardize interpretation and reporting of

NA inhibitor susceptibility, criteria were defined by the WHO-AVWG using IC_{50} fold-change thresholds, compared to the median for viruses of the same type, subtype, and lineage showing normal inhibition (NI) [11]. Viruses showing reduced inhibition (RI) are influenza A viruses that have a 10- to 100-fold increase in IC_{50}, or influenza B viruses with a 5- to 50-fold increase in IC_{50}. Viruses showing highly reduced inhibition (HRI) are influenza A viruses with a greater than 100-fold increase in IC_{50} or influenza B viruses with a greater than 50-fold increase in IC_{50}.

The WHO-AVWG has summarized the NA amino acid substitutions that are associated with NA inhibitor resistance [12]. NA H275Y in A(H1N1) or A(H1N1)pdm09 viruses and NA E119V and NA R292K in A(H3N2) viruses are the most common substitutions [3]. A(H1N1) and A(H1N1)pdm09 viruses carrying the NA H275Y substitution show HRI to oseltamivir and peramivir but are susceptible to zanamivir and laninamivir (Table 22.2). A(H3N2) viruses carrying the NA E119V substitution show HRI to oseltamivir but are susceptible to the other three NA inhibitors, and A(H3N2) viruses carrying the NA R292K substitution show HRI to oseltamivir, peramivir, and zanamivir, but are susceptible to laninamivir [12].

A(H1N1) viruses carrying the NA H275Y substitution, which confers cross-resistance to oseltamivir and peramivir, emerged in Europe during the 2007–2008 influenza season and spread globally within a year despite infrequent use of NA inhibitors. These results indicate that antiviral selective pressure is not the only factor that determines the spread of resistant viruses, although it may have been involved in their initial emergence. In 2009, A(H1N1)pdm09 viruses emerged and replaced A(H1N1) viruses. The A(H1N1)pdm09 virus NA protein was derived from the Eurasian lineage of swine viruses [8] and did not contain the NA H275Y substitution. Therefore, currently circulating A(H1N1)pdm09 viruses have been susceptible to the NA inhibitors. Nevertheless, the first widespread community cluster of A(H1N1)pdm09 viruses carrying the NA H275Y substitution was detected in Newcastle, Australia in 2011 [13], and then a large community cluster of NA H275Y mutant A(H1N1)pdm09 viruses occurred in Hokkaido, Japan during the 2013–2014 season [14]. The detection rate for these oseltamivir and peramivir cross-resistant viruses reached 29% in Hokkaido during this season; however, the resistant viruses were replaced by the wild-type viruses and disappeared.

The A(H1N1) viruses carrying the NA H275Y substitution circulated worldwide and possessed some permissive substitutions such as R222Q, V234M, and D344N in their NA and T82K, K141E, and R189K in their hemagglutinin (HA) proteins [14]. These substitutions were shown to enhance the replication and transmission fitness of the NA H275Y mutant A(H1N1) viruses, thereby making the mutant viruses more transmissible than the wild-type viruses. The pathogenicity of these mutant viruses was significantly higher than that of the wild-type viruses [15]. Antigenic changes of circulating A(H1N1) viruses were accompanied by the NA H275Y substitution, which may have allowed the rapid spread of the mutant viruses [16]. The V241I and N369K substitutions in the A(H1N1)pdm09 virus NA protein were reported to increase the replication and transmission fitness of the NA H275Y mutant A(H1N1)pdm09 viruses [14]. These substitutions contribute to efficient transmission of the mutant viruses but are not enough to replace the wild-type

Table 22.2 NA inhibitor susceptibility of influenza A(H1N1)pdm09 viruses carrying the H275Y amino acid substitution in the NA protein

			IC_{50}, nM (fold-change)[a]			
Isolate name	NA substitution	GISAID isolate ID	Oseltamivir	Peramivir	Zanamivir	Laninamivir
A/OKINAWA/97/2019	H275Y	EPI ISL 394161	437.57 (1300)	26.58 (300)	0.55 (2)	1.03 (2)
A/KANAGAWA/ZC1905/2019	H275Y	EPI ISL 398281	393.60 (1200)	27.47 (310)	0.23 (1)	0.46 (1)
A/YOKOHAMA/269/2019	H275Y	EPI ISL 408557	407.31 (1200)	25.68 (290)	0.73 (2)	1.40 (3)
A/KANAGAWA/193/2019	H275Y	EPI ISL 411923	374.10 (1100)	20.32 (230)	0.17 (1)	0.30 (1)
A/MIE/2/2020	H275Y	EPI ISL 410506	414.40 (1200)	20.60 (230)	0.31 (1)	1.46 (3)
Median IC_{50} values[b]	None (wild type)		0.34	0.09	0.30	0.46

NA neuraminidase, *GISAID* Global Initiative on Sharing All Influenza Data, IC_{50} 50% inhibitory concentration

[a] IC_{50} values were determined by use of a fluorescence NA inhibition assay. Fold-change in IC_{50} values compared with the median IC_{50} values

[b] Median IC_{50} values of A(H1N1)pdm09 viruses isolated during the 2019–2020 influenza season in Japan

viruses. However, currently circulating A(H1N1)pdm09 viruses possess these permissive substitutions, suggesting an increased risk for oseltamivir and peramivir cross-resistant viruses to emerge and spread globally.

The duration of fever was significantly longer in patients infected with the NA H275Y mutant A(H1N1) viruses than those infected with the wild-type viruses [17–19]. Children aged 0–6 years infected with these mutant viruses showed a significant recurrence of fever [19]. The NA inhibitor-resistant viruses can thus lead to clinical resistance to NA inhibitors.

4 Polymerase Inhibitors

The influenza virus RNA-dependent RNA polymerase consists of three subunits: polymerase basic protein 1 (PB1), polymerase basic protein 2 (PB2), and polymerase acidic protein (PA) in influenza A and B viruses or polymerase 3 protein (P3) in influenza C and D viruses. The polymerase inhibitors favipiravir and baloxavir target the PB1 and PA proteins, respectively [20]. Favipiravir acts as a chain terminator and inhibits RNA elongation, which is carried out by PB1. It also acts as a mutagen and causes lethal mutagenesis by increasing the G-to-A and C-to-U mutation frequency and generating nonviable progeny virus. Baloxavir binds to the PA endonuclease domain and inhibits RNA cleavage by the PA cap-dependent endonuclease activity. Since the influenza virus RNA-dependent RNA polymerase is highly conserved among influenza A, B, C, and D viruses, favipiravir and baloxavir inhibit the replication of all of these viruses.

The WHO-AVWG initiated global surveillance of baloxavir resistance in the 2017–2018 period [1]. Polymerase inhibitor susceptibility is evaluated based on the drug concentration required to inhibit virus growth by 50% (IC_{50}) in cell culture-based assays. The criteria to define polymerase inhibitor susceptibility have not yet been established; therefore, provisional criteria based on IC_{50} fold-change thresholds, compared to the median for viruses of the same type, subtype, and lineage, are used [21]. The provisional criteria define influenza virus inhibition as normal (<3-fold increase) or reduced (≥3-fold increase).

Favipiravir was approved in Japan for influenza pandemic preparedness in 2014, and baloxavir has now been approved in at least 16 countries for the treatment of influenza A and B virus infections. In clinical trials of favipiravir, no mutant viruses with reduced susceptibility to favipiravir emerged after favipiravir treatment; however, in vitro studies have shown that a K229R substitution in the PB1 protein confers about a 30-fold reduction in susceptibility to favipiravir [20]. I38 substitutions in the PA protein that were associated with baloxavir resistance emerged after baloxavir treatment during the Phase II and III clinical trials of baloxavir [22–25]. In children aged <6 years infected with A(H3N2) viruses, the frequency of the PA I38 substitutions reached 52.2% [20]. The PA I38T mutant viruses isolated during the 2018–2019 season showed about 50- to 230-fold reduced susceptibility to baloxavir but remained susceptible to favipiravir [26–29] (Table 22.3). These results demonstrate that higher concentrations of baloxavir are required to inhibit the replication

Table 22.3 Polymerase inhibitor susceptibility of influenza A(H3N2) viruses carrying the I38T amino acid substitution in the PA protein

Isolate name	PA substitution	GISAID Isolate ID	IC_{50}, nM (fold-change)[a]	
			Favipiravir	Baloxavir
A/KOBE/18578/2019	I38T	EPI ISL 356751	27.24 (2)	313.65 (170)
A/KANAGAWA/AC1878/2019	I38T	EPI ISL 356753	14.14 (1)	161.21 (87)
A/HIROSHIMA-C/30/2019	I38T	EPI ISL 363718	21.88 (1)	163.18 (88)
Median IC_{50} values[b]	None (wild type)		15.77	1.85

PA polymerase acidic protein, *GISAID* Global Initiative on Sharing All Influenza Data, *IC_{50}* 50% inhibitory concentration

[a]IC_{50} values were determined by use of a focus reduction assay. Fold-change in IC_{50} values compared with the median IC_{50} values

[b]Median IC_{50} values of A(H3N2) viruses isolated during the 2018–2019 influenza season in Japan

of the baloxavir-resistant viruses. Indeed, the emergence of PA I38T mutant viruses was correlated with decreasing plasma concentrations of baloxavir [23, 25].

During the 2018–2019 season, several cases of human-to-human transmission of the PA I38T mutant A(H3N2) viruses were observed in Japan [26, 27, 29]. A(H1N1) pdm09 and A(H3N2) viruses carrying the PA I38T substitution that were isolated during this season showed similar pathogenicity, transmissibility, and replication fitness to that of baloxavir-susceptible wild-type viruses [26]. However, a widespread cluster of these baloxavir-resistant viruses has not been detected. Antigenic changes of circulating viruses accompanied by the PA I38T substitution may be one of the factors that will determine the spread of the PA I38T mutant viruses as well as that of the M2 S31N mutant viruses and the NA H275Y mutant viruses.

Patients infected with the PA I38T/M/S mutant viruses exhibited prolonged virus shedding, a rebound in virus titers, and delayed symptom alleviation [22, 23, 25, 30]. Among these patients, symptom alleviation was longer in those with low baseline HA inhibition antibody titers than in those with higher antibody titers [23]. These results indicate that baloxavir-resistant viruses can lead to clinical resistance to baloxavir.

5 Conclusion

Antiviral-resistant viruses possess characteristic amino acid substitutions associated with antiviral resistance and exhibit reduced antiviral susceptibility. The clinical significance of antiviral-resistant viruses likely depends on numerous factors including their frequency of emergence, genetic stability, pathogenicity, transmissibility, and replication fitness. The clinical efficacy of antiviral drugs can be inadequate in patients infected with antiviral-resistant viruses, compared with those infected with wild-type viruses, which then fosters clinical resistance to the antiviral drug.

References

1. Takashita E, Daniels RS, Fujisaki S, Gregory V, Gubareva LV, Huang W, et al. Global update on the susceptibilities of human influenza viruses to neuraminidase inhibitors and the cap-dependent endonuclease inhibitor baloxavir, 2017–2018. Antiviral Res. 2020;175:104718. https://doi.org/10.1016/j.antiviral.2020.104718.
2. Hayden FG, Hay AJ. Emergence and transmission of influenza A viruses resistant to amantadine and rimantadine. Curr Top Microbiol Immunol. 1992;176:119–30. https://doi.org/10.1007/978-3-642-77,011-1_8.
3. Tisdale M. Influenza M2 ion-channel and neuraminidase inhibitors. In: Mayers DL, Lerner SA, Ouellette M, Sobel JD, editors. Antimicrobial drug resistance; clinical and epidemiological aspects. New York: Springer; 2009;421–47. https://doi.org/10.1007/978-1-59745-180-2_31.
4. Cochran KW, Maassab HF, Tsunoda A, Berlin BS. Studies on the antiviral activity of amantadine hydrochloride. Ann N Y Acad Sci. 1965;130(1):432–9. https://doi.org/10.1111/j.1749-6632.1965.tb12579.x.
5. Appleyard G. Amantadine-resistance as a genetic marker for influenza viruses. J Gen Virol. 1977;36(2):249–55. https://doi.org/10.1099/0022-1317-36-2-249.
6. Lubeck MD, Schulman JL, Palese P. Susceptibility of influenza A viruses to amantadine is influenced by the gene coding for M protein. J Virol. 1978;28(3):710–6. https://doi.org/10.1128/JVI.28.3.710-716.1978.
7. Bright RA, M-j M, Xu X, Perez-Oronoz G, Wallis TR, Davis XM, et al. Incidence of adamantane resistance among influenza A (H3N2) viruses isolated worldwide from 1994 to 2005: a cause for concern. Lancet. 2005;366(9492):1175–81. https://doi.org/10.1016/s0140-6736(05)67338-2.
8. Smith GJ, Vijaykrishna D, Bahl J, Lycett SJ, Worobey M, Pybus OG, et al. Origins and evolutionary genomics of the 2009 swine-origin H1N1 influenza A epidemic. Nature. 2009;459(7250):1122–5. https://doi.org/10.1038/nature08182.
9. Hayden FG, Couch RB. Clinical and epidemiological importance of influenza a viruses resistant to amantadine and rimantadine. Rev. Med Virol. 1992;2(2):89–96. https://doi.org/10.1002/rmv.1980020205.
10. Shobugawa Y, Saito R, Sato I, Li D, Suzuki Y, Sasaki A, et al. Recurrence and persistence of fever in children who developed amantadine-resistant influenza viruses after treatment. Tohoku J Exp Med. 2008;214(2):129–38. https://doi.org/10.1620/tjem.214.129.
11. World Health Organization. Meetings of the WHO working group on surveillance of influenza antiviral susceptibility - Geneva, November 2011 and June 2012. Wkly Epidemiol Rec. 2012;87(39):369–74. https://apps.who.int/iris/handle/10665/241965. Accessed 24 Sep 2020.
12. World Health Organization. Laboratory methodologies for testing the antiviral susceptibility of influenza viruses. https://www.who.int/influenza/gisrs_laboratory/antiviral_susceptibility/en/. Accessed 24 Sep 2020.
13. Hurt AC, Hardie K, Wilson NJ, Deng YM, Osbourn M, Leang SK, et al. Characteristics of a widespread community cluster of H275Y oseltamivir-resistant A(H1N1)pdm09 influenza in Australia. J Infect Dis. 2012;206(2):148–57. https://doi.org/10.1093/infdis/jis337.
14. Takashita E, Kiso M, Fujisaki S, Yokoyama M, Nakamura K, Shirakura M, et al. Characterization of a large cluster of influenza A(H1N1)pdm09 viruses cross-resistant to oseltamivir and peramivir during the 2013–2014 influenza season in Japan. Antimicrob Agents Chemother. 2015;59(5):2607–17. https://doi.org/10.1128/AAC.04836-14.
15. Baz M, Abed Y, Simon P, Hamelin ME, Boivin G. Effect of the neuraminidase mutation H274Y conferring resistance to oseltamivir on the replicative capacity and virulence of old and recent human influenza A(H1N1) viruses. J Infect Dis. 2010;201(5):740–5. https://doi.org/10.1086/650464.
16. Kelso A, Hurt AC. The ongoing battle against influenza: drug-resistant influenza viruses: why fitness matters. Nat Med. 2012;18(10):1470–1. https://doi.org/10.1038/nm.2954.

17. Kawai N, Ikematsu H, Hirotsu N, Maeda T, Kawashima T, Tanaka O, et al. Clinical effectiveness of oseltamivir and zanamivir for treatment of influenza A virus subtype H1N1 with the H274Y mutation: a Japanese, multicenter study of the 2007–2008 and 2008–2009 influenza seasons. Clin Infect Dis. 2009;49(12):1828–35. https://doi.org/10.1086/648424.
18. Matsuzaki Y, Mizuta K, Aoki Y, Suto A, Abiko C, Sanjoh K, et al. A two-year survey of the oseltamivir-resistant influenza A(H1N1) virus in Yamagata, Japan and the clinical effectiveness of oseltamivir and zanamivir. Virol J. 2010;7:53. https://doi.org/10.1186/1743-422X-7-53.
19. Saito R, Sato I, Suzuki Y, Baranovich T, Matsuda R, Ishitani N, et al. Reduced effectiveness of oseltamivir in children infected with oseltamivir-resistant influenza A (H1N1) viruses with His275Tyr mutation. Pediatr Infect Dis J. 2010;29(10):898–904. https://doi.org/10.1097/INF.0b013e3181de9d24.
20. Takashita E. Influenza polymerase inhibitors: mechanisms of action and resistance. In: Neumann G, Kawaoka Y, editors. Influenza: The Cutting Edge. New York: Cold Spring Harbor Laboratory Press; 2020. a038687. https://doi.org/10.1101/cshperspect.a038687.
21. Gubareva LV, Mishin VP, Patel MC, Chesnokov A, Nguyen HT, De La Cruz J, et al. Assessing baloxavir susceptibility of influenza viruses circulating in the United States during the 2016/17 and 2017/18 seasons. Euro Surveill. 2019;24(3):1800666. https://doi.org/10.2807/1560-7917.ES.2019.24.3.1800666.
22. Hayden FG, Sugaya N, Hirotsu N, Lee N, de Jong MD, Hurt AC, et al. Baloxavir marboxil for uncomplicated influenza in adults and adolescents. N Engl J Med. 2018;379(10):913–23. https://doi.org/10.1056/NEJMoa1716197.
23. Hirotsu N, Sakaguchi H, Sato C, Ishibashi T, Baba K, Omoto S, et al. Baloxavir marboxil in Japanese pediatric patients with influenza: safety and clinical and virologic outcomes. Clin Infect Dis. 2020;71(4):971–81. https://doi.org/10.1093/cid/ciz908.
24. Omoto S, Speranzini V, Hashimoto T, Noshi T, Yamaguchi H, Kawai M, et al. Characterization of influenza virus variants induced by treatment with the endonuclease inhibitor baloxavir marboxil. Sci Rep. 2018;8(1):9633. https://doi.org/10.1038/s41598-018-27,890-4.
25. Uehara T, Hayden FG, Kawaguchi K, Omoto S, Hurt AC, De Jong MD, et al. Treatment-emergent influenza variant viruses with reduced baloxavir susceptibility: impact on clinical and virologic outcomes in uncomplicated influenza. J Infect Dis. 2020;221(3):346–55. https://doi.org/10.1093/infdis/jiz244.
26. Imai M, Yamashita M, Sakai-Tagawa Y, Iwatsuki-Horimoto K, Kiso M, Murakami J, et al. Influenza A variants with reduced susceptibility to baloxavir isolated from Japanese patients are fit and transmit through respiratory droplets. Nat Microbiol. 2020;5(1):27–33. https://doi.org/10.1038/s41564-019-0609-0.
27. Takashita E, Ichikawa M, Morita H, Ogawa R, Fujisaki S, Shirakura M, et al. Human-to-human transmission of influenza A(H3N2) virus with reduced susceptibility to baloxavir, Japan, February 2019. Emerg Infect Dis. 2019;25(11):2108–11. https://doi.org/10.3201/eid2511.190757.
28. Takashita E, Kawakami C, Morita H, Ogawa R, Fujisaki S, Shirakura M, et al. Detection of influenza A(H3N2) viruses exhibiting reduced susceptibility to the novel cap-dependent endonuclease inhibitor baloxavir in Japan, December 2018. Euro Surveill. 2019;24(3):1800698. https://doi.org/10.2807/1560-7917.ES.2019.24.3.1800698.
29. Takashita E, Kawakami C, Ogawa R, Morita H, Fujisaki S, Shirakura M, et al. Influenza A(H3N2) virus exhibiting reduced susceptibility to baloxavir due to a polymerase acidic subunit I38T substitution detected from a hospitalised child without prior baloxavir treatment, Japan, January 2019. Euro Surveill. 2019;24(12):1900170. https://doi.org/10.2807/1560-7917.ES.2019.24.12.1900170.
30. Sato M, Takashita E, Katayose M, Nemoto K, Sakai N, Hashimoto K, et al. Detection of variants with reduced baloxavir marboxil susceptibility after treatment of children with influenza A during the 2018/2019 influenza season. J Infect Dis. 2020;222(1):121–5. https://doi.org/10.1093/infdis/jiaa061.

Correction to: Influenza

Jiro Fujita

Correction to:
J. Fujita (ed.), Influenza, Respiratory Disease Series: Diagnostic Tools and Disease Managements, https://doi.org/10.1007/978-981-15-9109-9

The book was inadvertently published with the below corrections. These changes have been updated.

In Chapter 14, the author name has been corrected from "Yosule Aoki" to "Yosuke Aoki".

In chapter 18, the first author name in reference 10 has been corrected from "Nobuo N" to "Hirotsu N".

The updated version of these chapters can be found at
https://doi.org/10.1007/978-981-15-9109-9_14
https://doi.org/10.1007/978-981-15-9109-9_18

J. Fujita (ed.), *Influenza*, Respiratory Disease Series: Diagnostic Tools
and Disease Managements, https://doi.org/10.1007/978-981-15-9109-9_23

GPSR Compliance

The European Union's (EU) General Product Safety Regulation (GPSR) is a set of rules that requires consumer products to be safe and our obligations to ensure this.

If you have any concerns about our products, you can contact us on ProductSafety@springernature.com

In case Publisher is established outside the EU, the EU authorized representative is:

Springer Nature Customer Service Center GmbH
Europaplatz 3
69115 Heidelberg, Germany

Batch number: 10732090

Printed by Printforce, the Netherlands